Also Available

Borderline Personality Disorder: Clinical and Empirical Perspectives
Edited by John F. Clarkin, Elsa Marziali, and Heather Munroe-Blum

Handbook of Personality Disorders: Theory, Research, and Treatment
Edited by W. John Livesley

Journal of Personality Disorders: Official Journal of the International Society for the Study of Personality Disorders
Edited by Robert F. Krueger and W. John Livesley

Major Theories of Personality Disorder, Second Edition
Edited by Mark F. Lenzenweger and John F. Clarkin

Practical Management of Personality Disorder
W. John Livesley

INTEGRATED TREATMENT FOR PERSONALITY DISORDER

INTEGRATED TREATMENT FOR PERSONALITY DISORDER

A Modular Approach

edited by

W. JOHN LIVESLEY
GIANCARLO DIMAGGIO
JOHN F. CLARKIN

THE GUILFORD PRESS
New York London

© 2016 The Guilford Press
A Division of Guilford Publications, Inc.
370 Seventh Avenue, Suite 1200, New York, NY 10001
www.guilford.com

Printed in the United States of America

This book is printed on acid-free paper.

Last digit is print number: 9 8 7 6 5 4 3 2 1

The authors have checked with sources believed to be reliable in their efforts to provide information that is complete and generally in accord with the standards of practice that are accepted at the time of publication. However, in view of the possibility of human error or changes in behavioral, mental health, or medical sciences, neither the authors, nor the editors and publisher, nor any other party who has been involved in the preparation or publication of this work warrants that the information contained herein is in every respect accurate or complete, and they are not responsible for any errors or omissions or the results obtained from the use of such information. Readers are encouraged to confirm the information contained in this book with other sources.

Library of Congress Cataloging-in-Publication Data

Integrated treatment for personality disorder : a modular approach / edited by W. John Livesley, Giancarlo Dimaggio, John F. Clarkin.
p. ; cm.
Includes bibliographical references and index.
ISBN 978-1-4625-2288-0 (hardcover : alk. paper)
I. Livesley, W. John, editor. II. Dimaggio, Giancarlo, editor. III. Clarkin, John F., editor.
[DNLM: 1. Personality Disorders—therapy. 2. Psychotherapy—methods. WM 190]

RC554
616.85′81—dc23

2015009843

About the Editors

W. John Livesley, MD, PhD, is Professor Emeritus in the Department of Psychiatry at the University of British Columbia, Canada. His research focuses on the structure, classification, and origins of personality disorder, and on constructing an integrated framework for describing and conceptualizing personality pathology. His clinical interests are directed toward developing a unified approach to treatment. Dr. Livesley is a Fellow of the Royal Society of Canada. He is coeditor of the *Journal of Personality Disorders.*

Giancarlo Dimaggio, MD, is a co-founding member of the Centre for Metacognitive Interpersonal Therapy in Rome, Italy. His primary interest is in metacognitive processes and mental disorders. Dr. Dimaggio has published four books, including the coauthored *Metacognitive Interpersonal Therapy for Personality Disorders*, and more than 120 papers in scientific journals. He is an associate editor of *Psychology and Psychotherapy* and the *Journal of Psychotherapy Integration*, and serves on the editorial board of the *Journal of Personality Disorders.* He has guest-edited many journal special issues on research and treatment for personality disorder.

John F. Clarkin, PhD, is Clinical Professor of Psychology in Psychiatry at Weill Cornell Medical College and Co-Director of the Personality Disorders Institute at New York Presbyterian Hospital. His research focuses on the phenomenology of personality disorder and treatment of patients with borderline personality disorder and bipolar disorder. Past president of the Society for Psychotherapy Research, Dr. Clarkin has published numerous articles and books on psychopathology, differential treatment planning, and personality disorder.

Contributors

Anthony W. Bateman, MA, FRCPsych, The Anna Freud Centre and Research Department of Clinical, Educational and Health Psychology, University College London, London, United Kingdom

Yvonne Bergmans, MSW, RSW, Suicide Studies Unit, St. Michael's Hospital, and Department of Psychiatry, Faculty of Medicine, University of Toronto, Toronto, Ontario, Canada

Nicole M. Cain, PhD, Department of Psychology, Long Island University Brooklyn, Brooklyn, New York

Antonino Carcione, MD, Third Center of Cognitive Psychotherapy, Rome, Italy

Lee Anna Clark, PhD, Department of Psychology, University of Notre Dame, Notre Dame, Indiana

John F. Clarkin, PhD, Department of Psychiatry, New York Presbyterian Hospital–Westchester Division, Weill Cornell Medical College, White Plains, New York

Chiara De Panfilis, PhD, Department of Neuroscience, University of Parma, Parma, Italy

Giancarlo Dimaggio, MD, Centre for Metacognitive Interpersonal Therapy, Rome, Italy

Peter Fonagy, PhD, FBA, FMedSci, Research Department of Clinical, Educational and Health Psychology, University College London, London, United Kingdom

Robert O. Friedel, MD, Department of Psychiatry, Virginia Commonwealth University, Richmond, Virginia

Roelie J. Hempel, PhD, School of Psychology, University of Southampton, Southampton, United Kingdom

Robert L. Leahy, PhD, American Institute for Cognitive Therapy, New York, New York

Kenneth N. Levy, PhD, Department of Psychology, The Pennsylvania State University, University Park, Pennsylvania

Paul S. Links, MD, FRCPC, Department of Psychiatry, University of Western Ontario, London, Ontario, Canada

W. John Livesley, MD, PhD, Department of Psychiatry, University of British Columbia, Vancouver, British Columbia, Canada

Thomas R. Lynch, PhD, FBPsS, School of Psychology, University of Southampton, Southampton, United Kingdom

Deanna Mercer, MD, FRCPC, Department of Psychiatry, University of Ottawa, Ottawa, Ontario, Canada

J. Christopher Muran, PhD, Derner Institute of Advanced Psychological Studies, Adelphi University, Garden City, New York

Jon S. Novick, MD, FRCPC, Department of Psychiatry, University of Toronto, Toronto, Ontario, Canada

Paolo Ottavi, PhD, Centre for Metacognitive Interpersonal Therapy, Rome, Italy

Tiziana Passarella, PhD, Centre for Metacognitive Interpersonal Therapy, Rome, Italy

Manuela Pasinetti, PhD, Centre for Metacognitive Interpersonal Therapy, Rome, Italy

Aaron L. Pincus, PhD, Department of Psychology, The Pennsylvania State University, University Park, Pennsylvania

Raffaele Popolo, MD, Centre for Metacognitive Interpersonal Therapy, Rome, Italy

Giampaolo Salvatore, MD, Centre for Metacognitive Interpersonal Therapy, Rome, Italy

Kenneth R. Silk, MD, Department of Psychiatry, University of Michigan Health System, Ann Arbor, Michigan

William B. Stiles, PhD, Department of Psychology, Miami University, Oxford, Ohio

Sumru Tufekcioglu, PhD, Derner Institute of Advanced Psychological Studies, Adelphi University, Garden City, New York

Stephen C. P. Wong, PhD, Department of Psychology, University of Saskatchewan, Saskatoon, Saskatchewan, Canada; School of Medicine, University of Nottingham, Nottingham, United Kingdom; and Centre of Forensic Behavioural Science, Swinburne Uniersity of Technology, Melbourne, Australia

Frank Yeomans, MD, PhD, Department of Psychiatry, Weill Cornell Medical College, New York, New York

Preface

This volume reflects our conviction that it is time to rethink how personality disorder is treated. Over the last 25 years, the development of specific therapies for personality disorders, most notably borderline personality disorder, has radically changed our understanding of these disorders and their treatment. The therapeutic nihilism that prevailed little more than 20 years ago has given way to greater optimism. At the same time, it is clear that personality disorder is not as static as previously thought. Not only are treatments effective, but also outcome does not look to be very different from that for most other mental disorders. During this time, more than a handful of treatment protocols based on very different theoretical models have gained empirical support, opening the way for evidence-based care. However, although all therapies evaluated to date produce considerable improvement, none stands out as demonstrably more effective than the rest. Nevertheless, the prevailing opinion is that treatment should be based on one or more of these specialized therapeutic models. We think differently—that these findings provide a solid foundation for developing a more integrated and transtheoretical approach that combines principles and methods from all effective therapies to establish a treatment model that is sufficiently comprehensive and flexible to accommodate the diverse pathology and protean forms that personality disorder takes. Why choose among different treatments that do not differ in outcome when each contains effective treatment strategies and methods that could be combined to provide a more comprehensive treatment?

A transtheoretical treatment model opens up the prospect of more cost-effective treatments that could be made more widely available because they can be delivered by staff without the extensive training needed to deliver most forms of specialized therapy for treating personality disorder. A unified approach would also allow therapists to use any effective intervention that they consider to be potentially beneficial to their patients rather than being forced to confine interventions to those recommended by a given treatment protocol. The challenge is how to do this in an efficient and straightforward way that is readily implemented by both seasoned practitioners and those just learning their craft.

The idea of an integrated treatment is not new, nor is our approach novel. Our ideas build upon the many thoughtful and innovative contributions to the literature on psychotherapy integration over the years. Our approach incorporates a broad perspective on integration that emphasizes both (1) the importance of principles of therapeutic change common to all effective therapies and (2) the use of an eclectic array of interventions that are more specific to the various forms of therapy. Interventions based on common principles form the core of therapy—the scaffolding to support more specific interventions drawn from all effective therapies according to the needs of individual patients. Whereas a number of specialized treatments for personality disorder tend to use fixed protocols, we believe that an integrated approach offers greater opportunity to accommodate the diversity of personality pathologies and to tailor treatment to the specific needs and problems of individual patients, while at the same time providing the structure needed for successful outcomes.

Consistent with our emphasis on integration and eclecticism, we have sought contributions from authors from diverse perspectives and theoretical schools to describe the methods that they find useful in treating personality disorder and to consider how to deliver those methods in the context of integrated therapy. We are grateful to the authors who responded to our request, because integration is challenging. It requires that we move outside the comfort zone provided by our usual treatment model to begin embracing different perspectives and intervention strategies from those that are familiar to us. The varied chapters describing the treatment of major domains of personality pathology are not intended to provide a comprehensive account of all possible interventions, nor to cover all components of personality disorder. Rather, our goal is to demonstrate the feasibility of a unified approach and to show how theoretically diverse interventions may be used as part of a more comprehensive treatment plan. We recognize that the challenge is to ensure that a conceptually diverse combination of strategies and interventions is seen to be coherent and to provide sufficient guidelines to help therapists to deliver eclectic treatment methods in a coordinated way. We have sought to facilitate this understanding and application by including a case description of integrated treatment and by attempting to draw things together in a final overview chapter.

W. John Livesley
Giancarlo Dimaggio
John F. Clarkin

Contents

PART I. CONCEPTUAL FRAMEWORK AND TREATMENT PRINCIPLES

PART II. ASSESSMENT, TREATMENT PLANNING, AND THE TREATMENT CONTRACT

PART III. GENERAL CHANGE PRINCIPLES AND MECHANISMS

PART VI. INTEGRATION

part one

CONCEPTUAL FRAMEWORK AND TREATMENT PRINCIPLES

chapter 1

Why Integrated Treatment?

General Principles of Therapeutic Change

W. John Livesley, Giancarlo Dimaggio, and John F. Clarkin

There is now solid evidence that personality disorders can be treated effectively. Prior to about 1990, treatment was dominated by various psychoanalytical therapies. Studies of treatment outcome were sparse, and therapeutic nihilism prevailed. Therapeutic developments were largely derived from observations of patients in long-term psychoanalytical therapy. Although these observations yielded a valuable understanding of the importance of such factors as a structured approach, the treatment contract, consistency, and the treatment alliance, there were few methodologically sound outcome studies to help the clinician to plan treatment. The situation changed in the 1990s with the development of a several manualized therapies.

Although this second phase in the evolution of personality disorder treatment was characterized by the emergence of specialized therapies for borderline personality disorder (BPD) and their systematic evaluation in randomized controlled trials (RCTs), the phase was ushered in with the publication of a more general work—Beck and colleagues' volume on cognitive therapy (Beck, Freeman, & Associates, 1990), which paved the way for new treatment options. Shortly afterward, randomized controlled outcome studies began to appear, led by Linehan, Armstrong, Suarez, Allmon, and Heard's (1991) investigation of dialectical behavior therapy (DBT), a landmark development that demonstrated the feasibility of evidence-based treatments for personality disorder. Other therapies rapidly became available so that, as we write, at least seven specific manualized therapies have been shown to be effective in at least one reasonably methodologically sound evaluation. These include DBT (Linehan, 1993), cognitive therapy (Davidson, 2008), cognitive analytic therapy (Ryle, 1997), mentalizing-based therapy (MBT; Bateman & Fonagy, 1999, 2001), transference-focused psychotherapy (TFP; Clarkin, Yeomans, & Kernberg, 1999, 2006), schema-focused therapy (SFT; Young, Klosko, & Weishaar, 2003), and systems training for predictability and problem solving (STEPPS; Blum et al., 2008).

These developments are cause for optimism. Now a rich array of therapies apparently provide the clinician with a range of treatment options, although most studies were on patients with BPD—with the exception of a few studies on DSM-IV Cluster C disorders (Arnevik et al., 2008; Muran, Safran, Samstag, & Winston, 2005) and some recent studies dealing with all forms of personality disorder (Bamelis, Evers, Spinhoven, & Arntz, 2014; Clarke, Thomas, & James, 2013). The current *zeitgeist* tends to imply that therapists should use one or more of these evidence-based therapies. This approach is encouraged by advocates of specific treatments, who often argue that their treatment is the most empirically validated or in some way more comprehensive than the rest. This volume was motivated by a different perspective: the conviction that the treatment of personality disorders is entering a third phase characterized by greater concern with integrating treatment principles and methods across therapies, the use of eclectic and pragmatic treatment strategies, and the emergence of more modular and transdiagnostic approaches focusing on specific domains of personality pathology rather than global diagnoses. For want of a better term, we refer to this approach as *integrated modular treatment* (IMT). We suggest that individual patients present with a unique array of problems spanning multiple domains of functioning and that treatment should utilize an integrated array of strategies and techniques to address these diverse impairments. With this approach, domains of impairment such as symptoms, problems with emotion and impulse regulation, interpersonal patterns and self-identity problems, and overall severity of dysfunction are the focus of intervention, rather than a more globally conceptualized categorical disorder.

We recognize that integrated therapy is a rather soft and overused term; the proponents of various specialized therapies commonly claim that theirs is an integrated approach despite the fact that most are based on a single theoretical model and a relatively limited repertoire of interventions that reflect the assumptions of the underlying model. Here we use the term *integrated* to refer to an approach that combines an eclectic array of treatment principles, strategies, and methods drawn from all effective treatments and uses them in a targeted way to treat specific impairments. Later, we discuss the idea of integrated treatment in more detail. For now, we note our conviction that the time is ripe to integrate treatments: Outcome does not differ substantially across therapies, and the field is recognizing that personality disorders are complex conditions with a multifaceted psychopathology and a multidimensional biopsychological etiology. These developments challenge continued reliance on treatments based on one-dimensional models of specific personality disorders that assume a single impairment and hence rely upon a limited set of treatment methods.

THE IMPLICATIONS OF OUTCOME STUDIES

The RCTs of specialized treatments that radically changed the treatment landscape have several shortcomings that need to be considered when applying their findings to treatment planning. Because evaluations are largely confined to treatments of BPD, findings have to be extrapolated to other disorders, although there is evidence that some treatments, such as SFT, are effective with other disorders (Bamelis et al., 2014). Nevertheless, even with BPD, most RCTs used small samples, which limit the generalizability of their findings (Davidson et al., 2006). Also, in some studies information on follow-up is limited, so it is not clear whether the effects observed at the end of treatment are lasting, although a few studies show that outcomes are stable (see Bateman & Fonagy, 2008). In all trials, a significant number of patients did not respond to treatment, raising the question as to whether they would respond to an alternative treatment or to integrated treatment tailored to their individual needs. Finally, randomized trials do not normally provide information about the mechanisms of change, especially whether change is due to methods and strategies specific to the treatments being investigated.

With respect to treatment selection, the important finding of these studies is the lack of evidence of clinically significant differences in outcome across therapies (Bartak, Soeteman, Verheul, & Busschbach, 2007; Budge et al., 2014; Leichsenring & Leibing, 2003; Leichsenring, Leibing, Kruse, New, & Leweke, 2011; Mulder & Chanen, 2013). Significant differences are sometimes reported, but these are often difficult to interpret. For example, a comparison of TFP (Clarkin et al., 1999) and schema-focused therapy (Young et al., 2003) suggested that schema-focused therapy produced fewer dropouts (a significant problem in the treatment of personality disorder) and better outcomes (Giesen-Bloo et al., 2006). However, differences were modest, the sample size was small, and questions have been raised about whether the two treatments were delivered in comparable ways (Yeomans, 2007). Overall, outcome studies suggest that there are few empirical grounds for selecting one evidence-supported approach over another. However, the specialized therapies are more efficacious than treatment as usual or treatment delivered by expert clinicians (Budge et al., 2014; Doering et al., 2010; Linehan, Comtois, et al., 2006). Although this finding appears to suggest that advantages accrue from using a specialized therapy, there are reasons to question this conclusion. Treatment as usual is a rather modest standard because it is limited to whatever routine care is available in the setting in which the study occurred, and in some settings this care may be limited. Differences between specialized treatments and treatment as usual are also decreasing with time, presumably because treatment as usual is improving. Moreover, when specialized therapies are compared with well-specified, manualized general psychiatric care tailored to BPD, the results are different.

The four studies that have examined this issue failed to find substantial differences. Clarkin, Levy, Lenzenweger, and Kernberg (2007) compared TFP, DBT, and a supportive dynamic treatment over 1 year and found few differences across multiple outcome measures. A limitation of this study was a small number of participants. This limitation was overcome in a study by McMain and colleagues (2009), who compared DBT with general psychiatric management that included a combination of psychodynamically informed therapy and symptom-targeted medication management based on APA guidelines for treating BPD (American Psychiatric Association, 2001). The two treatments did not differ significantly in outcome. This finding is especially important because DBT is the most studied treatment for BPD and considered by many to be the treatment of choice. It should also be noted that at the end of each treatment, patients still had substantial problems (McMain et al., 2009; see also Kröger, Harbeck, Armbrust, & Kliem, 2013).

A comparison of MBT and structured clinical management also reported similar outcomes for the two therapies, although problems decreased slightly faster with MBT (Bateman & Fonagy, 2009). Subsequently, the same investigators (Bateman & Fonagy, 2013) examined whether severity, variously assessed as severity of comorbid psychiatric syndromes, severity of BPD (number of criteria met), number of co-occurring Axis II disorders, and severity of symptom distress, influenced outcome for MBT and structured clinical management. Although none of the severity criteria predicted outcome at the end of treatment, patients with more severe disorder indicated by two of the severity criteria (multiple Axis II diagnoses and symptom distress) did better with MBT. The other severity criteria did not have a differential effect on outcome. The authors cautiously raise the possibility that greater severity of personality pathology and symptom distress may predict greater benefit of MBT over structured clinical management. An interesting feature of this finding in terms of its implications for a unified treatment model is how the authors characterize the distinction between MBT and structured management. They state that structured clinical management is based on routine psychiatric practice that matches "the non-specialized features of MBT in terms of intensity, organization and pharmacological treatment" (Bateman & Fonagy, 2013, p. 221). Presumably, they consider the specialized features of MBT to be strategies and interventions that enhance mentalization capacity. However, it could be argued that mentalizing interventions of MBT are not specialized interventions confined to this mode of therapy but rather a highly effective way to operationalize an essential set of generic change mechanisms in the context of treating BPD. These generic mechanisms include change mechanisms that have consistently been shown to be critical components of effective therapies such as self-reflection, perspective taking, psychological mindedness, empathy, and various metacognitive processes. This raises the possibility that the demonstrated efficacy of MBT arises from the consistent and structured application of an array of generic interventions rather than the use of mechanisms specific to the approach.

Finally, Chanen and colleagues (2008) reported that cognitive analytic therapy was not significantly better than manualized good clinical care—a modular treatment package based on standard psychiatric management and a problem-solving approach combined with specific modules to address specific symptom clusters. The interesting feature of these studies is that they were conducted by investigators with different theoretical orientations using three different specialized treatments that were compared with three forms of general clinical care in three countries, Canada, the United Kingdom, and Australia. This lends confidence to the generalizability of the findings. Consistent with this interpretation is evidence that some specialized therapies are not more effective than supportive therapy. Jorgensen and colleagues (2013) compared the outcome of MBT and supportive psychotherapy in patients with BPD. Outcome assessed using multiple self-report measures and the Structured Clinical Interview for DSM-IV Axis II Personality Disorders (SCID-II) did not differ across groups. The only significant difference observed between groups was in therapist-rated global assessment of functioning, which was open to bias as it was not a blind rating. The failure to demonstrate greater efficacy for MBT was especially notable because treatment intensity differed substantially across groups, with the MBT group receiving 45 minutes of individual therapy and 90 minutes of group therapy per week, whereas the supportive therapy condition received only 90 minutes of group therapy every 2 weeks. In contrast, Bales and colleagues (in press) did not find differences in favor of day-hospital MBT versus other specialized psychotherapeutic treatments.

Evidence that the specialized therapies do not differ substantially in outcome either from each other or from good clinical care that largely relies on generic change factors and that supportive therapy is as effective as MBT suggests that nothing is gained by using a specialized treatment, a conclusion with major implications for conceptualizing and implementing treatment. It suggests that positive outcome is more a function of a structured approach and change mechanisms common to all effective treatments than to treatment-specific interventions. In this sense, the results of outcome of treatments for BPD converge with the results of psychotherapy outcomes generally: we have known for more than 40 years that outcome is similar across therapies (Beutler, 1991; Luborsky, Singer, & Luborsky, 1975), which suggests that different therapies share common elements associated with successful outcome (Castonguay & Beutler, 2006a, 2006b; Norcross & Newman, 1992). Personality disorders are unlikely to show a different pattern.

Nevertheless, the general factors may not be the whole story. Some treatment methods specific to a given therapeutic approach are also likely contribute to positive outcomes. The evidence on this point is not strong because outcome studies do not evaluate mechanisms of action. However, some older studies show evidence of domain specificity. Piper and Joyce (2001), reviewing the literature on psychotherapy for personality disorder, noted evidence of differential effectiveness: Treatment methods that work for one domain do not necessarily work for another. Consistent with this conclusion is evidence that some therapies are better than others in treating specific impairments. For example, TFP appears to significantly increase reflective functioning compared with either MBT or supportive therapy. These considerations suggest that integrated treatment should not rely solely on a common-factors approach but also needs to incorporate specific methods to treat specific impairments or domains of psychopathology. Hence a guiding principle behind this volume is that treatment should start not from a narrowly focused, disorder-specific manual but from a detailed analysis or deconstruction of the patient's psychopathology into domains of dysfunction and that treatment methods should be selected on the basis of what works for the specific problems and domains that are the focus of therapeutic attention.

CONCEPTUAL AND PRACTICAL LIMITATIONS OF SPECIALIZED THERAPIES

Thus far we have argued for integrated treatment based on the results of outcome research. However, an examination of the specialized treatments provides a second reason for pursuing integration: None of these treatments offer the range of interventions needed to treat all components of personality disorder. Each specialized treatment is based on a theory of personality disorder that is largely speculative but nevertheless determines the primary focus of treatment and the interventions used. A general limitation of these theories is the tendency to explain the diverse psychopathology of personality disorders in terms of a single primary impairment. Although this assumption has the advantage of providing the therapist with a clear conceptual approach, it neglects the contribution of other explanatory factors and runs the risk of neglecting other important intervention strategies. For example, the proposed impairments associated with BPD include affect dysregulation, maladaptive thinking, maladaptive schemas, conflicted relationships, primary problems with impulsivity, fragmented object relationships, impaired mentalizing capacity, and identity pathology. Because therapies differ in the assumed impairment, they emphasize different strategies and interventions. For example, because cognitive therapy emphasizes dysfunctional beliefs and maladaptive thinking, treatment primarily focuses on cognitive restructuring and the development of new beliefs and associated behaviors. In contrast, DBT (Linehan, 1993) assumes that affect regulation is the critical feature and hence focuses on developing emotional regulation skills. MBT (Bateman & Fonagy, 2004), on the other hand, considers impaired mentalizing to be the central problem and hence focuses primarily on enhancing mentalizing capacity on the assumption that this will promote affect regulation and more adaptive cognitive functioning.

However, even a cursory consideration of borderline pathology indicates that it involves maladaptive cognitions, emotion dysregulation, impaired mentalizing, and more. Personality pathology is complex spanning multiple domains of problems that include symptoms, emotion and impulse regulation, interpersonal pathology, maladaptive traits, situational or environmental problems, identity problems, and impaired metacognitive processes (Clarkin, 2008; Livesley, 2003). This suggests that evidence-based treatment needs to adopt a multidimensional model of personality disorder and a comprehensive array of interventions.

Our discussion of outcome studies and the limitations of contemporary treatments points to the need for a more unified approach that incorporates interventions based on change mechanisms common to all effective treatments and more specific interventions targeted to specific domains of psychopathology. This structure has implications for assessment. It implies that a global diagnosis based on current diagnostic categories is insufficient. In order to select appropriate interventions, personality disorder needs to be decomposed into different functional domains (see Livesley & Clarkin, Chapter 3, this volume). This reveals an additional benefit of integration: It accommodates the considerable heterogeneity among patients with a given disorder and permits treatment to be tailored to the individual (Livesley, 2012; Stone, 2010). The importance of tailoring treatment to the individual is illustrated by a recent outcome study of borderline and avoidant personality disorders (Gullestad et al., 2012) that assessed pretreatment mentalizing abilities. Patients with lower pretreatment mentalizing skills fared worst in day-hospital treatment than in individual therapy. The authors noted that poor understanding of mental states may make group therapy and day-hospital treatment too distressing and confusing, leading to poor outcome. Individual therapy was more effective because the use of individual therapy made it easier to manage the impaired mentalizing by providing a safer and more predictable environment (Gullestad, Johansen, Høglend, Karterud, & Wilberg, 2013).

PATHWAYS TO INTEGRATION

Integrated treatment may be organized in various ways depending on how integration is conceptualized and the way interventions from different therapies are combined. The model proposed here incorporates to varying degrees the three routes to integration that have traditionally been described in the general psychotherapy literature: common factors, technical eclecticism, and theoretical integration (Arkowitz, 1989; Norcross & Grencavage, 1989; Norcross & Newman, 1992). The common-factors approach seeks to identify principles of change common to all therapies and uses these principles to establish the basic structure of treatment. Technical eclecticism uses treatment methods from diverse treatment models without adoption of their associated theories. Most experienced clinicians show a degree of technical eclecticism—they use methods that they have found to work even though they may not subscribe to the theoretical position on which they are based, an approach that Stricker (2010) calls *assimilative integration*. Theoretical integration is more complex. It seeks to combine the major components of two or more therapies to create a more effective model. The concern is not just to identify common change principles and blend diverse interventions to integrate underlying theories of therapeutic change (Norcross & Newman, 1992; Stricker, 2010).

We emphasize the common-factors approach based on similarity in outcome across specialized treatments and evidence that the common factors account for much of the change we see in patients. Within the current framework, interventions implementing generic change mechanisms form the basic structure of treatment that provides the consistency and structure needed for effective treatment. It will be apparent from earlier comments that we also espouse technical eclecticism and consider it necessary to comprehensive treatment of personality pathology. Hence we propose using a wide range of interventions drawn from all therapies without adopting the theories on which they are based. The challenge for eclecticism is how to select and combine diverse and even theoretically incompatible interventions. The solution that we advocate is to decompose personality disorder into different problem domains and select specific interventions to treat each domain based on empirical and rational considerations. We believe this provides a more effective and parsimonious way to treat personality disorder than to use a combination of specialized therapies. Theoretical integration involving the melding of different therapies is probably not feasible given current knowledge. As an alternative, a descriptive scheme is offered for decomposing personality disorder into components for treatment purposes (see Livesley & Clarkin, Chapters 2 and 3, this volume).

The combination of general factors and technical eclecticism determines the basic structure of treatment. It implies the use of two broad kinds of intervention modules: general modules based on interventions that operationalize general change mechanisms common to all therapies and more specific modules composed of interventions that target more specific impairments, such as emotion dysregulation, violent behavior, deliberate self-harm, and submissiveness.

OVERVIEW OF THE VOLUME

The overarching goals of this book are to foster integrated treatments for personality disorders and to stimulate a professional climate and discussion of clinical integration because we think such a development is timely. Outcome research points to the feasibility of integration, and nosological research increasingly emphasizes the general features of personality disorder and its severity as opposed to particular personality disorder types. At the same time, interest is growing in transdiagnostic approaches to diagnostic classification based on domains of impairment that cut across traditional diagnostic entities (Cuthbert & Insel, 2013; Doherty & Owen, 2014), an approach that is congenial to our emphasis on domains of personality dysfunction and the selection of interventions based on domains rather than global diagnoses. The authors we approached to contribute to this volume were all willing to abandon the idea that their approach is the best and to contribute to a larger enterprise of exploring the domains of dysfunction in patients with personality disorder and exploring various treatment approaches. This willingness suggests to us that the spirit of integration is alive and well. We also attempt to provide a template to guide clinicians in applying an integrated approach to assessment and treatment and to facilitate the teaching of an integrated treatment approach in training programs for mental health professionals.

We have organized this book with these ideas in mind. Part I, "Conceptual Framework and Treatment Principles," provides the reader with the rationale for integration and a general framework for organizing treatment. In Chapter 2, W. John Livesley and John F. Clarkin describe a general framework that distinguishes between general treatment modules based on the common-factors approach to integration and specific treatment modules. Each module consists of a set of interventions for treating a specific problem or problem domain.

Part II, "Assessment, Treatment Planning, and the Treatment Contract," deals with assessment, formulation, treatment planning, and establishing the treatment contract. The emphasis that IMT places on tailoring treatment to the problems and impairments of individual patients and on linking interventions to specific problems requires a more detailed evaluation than a simple categorical diagnosis. These issues are addressed in Chapter 3 by W. John Livesley and John F. Clarkin, who describe a three-stage diagnostic assessment covering severity, clinically important traits, and domains of personality impairment. In Chapter 4, Clarkin and Livesley then discuss how this information can be used to construct a formulation and plan treatment. This chapter also deals with the important problem of how to match domains of personality pathology with treatment modules and how to sequence the use of specific intervention modules. The chapter also introduces the important point that integration is ultimately something that occurs in the mind of the therapist, who arrives at a comprehensive formulation that is used to select appropriate treatment methods based largely on clinical judgment. In Chapter 5, Paul S. Links, Deanna Mercer, and Jon Novick set the stage for treatment by examining strategies for developing a treatment contract, a crucial issue in treating personality disorder: All effective therapies stress the importance of the contract as something that is essential to providing the structure needed to establish a consistent treatment process.

In Part III, "General Change Principles and Mechanisms," Sumru Tufekcioglu and J. Christopher Muran (Chapter 6) discuss diverse aspects of the therapeutic relationship in treating personality disorder. They offer a relational theory of the person as a context for understanding the therapeutic alliance and explore in depth the critical issue of how to manage breakdowns to the therapeutic alliance. The next two chapters explore different aspects of the treatment of impaired metacognitive functioning and the role these problems play in disordered personality. In Chapter 7, Anthony W. Bateman and Peter Fonagy discuss mentalization as a core impairment of personality disorder and show how enhancing mentalizing capacity is fundamental to effective therapy. This theme of metacognitive processes generally is continued in Chapter 8 by Giancarlo Dimaggio, Raffaele Popolo, Antonino Carcione, and Giampaolo Salvatore. In describing the nature and treatment of impaired metacognitive functions, they introduce the important idea of using analysis of specific events or scenarios to facilitate different aspects of change. The first three sections flesh out a broad framework for implementing integrated treatment by providing an approach to treatment that can readily be structured to meet the needs of individual patients and the clinician's preferred mode of working.

Part IV, "Treating Symptoms and Dysregulated Emotions," covers strategies for treating diverse aspects of personality pathology. This section is not intended to provide comprehensive coverage of all components of personality disorder but rather to illustrate how different methods can be used within an integrated framework. To this end, we invited authors to describe their approach to treatment and to show how this could be delivered within a unified model. The sequence of these chapters roughly approximates the sequence in which different problems and impairments are treated.

The section begins with Chapter 9, in which Paul S. Links and Yvonne Bergmans discuss the management of suicidal and other crises. They develop a practical and integrated framework by comparing and contrasting the way crises are managed in DBT and general psychiatric management. Kenneth R. Silk and Robert O. Friedel then address the use of medication in treating personality disorder in Chapter 10. After reviewing the evidence on the benefits of medication, they discuss strategies for integrating the use of medication with psychotherapy. This is an important issue because many patients with personality disorder also receive medication, and it is important that this is delivered in a way that is consistent with an integrative approach and that facilitates psychotherapeutic work.

Chapter 11, by W. John Livesley, describes the treatment of emotional dysregulation using a modular strategy that is based on an analysis of the structure of emotional dysregulation and the patient's subjective experience of intense, unstable emotions. A four-module strategy is proposed, with each module consisting of an eclectic set of interventions that target an component of emotional dysregulation from different perspectives with the aim of increasing understanding of emotions and the nature of emotional experiences, enhancing emotional awareness, improving emotional self-regulation, and increasing emotion processing capacity. The following two chapters discuss other aspects of treating emotional dysregulation, providing additional perspectives that may contribute to a more unified framework. Robert L. Leahy, in Chapter 12, describes a metacognitive model of emotion and introduces the idea of emotional schemas—thoughts and ideas about the emotion aroused by events and how these schemas influence both the appraisal of events and the subsequent processing of emotional responses. Strategies and techniques for restructuring emotional schemas are discussed in the context of different forms of personality disorder. The chapter concludes by illustrating the use of these strategies in treating a case of BPD. In Chapter 13, Paolo Ottavi, Tiziana Passarella, Manuela Pasinetti, Giampaolo Salvatore, and Giancarlo Dimaggio consider the role of mindfulness in treating personality disorder, especially its value in treating the ruminative tendencies observed in many patients. After considering the ways standard mindfulness protocols need to be modified for use with patients with severe personality pathology, they outline specific strategies and techniques and discuss their applications in specific cases.

In Part V, "Treating Interpersonal and Self Functioning," the focus changes. The section begins with Chapter 14, in which Nicole M. Cain and Aaron L. Pincus discuss the management of interpersonal pathology. They use interpersonal theory as the basis for proposing the concept of interpersonal signature to describe and explain adaptive and maladaptive social behavior and then consider how this framework can be applied to to identifying and treating the disturbed interpersonal relationships that characterize personality disorder. In Chapter 15, Thomas R. Lynch, Roelie J. Hemple, and Lee Anna Clark discuss the treatment of a less commonly treated form of disorder—social withdrawal and emotional constriction. They argue that treatments should not assume that patients have the capability for effective emotional responding and hence emphasize the need for skills-based approaches, suggesting that the overcontrolled forms of emotional dysregulation are likely to benefit from interventions designed to reduce inhibitory control and increase flexible responding. Their perspective complements Dimaggio and colleagues' earlier discussion of the management of the treatment narrative in emotionally constricted individuals (see Chapter 8). Stephen C. P. Wong discusses the challenging problem of treating aggression and violent behavior in individuals with psychopathic traits. The two-component structure of psychopathy is used to discuss treatment of the interpersonal and more behavioral components of psychopathy using an integrated approach that combines elements of both the treatment of personality disorder and the more structured approaches to treating risk commonly used by forensic and correctional treatment services.

The subsequent three chapters offer different perspectives on treating the self and identity problems associated with personality disorder. This is an important domain of personality pathology that has not always received the attention it warrants, although it has recently been given greater prominence by the current emphasis on the general features of personality disorder as opposed to specific diagnoses. This prominence is reflected in the DSM-5, Section 3, proposed definition of personality disorders as a combination of chronic interpersonal dysfunction and self-identity problems. The theme is introduced in Chapter 17, by Giancarlo Dimaggio, Raffaele Popolo, Antonino

Carcione, Giampaolo Salvatore, and William B. Stiles, who discuss ways to elaborate and enrich patients' self-narratives. This is an important topic. The self-systems of most patients are poorly developed, and many lack an adaptive self-narrative to guide action and give direction and purpose to their lives and to help promote more adaptive personality functioning. The chapter discusses the importance of self-narratives or scripts to place the issue in the broader context of overall personality functioning before examining the kinds of problems observed in the life scripts of patients with personality disorder. This discussion sets the stage for presenting strategies for constructing more adaptive scripts. An eclectic approach is used that combines narrative methods, metacognitive strategies, and behavioral exposure and behavioral experiments.

Chapter 18, by John F. Clarkin, Frank Yeomans, Chiara De Panfilis, and Kenneth N. Levy, examines the challenge of constructing a more adaptive self-system from a different perspective—that of object relations theory—that conceptualizes identity and interpersonal functioning as intertwined structures and processes arising from the same interactional matrix. The authors suggest that some of the concepts and procedures emphasized by object relations therapy, including a focus on the patient–therapist relationship, could be useful components of an integrated treatment that addresses both the disturbed behavior and the disturbed internal world associated with severe self-pathology. In the final chapter to examine self and identity problems, Giampaolo Salvatore, Raffaele Popolo, and Giancarlo Dimaggio offer a complementary approach to integrating the disjunctions existing in the self-states and inner experience of patients with severe personality disorder. Rather than focusing on the use of the patient–therapist relationship as a vehicle for integration, Salvatore and colleagues examine the way the ongoing reformulation of a case during treatment may be used to promote integration of separate and disparate self-states. Throughout the volume, reference has been made to the importance of formulation in planning and delivering treatment and the need to revise the formulation throughout therapy as new information becomes available. Viewed from this perspective, the formulation is a blueprint both for therapy and for constructing a more adapive self-script. Collaborative work in reformulation allows the patient to revise and reconstruct the formulation so that it becomes the basis for an autobiographical self-narrative.

Our experience in editing this volume and working with authors with diverse theoretical orientations and interests is that psychotherapy integration is difficult and challenging. We anticipate that the reader who wishes to practice integrated treatment will also find it challenging, at least initially. However, we also believe it necessary to improving treatments for personality disorder. Consequently, we gave considerable thought to what else we could do as editors to help the reader to assimilate the ideas discussed. This deliberation led to the inclusion of a case, in Part VI, "Integration," that illustrates an integrated approach in the treatment of a specific patient with multiple problems so that the reader can see how the therapist struggled with integrating different intervention strategies (Chapter 20). Although we have placed this at the end of the book, the reader may find it helpful to peruse this earlier. Finally, in Chapter 21, we attempt to synthesize the main ideas.

There are similarities but also major differences between what we are advocating here and what the major empirically supported treatments have done for patients with personality disorders. We are suggesting a unified approach to any patient with a personality disorder, not just one of the specific categories of personality disorder. We agree with the major treatment designers about the need to provide the therapist with a unified conception of psychopathology to guide treatment. In contrast to the major treatments that focus on a single concept (e.g., affect dysregulation, mentalization, internal object relations, or interpersonal schemas), we use a framework based on domains of dysfunction in these patients. The authors in this volume have indicated the major domains of dysfunction that they encounter in their work. Although the logical empirical approach to the single-focus therapies is to compare their approaches with treatment as usual or with a competing treatment, our approach would have to be examined at the level of the individual patient and the success or failure with the domains of dysfunction relevant to that patient.

We have considered the integration of multiple strategies and techniques for domains of dysfunction in patients with a personality disorder diagnosis limited to the individual-treatment format. We have not examined integration as applied to marital, family, or group treatment formats, nor to treatments with multiple modalities, such as a day-hospital approach. This first focus seemed appropriate, as the individual format alone or combined with group format (e.g., DBT) has enjoyed the most empirical investigation. Finally, in the spirit of what has been articulated so far, we are not intending to develop a manualized treatment (with a three-letter name) leading to a randomized clinical trial with dedicated followers for our approach.

REFERENCES

American Psychiatric Association. (2001). *Practice guidelines for the treatment of patients with borderline personality disorder*. Washington, DC: Author.

Arkowitz, H. (1989). The role of theory in psychotherapy integration. *Journal of Integrative and Eclectic Psychotherapy, 8*, 8–16.

Arnevik, E., Wilberg, T., Urnes, O., Johansen, M., Monsen, J., & Karterud, S. (2009). Psychotherapy for personality disorders: Short term day hospital psychotherapy versus outpatient individual therapy: A randomized controlled study. *European Psychiatry, 24*, 71–78.

Bales, D. L., Timman, R., Andrea, H., Busschbach, J. J., Verheul, R., & Kamphuis, J. H. (in press). Effectiveness of day hospital mentalization-based treatment for patients with severe borderline personality disorder: A matched control study. *Clinical Psychology and Psychotherapy.*

Bamelis, L. L. M., Evers, S. M. A. A., Spinhoven, P., &, Arntz, A. (2014). The results of a multicenter randomized controlled trial on the clinical effectiveness of schema therapy for personality disorders. *American Journal of Psychiatry, 171*, 305–322.

Bartak, A., Soeteman, D. I., Verheul, R., & Busschbach, J. J. V. (2007). Strengthening the status of psychotherapy for personality disorders: An integrated perspective on effects and costs. *Canadian Journal of Psychiatry, 52*, 803–810.

Bateman, A. W., & Fonagy, P. (1999). The effectiveness of partial hospitalization in the treatment of borderline personality disorder—a randomized controlled trial. *American Journal of Psychiatry, 156*, 1563–1569.

Bateman, A. W., & Fonagy, P. (2001). The treatment of borderline personality disorder with psychoanalytically oriented partial hospitalization: An 18-month follow-up. *American Journal of Psychiatry, 158*, 36–42.

Bateman, A. W., & Fonagy, P. (2004). *Psychotherapy for borderline personality disorder.* Oxford, UK: Oxford University Press.

Bateman, A. [W.], & Fonagy, P. (2008). 8-year follow-up of patients treated for borderline personality disorder: Mentalization-based treatment versus treatment as usual. *American Journal of Psychiatry, 165*, 631–638.

Bateman, A. [W.], & Fonagy, P. (2009). Randomly controlled trial of outpatient mentalizing-based therapy versus structured clinical management for borderline personality disorder. *American Journal of Psychiatry, 166*, 1355–1364.

Bateman, A. [W.], & Fonagy, P. (2013). Impact of clinical severity on outcomes of mentalisation-based treatment for borderline personality disorder. *British Journal of Psychiatry, 203*, 221–227.

Beck, A. T., Freeman, A., & Associates. (1990). *Cognitive therapy of personality disorders.* New York: Guilford Press.

Beutler, L. E. (1991). Have all won and must all have prizes? Revisiting Luborsky et al.'s verdict. *Journal of Consulting and Clinical Psychology, 59*, 226–232.

Blum, N., St. John, D., Pfohl, B., Stuart, S., McCormick, B., Allen, J., et al. (2008). Systems training for emotional predictability and problem solving (STEPPS) for outpatients with borderline personality disorder: A randomized controlled trial and 1-year follow-up. *American Journal of Psychiatry, 165*, 468–478.

Budge, S. L., Moore, J. T., Del Re, A. C., Wampold, B. E., Baardseth, T. P., & Nienhaus, J. B. (2014). The effectiveness of evidence-based treatments for personality disorders when comparing treatment-as-usual and bona fide treatments. *Clinical Psychology Review, 34*(5), 451–452.

Castonguay, L. G., & Beutler, L. E. (2006a). Common and unique principles of therapeutic change: What do we know and what do we need to know? In L. G. Castonguay & L. E. Beutler (Eds.), *Principles of therapeutic change that work* (pp. 353–369). New York: Oxford University Press.

Castonguay, L. G., & Beutler, L. E. (Eds.). (2006b). *Principles of therapeutic change that work.* New York: Oxford University Press.

Chanen, A. M., Jackson, H. J., McCutcheon, L. K., Jovev, M., Dudgeon, P., Yuen, H. P., et al. (2008). Early intervention for adolescents with borderline personality disorder using cognitive analytic therapy: Randomised controlled trial. *British Journal of Psychiatry, 193*, 477–484.

Clarke, S., Thomas, T., & James, K. (2013). Cognitive analytic therapy for personality disorder: Randomized controlled trial. *British Journal of Psychiatry, 202*, 129–134.

Clarkin, J. F. (2008). Clinical approaches to Axis II comorbidity: Commentary. *Journal of Clinical Psychology: In Session, 64*, 1–9.

Clarkin, J. F., Levy, K. N., Lenzenweger, M. F., & Kernberg, O. F. (2007). Evaluating three treatments for borderline personality disorder: A multiwave study. *American Journal of Psychiatry, 164,* 922–928.

Clarkin, J. F., Yeomans, F. E., & Kernberg, O. (1999). *Psychotherapy for borderline personality disorder.* New York: Wiley.

Clarkin, J. F., Yeomans, F. E., & Kernberg, O. F. (2006). *Psychotherapy for borderline disorder: Focusing on object relations.* Washington, DC: American Psychiatric Publishing.

Cuthbert, B. N., & Insel, T. R. (2013). Toward the future of psychiatric diagnosis: The seven pillars of RDoC. *BMC Medicine, 11,* 126.

Davidson, K. (2008). *Cognitive therapy for personality disorders.* London: Routledge.

Davidson, K., Norrie, J., Tyrer, P., Gumley, A., Tata, P., Murray, H., et al. (2006). The effectiveness of cognitive behavior therapy for borderline personality disorder: Results from the BOSCOT trial. *Journal of Personality Disorders, 20,* 450–465.

Doering, S., Hörz, S., Rentrop, M., Fischer-Kern, M., Schuster, P., Benecke, C., et al. (2010). Transference-focused psychotherapy v. treatment by community psychotherapists for borderline personality disorder: Randomised controlled trial. *British Journal of Psychiatry, 196,* 389–395.

Doherty, J. L., & Owen, D. J. (2014). The research domain criteria: Moving the goalposts to change the game. *British Journal of Psychiatry, 204,* 171–173.

Giesen-Bloo, J., van Dyck, R., Spinhoven, P., van Tilberg, W., Dirksen, C., van Asselt, T., et al. (2006). Outpatient psychotherapy for borderline personality disorder: Randomized trial of schema-focused therapy vs. transference-focused therapy. *Archives of General Psychiatry, 63,* 649–658.

Gullestad, F. S., Johansen, M. S., Høglend, P., Karterud, S., & Wilberg, T. (2013). Mentalization as a moderator of treatment effects: Findings from a randomized clinical trial for personality disorders. *Psychotherapy Research, 23*(6), 674–689.

Gullestad, F. S., Wilberg, T., Klungsøyr, O., Johansen, M. S., Urnes, Ø., & Karterud, S. (2012). Is treatment in a day hospital step-down program superior to outpatient individual psychotherapy for patients with personality disorders?: 36 months follow-up of a randomized clinical trial comparing different treatment modalities. *Psychotherapy Research, 22,* 426–441.

Jorgensen, C. R., Freund, C., Boye, R., Jordet, H., Andersen, D., & Kjolbye, M. (2013). Mentalizing-based therapy versus psychodynamic supportive therapy. *Acta Psychiatrica Scandinavica, 127,* 305–317.

Kröger, C., Harbeck, S., Armbrust, M., & Kliem, S. (2013). Effectiveness, response, and dropout of dialectical behavior therapy for borderline personality disorder in an inpatient setting. *Behaviour Research and Therapy, 51,* 411–416.

Leichsenring, F., & Leibing, E. (2003). The effectiveness of psychodynamic therapy and cognitive behavior therapy in the treatment of personality disorders: A meta-analysis. *American Journal of Psychiatry, 160,* 1223–1232.

Lenzenweger, M. F., & Clarkin, J. F. (Eds.). (2005). *Major theories of personality disorder* (2nd ed.). New York: Guilford Press.

Linehan, M. M. (1993). *Cognitive-behavioral treatment of borderline personality disorder.* New York: Guilford Press.

Linehan, M. M., Armstrong, H. E., Suarez, A., Allmon, D., & Heard, H. (1991). Cognitive-behavioural treatment of chronically parasuicidal borderline patients. *Archives of General Psychiatry, 48,* 1060–1064.

Linehan, M. M., Comtois, K. A., Murray, A. M., Brown, M. Z., Gallop, R. J., Heard, H. L., et al. (2006). Two-year randomized controlled trial and follow-up of dialectical behavior therapy vs therapy by experts for suicidal behaviors and borderline personality disorder. *Archives of General Psychiatry, 63*, 757–766.

Livesley, W. J. (2003). *Practical management of personality disorder.* New York: Guilford Press.

Livesley, W. J. (2007). Integrated therapy for complex cases of personality disorder. *Journal of Clinical Psychology: In Session, 64*, 207–221.

Livesley, W. J. (2012). Moving beyond specialized therapies for borderline personality disorder: The importance of integrated domain-focused treatment. *Psychodynamic Psychiatry, 40*(1), 47–74.

Luborsky, L., Singer, B., & Luborsky, L. (1975). Comparative studies of psychotherapies. *Archives of General Psychiatry, 32*, 995–1008.

McMain, S. F., Links, P. S., Gnam, W. H., Guimond, T., Cardish, R. J., Korman, L., et al. (2009). A randomized trial of dialectical behavior therapy versus general psychiatric management for borderline personality disorder. *American Journal of Psychiatry, 166*, 1365–1374.

Mulder, R., & Chanen, A. M. (2013). Effectiveness of cognitive analytic therapy for personality disorders. *British Journal of Psychiatry, 202*, 89-90.

Muran, J., Safran , J., Samstag, L., & Winston, A. (2005). Evaluating an alliance-focused treatment for personality disorders. *Psychotherapy: Theory, Research, Practice, Training, 42*, 532–545.

Norcross, J. C., & Grencavage, L. M. (1989). Eclecticism and integration in counselling and psychotherapy: Major themes and obstacles. *British Journal of Guidance and Counselling, 17*, 117–247.

Norcross, J. C., & Newman, J. C. (1992). Psychotherapy integration: Setting the context. In J. C. Norcross & M. R. Goldfried (Eds.), *Handbook of psychotherapy integration* (pp. 3–45). New York: Basic Books.

Piper, W. E., & Joyce, A. S. (2001). Psychosocial treatment outcome. In W. J. Livesley (Ed.), *Handbook of personality disorders: Theory, research, and treatment* (pp. 323–343). New York: Guilford Press.

Ryle, A. (1975). *Cognitive analytic therapy and borderline personality disorder.* Chichester, UK: Wiley.

Stone, M. H. (2010). On the diversity of borderline syndromes. In T. Millon, R. F. Krueger, & E. Simonsen (Eds.), *Contemporary directions in psychopathology: Scientific foundations of the DSM-V and ICD-10* (pp. 577–594). New York: Guilford Press.

Stricker, G. (2010). A second look at psychotherapy integration. *Journal of Psychotherapy Integration, 20*, 397–405.

Yeomans, F. (2007). Questions concerning the randomized trial of schema-focused therapy vs. transference-focused psychotherapy. *Archives of General Psychiatry, 64*, 609–610.

Young, J. E., Klosko, J. S., & Weishaar, M. E. (2003). *Schema therapy: A practitioner's guide.* New York: Guilford Press.

chapter 2

A General Framework for Integrated Modular Treatment

W. John Livesley and John F. Clarkin

As discussed by Livesley, Dimaggio, and Clarkin (Chapter 1, this volume), rational and empirical considerations point to the value of a unified treatment approach based on a comprehensive array of interventions culled from all effective therapies targeted to the specific problems of individual cases. The challenge confronting this approach is how to deliver such an eclectic array of interventions in an organized and coordinated way while avoiding disorganized treatment resulting from therapist struggles to accommodate the diverse and ever-changing problems presented by patients. This eventuality is reduced if the therapist has a clear and explicit understanding of both the nature of personality disorder and the structure of therapy. Consequently, integrated modular treatment (IMT) has an explicit conceptual structure consisting of two empirically informed frameworks. The first specifies the nature of personality disorder and the impairments that are the focus of treatment. The second conceptualizes treatment in terms of the interventions required to treat these impairments and the sequence with which problems are typically addressed. This sequence provides that structure needed to coordinate and sequence the use of multiple interventions. Table 2.1 provides a schematic overview of the structure of IMT and shows the components of the two conceptual frameworks to help guide the reader through a more detailed discussion of the overall structure of therapy.

TABLE 2.1. The Structure of Integrated Modular Treatment (IMT)

Framework for conceptualizing personality disorder

1. General and specific features of personality disorder
   a. General features
      i. Chronic interpersonal problems
      ii. Self/identify problems
   b. Specific features

2. The personality as a system giving rise to four domains of personality impairment
   a. Symptoms
   b. Regulation and modulation
   c. Interpersonal
   d. Self-identity

3. Cognitive–emotional personality schemas

Framework for conceptualizing treatment

1. Treatment modules
   a. General treatment modules
      i. Structure
      ii. Relationship
      iii. Consistency
      iv. Validation
      v. Motivation
      vi. Metacognition
   b. Specific modules

2. Phases of change
   a. Safety
   b. Containment
   c. Regulation and modulation
   d. Exploration and change
   e. Integration and synthesis

A FRAMEWORK FOR CONCEPTUALIZING PERSONALITY DISORDER

To treat any pathology, the clinician needs a practical conception of the disorder and the dysfunctions that are the focus of intervention. The conception we propose has three components. First, a distinction is drawn between impairments common to all forms of personality disorder and features that delineate different disorders, such as borderline and antisocial personality disorders (Livesley, 2003a, 2003b). Second, personality is conceptualized as a loosely organized system consisting of trait, regulatory, interpersonal, and self-identity subsystems, each defining impairments that are addressed in treatment. Third, the different personality subsystems are assumed to involve cognitive–emotional–personality schemas that are used to encode and appraise environmental inputs and initiate a response. These schemas are a primary focus of intervention.

Two-Component Structure of Personality Disorder

Recent developments in diagnostic classification draw a distinction between features common to all personality disorders and the specific features of different disorders, an idea that is incorporated in both DSM-5 (American Psychiatric Association, 2013) and the proposed revisions to the *International Classification of Diseases* (ICD-11; Tyrer et al., 2011). The distinction expands the traditional focus on diagnosing specific disorders to include assessment of general personality disorder and severity of personality impairment. These are clinically useful developments because the general features of personality disorder have a substantial impact on treatment and severity predicts outcome better than specific categorical diagnoses (Crawford, Koldobsky, Mulder, & Tyrer, 2011). The distinction also helps to organize treatment: It implies that treatment methods may be divided into general methods used with all patients to manage and treat general personality disorder and specific methods needed to treat the specific features of different disorders and impairments of individual patients. The specific methods used will vary across patients and during therapy as different problems become the targets for change.

Clinical descriptions of the general features typically refer to difficulty in establishing a coherent self or identity (e.g., Kernberg, 1984; Kohut, 1971) and chronic interpersonal dysfunction (e.g., Benjamin, 1993, 2003; Rutter, 1987; see Livesley & Clarkin, Chapter 3, this volume). Both features adversely affect treatment by hindering the establishment of a collaborative treatment alliance, creating boundary problems, impeding motivation for change, and causing difficulty setting and achieving long-term goals. Consequently, a fundamental issue for any therapy is to establish the basic strategy for treating core personality disorder pathology. This is where the common-factors approach discussed in the previous chapter is helpful: It highlights the importance of the treatment relationship in the change process (Castonguay & Beutler, 2006a, 2006b). A consistent emphasis on the relationship provides the support, empathy, and validation needed to manage core impairments while also reducing the risk of activating reactive emotions and maladaptive interpersonal behaviors in ways that hinder treatment. The common-factors approach also creates a therapeutic process that provides a continuous corrective experience that helps to modulate the maladaptive self and interpersonal schemas underlying core pathology.

Comprehensive treatment also requires an eclectic array of interventions to treat the specific impairments associated with the different personality disorders and the more idiosyncratic features of individual patients. The specific features of disordered personality are usually represented by the categorical diagnoses of the DSM systems. Consequently, many texts on treatment posit strategies for treating each DSM diagnosis. However, we do not find global diagnoses helpful in planning and delivering therapy. Most specific interventions are designed to treat specific problems, such as deliberate self-injury, anger, physical violence, rejection sensitivity, and so on. This means that global disorders need to be decomposed into their different components and interventions selected to target each component. The strategy we propose is based on the second part of our framework for conceptualizing personality disorder, the idea of personality as a system.

Personality System

IMT assumes that personality is a loosely organized set of subsystems that include the self- and interpersonal systems, a system of regulatory and modulatory processes, and traits. The personality system is assumed to develop around heritable predispositions that give rise to personality traits. Traits capture clinically important individual differences. The evidence suggests that personality disorder traits are organized into four clusters (Widiger & Simonsen, 2005): (1) anxious-dependent or emotional dysregulation; (2) dissocial behavior; (3) social avoidance; and (4) compulsivity (see Livesley & Clarkin, Chapter 3, this volume). The clusters represent the major dimensions of individual differences in personality disorder that need to be addressed in therapy. As traits emerge, they shape the development of the self- and interpersonal systems. These interrelated systems are essentially knowledge networks that organize information about the self and the interpersonal world into cognitive–emotional–personality schemas that are used to encode events, impose meaning on experience, and anticipate what is likely to happen. The connections established among self-schemas during development contribute to the subjective experience of coherence and personal unity that characterizes adaptive personality functioning (Livesley, 2003b; Toulmin, 1978). The more extensive and complex these connections are, the greater is the sense of personal unity and coherence (Horowitz, 1998).

The interpersonal system consists of schemas representing other people and beliefs and expectations about the interpersonal world. The emergence of the self- and interpersonal systems depends on an array of basic cognitive processes for combining and integrating information and on metacognitive processes used to understand the mental states of oneself and others (Dimaggio, Semerari, Carcione, Nicolò, & Procacci, 2007; Fonagy, Gergely, Jurist, & Target, 2002). The personality system also includes regulatory and modulatory mechanisms that control emotions and impulses and coordinate action.

The conception of personality as a system is useful in selecting and sequencing specific interventions in IMT. The impairments associated with personality disorder encompass all personality subsystems, giving rise to four major domains of functional impairment:

1. Symptoms such as dysphoria, self-harm, dissociative features, quasi-psychotic symptoms, and rage.
2. Regulation and modulation problems, including difficulty regulating emotions and impulses and impaired metacognitive processes, leading to problems with self-reflection and effortful control. Regulatory

impairments are manifested as either undercontrol of emotions and impulses, which leads to unstable emotions and impulsive behavior as seen in patients with borderline and antisocial pathology, or over-control, leading to emotional constriction as observed in patients with schizoid-avoidant and compulsive disorders.
3. Interpersonal problems, including difficulty establishing relationships, intimacy and attachment problems, conflicted interpersonal patterns, unstable relationships, and disregard for others.
4. Self- or identity impairments, involving difficulty regulating self-esteem, maladaptive self-schemas, unstable sense of self or identity, and a poorly developed self-system.

Decomposing personality disorder into domains helps to ensure that assessment and treatment address all aspects of personality pathology. We also use this scheme to select specific interventions and establish the sequence for using specific intervention modules. Domains differ in stability and the possibility for change either with or without treatment (Tickle, Heatherton, & Wittenberg, 2001). Hence treatment can be organized as a sequence in which the most changeable domains are addressed first because this increases the probability of progress early in therapy. Symptoms are the most variable and treatable domain; most symptoms fluctuate naturally, and many change early in treatment. This suggests that in both brief therapy and the early stages of longer-term treatment, the primary focus should be on symptom reduction and increasing emotion and impulse control, a focus that is consistent with evidence that giving priority to presenting symptoms and concerns enhances outcome (Critchfield & Benjamin, 2006), probably because early progress helps to improve enhance the alliance and motivation. Regulatory and modulatory mechanisms are somewhat more stable but also tend to change relatively early in treatment, as evidenced by the results of studies of cognitive-behavioral therapies and the impact of transference-focused psychotherapy (TFP; Clarkin, Yeomans, & Kernberg, 2006) and mentalizing-based therapy (MBT) on metacognitive impairments. The greater stability resulting from symptomatic improvement and increased self-regulation then permits more attention to the interpersonal domains. The most stable domain is self/identity, which appears to change relatively slowly.

This scheme applies particularly to more reactive patients, such as those with high levels of emotional dysregulation and dissocial behaviors (DSM-IV/DSM-5 borderline, antisocial, and narcissistic disorders). With patients who are more emotionally constricted and who tend to be socially avoidant, less time will be spent initially on containment and improving self-regulation and more on engaging the patient in treatment and increasing metacognitive functioning. Our emphasis on domains and domain-based selection of specific interventions contrasts with the approach of some specialized treatments for borderline personality disorder (BPD). We place less emphasis on formal DSM diagnoses and the use of relatively fixed treatment protocols and more emphasis on assessing functional capacities across domains and selecting the best interventions to treat each impairment, issues that are discussed further by Livesley and Clarkin (Chapters 3 and 4, this volume).

Cognitive–Emotional Structure of Personality

Most of the effective therapies for personality disorder share the idea that cognitive–emotional structures, variously referred to as object relationships (Kernberg, 1984), working models (Bowlby, 1980), self- and object representations (Gold, 1990a, 1990b, 1996; Ryle, 1997; Wachtel, 1991), and cognitive schemas (Beck, Freeman, Davis, & Associates, 2004), are basic units for understanding personality and that the goal of therapy is to restructure these units. IMT also shares this perspective: Personality is conceptualized as an information-processing–decision-making system that encodes and appraises events and initiates responses. Social-cognitive models of personality refer to these units as cognitive–affective personality systems (CAPS; Mischel & Shoda, 1995) and propose that personality is essentially a dynamic system of multiple cognitive–affective units (CAUs; see also Cervone, 2005; Mischel, 2004; Morf & Mischel, 2012). The CAPS model is used to conceptualize personality disorder in IMT with the additional assumption that cognitive–emotional schemas are based on heritable mechanisms that reflect the adaptive architecture of personality (Livesley, 2003b; Livesley & Jang, 2008).

As cognitive–emotional–personality structures (CEPS) underlie all domains of impairment, the concept is integral to understanding and treating personality pathology. For example, the self-identity system consists of multiple CEPS used to organize self-referential knowledge into a hierarchy of different representations of the self, culminating in an overarching autobiographical self (Angus & McLeod, 2004; Hermans & Dimaggio, 2004; Neimeyer, 2000). Personality disorder usually involves a poorly differentiated self with few self-schemas, leading to impoverished self-understanding as observed in those with schizoid or avoidant features, and poor integration of self-schemas, leading to a fragmented and unstable self, as occurs with emotionally dysregulated traits and BPD. Treatment of self-pathology involves promoting greater self-knowledge, leading to increasing differentiation of self-schemas and their integration that is achieved by continually linking events, thoughts, feelings, and actions.

The interpersonal system is similarly organized. A CEPS representing another person organizes information about that person's qualities, values, beliefs, and interests. With casual acquaintances, these schemas consist of a few salient qualities, such as whether the person is friendly or honest. In contrast, a schema representing a significant other is likely to be more detailed and recognize different facets of his or her personality. For example, a person may be thought to be friendly, kind, and cheerful on most occasions but irritable and disagreeable on others. Usually an attempt is made to integrate these apparent discrepancies—for example, by recognizing that a person is normally friendly but irritable when stressed. With personality disorder, schemas representing other people are often impoverished and poorly integrated. As with self-pathology, treatment goals include greater differentiation and integration of the person's conceptions of others.

There is also a substantial cognitive component to traits. Although traits are heritable, they are shaped during development by environmental events that come to influence how traits are expressed (Livesley & Jang, 2008). Developmental elaboration leads to a complex cognitive architecture that modulates the genetic predisposition and mediates between events and action. For example, anxiousness is probably based on an adaptive mechanism for managing threat (Gray, 1987; Livesley, 2008b). Experiences of threatening events give rise to knowledge about how threatening the world is that influences the evaluation of events and appraisal of the ability to handle them. Gradually, these cognitions affect the threshold for perceiving threat and, hence, the experience of anxiety and the intensity of fearful responses. These ideas guide treatment; they suggest that maladaptive traits can be managed by restructuring their associated schemas.

The conception of personality as an information-processing system and knowledge structure implies that a key treatment task is to increase the patient's understanding of how symptoms and problem behaviors are linked to maladaptive schemas and then to restructure these schemas and to encourage the acquisition of more adaptive alternatives. As Critchfield and Benjamin (2006) noted, this is a strategy employed by all effective treatments.

A FRAMEWORK FOR CONCEPTUALIZING THERAPEUTIC CHANGE

The second component of the conceptual foundation of IMT is a framework for describing treatment. This framework has two components: (1) treatment methods and (2) a model of the phases through which treatment progresses.

In IMT, interventions are nested under the concept of treatment module, each module consisting of interrelated interventions designed to achieve a given outcome. Modules are divided into *general treatment modules,* based on change mechanisms common to all effective therapies, and *specific treatment modules,* consisting of interventions selected from all therapies to treat the specific impairments associated with a given domain. General modules are used with all patients throughout treatment, whereas domain-based specific modules vary according to the needs of individual patients and the problems that are the focus of therapeutic effort at a given moment in therapy. The distinction between general and specific treatment modules implies a hierarchy of interventions. Priority is given to ensuring the safety of the individual and others (Clarkin, Yeomans, & Kernberg, 2006; Linehan, 1993). Once safety is ensured, interventions from the general treatment modules are used to build an effective alliance and patient motivation. When these conditions are met, specific intervention modules are used to treat the problem at hand.

IMT assumes that treatment typically progresses through five phases: (1) safety, (2) containment, (3) regulation and modulation, (4) exploration and change, and (5) integration and synthesis. The phases of change are closely related to domains of functional impairment and hence to specific intervention modules. The first two phases are basically concerned with managing the symptom domain. The main goals of these phases are to ensure safety, contain symptoms, establish a degree of stability, and engage the patient in therapy. As symptoms settle and the patient becomes more stable, the focus begins to shift to the regulation and modulation domain and improving self-management of emotions and impulses. Phase 4 focuses primarily on the interpersonal domain. The tasks are to enhance interpersonal functioning by modulating maladaptive interpersonal patterns, restructuring maladaptive interpersonal schemas, and resolving conflicted relationship patterns. The final phase focuses primarily on promoting more integrated personality functioning, especially the construction of a more adaptive sense of self. The following sections describe general treatment modules and the phases of change and the specific intervention appropriate for each phase. However, we first need to discuss the idea of treatment modules.

THE CONCEPT OF TREATMENT MODULES

A treatment module is an interconnected series of therapist interventions that have a specific dysfunctional target. The modules discussed in this book are interconnected techniques that have been used as part of larger intervention packages in empirical trials or that are recommended by authors with experience in treating specific domains of pathology in patients with personality disorders. A major aim of this chapter is to orient the reader to how domains of dysfunction in patients with personality disorders can be matched to specific modules of intervention.

Thinking in terms of modules of intervention rather than isolated techniques has several advantages. First, each patient with a personality disorder, even compared with others with the same personality disorder diagnosis, has a unique relationship to the environment and unique areas of dysfunction. An obvious example is that some but not all patients with borderline pathology exhibit suicidal behavior, and those who overcome the behavior are confronted with other domains of dysfunction. The careful clinician will focus treatment for the individual on only those domains of dysfunction present in that patient. Second, modules of intervention provide a way of thinking about intervention with a particular domain of dysfunction at various levels along the treatment pathway. Take suicidal behavior again as an example. One can use techniques to help the patient overcome suicidal urges in the moment by diversions and changing focus of attention (see Linehan, 1993; Links & Bergmans, Chapter 9, this volume). One can also help the patient understand the emotional upset that preceded the suicidal ideation and urges (see Livesley,

Chapter 11, this volume). One can also examine the motives for the suicidal thoughts in the present context of the patient, especially the interpersonal contexts in which the behavior is thought to have an impact on others, including the therapist (Clarkin et al., 2006). These different approaches to one behavior are often thought of as reflecting behavioral, cognitive-behavioral, and dynamic approaches and are sometimes presented as if they were exclusive approaches. A more inclusive, flexible, transtheoretical approach is to think of them as multiple techniques, parts of a module, that focus on a complex cognitive–affective–behavioral network.

The modular approach tailors the treatment to the individual patient, as opposed to using a treatment manual that dictates the same techniques for all patients with a given personality disorder diagnosis. A modular approach to treating symptoms and conduct problems in preadolescents has already shown superiority to empirically supported treatments (Weisz et al., 2012). Barlow and colleagues (2011) have articulated what they call a unified protocol for transdiagnostic treatment of emotional disorders, especially anxiety and depressive disorders. They articulate a number of treatment modules that are relevant to these conditions, including modules for motivation enhancement, understanding emotions, recognizing and tracking emotions, cognitive appraisal and reappraisal, and so forth. This approach to anxiety and depressive disorders is similar to the one espoused in this book for personality disorders, as it is transdiagnostic and focused on specific modules of treatment related to key dysfunctions. (It is dissimilar to our approach in that Barlow et al. [2011] focus only on cognitive-behavioral techniques, whereas we include all therapeutic approaches.)

We have conceptualized two overall modules of intervention: (1) general treatment modules based on common change mechanisms (i.e., structure of the treatment, relationship issues, consistency, validation, enhancing motivation for change, and encouraging mentalizing/metacognition) and (2) specific treatment modules targeted to specific domains of dysfunction such as symptoms, emotion regulation and modulation, interpersonal behavior, and self-functioning. The remainder of this book is organized around these two general treatment modules. Part III (Chapters 6–8) expands on aspects of general treatment modules, and Part IV (Chapters 9–13) offers a variety of perspectives on specific intervention modules.

The clinician using an integrated approach to the treatment of individuals with the essential features of personality disorder (dysfunctions in self- and interpersonal relations) will, in a planned and strategic way, choose from the entire range of therapeutic modules and related techniques based on the individual patient's personality difficulties, the focus of change, and the stages of recovery. Integration is a mental process that the therapist engages in as he or she conducts the assessment of the particular patient in that patient's unique environment, with an articulation of the clinical problem areas (reflected in the chapters in this book) and the therapists' vision of which areas to address sequentially using a unique combination of interventions. It must be emphasized that the locus of integration is in the individual therapist's mind. A complete formula for integration is ultimately impossible, as integration is a function of the clinician, who works over time with a specific patient who has difficulties in a unique set of environmental circumstances.

There are a number of elements in the mental process of integration: (1) a working conception of the problems/dysfunctional areas of the individual patient, (2) a vision of how this patient could achieve a more effective level of adjustment, (3) a conception of how the patient can improve sequentially over time (e.g., reducing suicidal behavior, followed by improvement in interpersonal relations), (4) therapeutic interventions (treatment modules) timed to the salient patient problems and the readiness of the patient to change, and (5) a changing conception of the therapist as perceived by the patient and the patient's growing conception of self.

GENERAL TREATMENT MODULES

Descriptions of common change mechanisms usually distinguish between treatment methods that are primarily relational and supportive and those that are more instrumental and provide new learning experiences and opportunities to apply new skills (Lambert, 1992; Lambert & Bergen, 1994). This structure is used here to delineate six general intervention modules that form the core components of IMT—four relationship-based modules and two more instrumental modules:

1. Structure: establish the basic structure of treatment by specifying the conceptual model on which treatment is based, delineating the frame of therapy, defining the therapeutic stance, and establishing an explicit treatment contract.
2. Treatment alliance: establish and maintain a collaborative treatment alliance.
3. Consistency: maintain a consistent treatment process.
4. Validation: promote validation.
5. Motivation: build motivation and a commitment to change.
6. Metacognition: promote self-observation, self-knowledge, and self-reflection.

Structure

All effective treatments for personality disorder are highly structured and attach importance to establishing an explicit therapeutic frame. The frame is defined by the therapeutic stance and treatment contract. Together they structure therapeutic activity, establish treatment boundaries, help to ensure a consistent process, and create conditions for change. The stance sets the tone of treatment and shapes intervention strategies by defining the responsibilities and activities that structure patient–therapist interaction. Given the importance of relationship factors for successful outcome, the most appropriate stance is assumed to involve support, empathy, and validation and fostering the patient's participation in a collaborative descriptive exploration of problems and the acquisition of more adaptive responses (Critchfield & Benjamin, 2006; Livesley, 2003b).

The treatment contract is a structured agreement that helps to contain emotional reactivity by creating a safe and consistent therapeutic environment. This issue is discussed in further detail by Links, Mercer, and Novick (Chapter 5, this volume). An important part of this process is agreement on the initial treatment goals. As Critchfield and Benjamin (2006) noted, positive outcomes are increased by a goal-oriented approach in which "a treatment frame (is) established in collaboration with the patient and structured to achieve clear and explicit goals" (p. 262). A discussion of goals forges the idea that treatment is a collaborative process for which patient and therapist share responsibility. This discussion includes agreement on the practical arrangements of therapy, such as frequency of sessions and duration of treatment, a clear explanation of the treatment process and how treatment will address patient problems and concerns, and a frank discussion of the therapist's contributions and limits (Critchfield & Benjamin, 2006).

Treatment Alliance

The alliance is given priority because it provides support and predicts outcome. Unfortunately, a collaborative relationship is not easily achieved; it is the result of treatment rather than a prerequisite for treatment. For this reason, careful attention needs to be given to building the alliance and promptly repairing any ensuring rupture to it. Two ideas are useful for this purpose: Luborsky's (1984) two-component description of the alliance and Safran and colleagues' (Safran, Muran, & Samstag, 1994; Safran, Muran, Samstag, & Stevens, 2002) work on repairing ruptures to the alliance (see Tufekcioglu & Muran, Chapter 6, this volume, for a detailed discussion). These ideas delineate three submodules: (1) promote credibility, (2) build collaboration, and (3) repair alliance ruptures.

Luborsky (1984) suggested that the alliance has a perceptual component, in which the patient sees the therapist as helpful and him- or herself as accepting help, and a relationship component, in which patient and therapist work cooperatively for the patient's benefit. The first component, involving the patient's perception of the credibility of therapy and therapist, is built through interventions that communicate hope, convey understanding and acceptance of the patient's problems, support treatment goals, acknowledge areas of competence, and recognize progress toward attaining treatment goals. The relationship component is built by encouraging the patient–therapist bond, promoting a joint search for understanding, facilitating the acquisition of new skills, and emphasizing the collaborative nature of treatment.

Deteriorations in the alliance need to be addressed promptly but supportively. Safran and colleagues (1994, 2002) described a five-stage process to repair alliance problems:

1. Changes in the alliance, such as decreased involvement, are noted.
2. The patient's attention is drawn to the event, the reasons for the rupture, and the way in which it was experienced; these things are explored, and the patient is encouraged to express any negative feelings about the event.
3. The therapist validates the patient's account of the experience.
4. If these steps are not effective, attention focuses on how the patient avoids recognizing and exploring the rupture.
5. The therapist acknowledges his or her contribution to the relationship problem and promotes joint reflection on the reasons that things went awry and how to reestablish a collaborative bond.

The value of this approach is that it uses a potentially negative event to identify and begin changing maladaptive schemas related to core self- and interpersonal impairments.

Consistency

A consistent treatment process is also associated with positive outcomes (Critchfield & Benjamin, 2006). Interestingly, patients who benefit from treatment mention therapist consistency as a major factor in their improvement (Livesley, 2008a). Consistency in this context is defined as adherence to the frame of therapy. This is the reason that the treatment contract is so important (see Links, Mercer, & Novick, Chapter 5, this volume). Consistency provides the structure needed to contain unstable emotions and impulses and offers the patient a stable experience of the self within the treatment relationship that helps in the formation of more adaptive conceptions of him- or herself and others. Maintenance of consistency is, however, a challenge because unstable self-states, labile emotions, distrust, difficulty with cooperation, hostility, and aggression often lead to recurrent attempts to alter the frame and to challenges to the therapist's resolve to be consistent. Success requires skill in setting limits in a supportive way that does not damage the empathic stance. This is best achieved by confronting attempts to change the frame by recognizing and thereby validating the reasons for violating the frame while pointing out how the violation could adversely affect therapy.

Validation

Therapies with widely different theoretical and philosophical perspectives agree that validation is crucial when treating personality disorder. Validation may be defined as the therapist's recognition and affirmation of the legitimacy of the patient's experience. This does not mean that the therapist agrees with these experiences or their causes; a therapist should not validate perspectives that are invalid (Linehan, 1993). Although affirmation of the patient's experience is the basic feature of validation, some therapies take validation a little further. For example, in DBT, validation also communicates to the patient that his or her responses—feelings and actions—make sense and are understandable given his or her life situation (Linehan, 1993).

Validation serves multiple functions: It strengthens the alliance and reduces the defensiveness that leads patients to spend time justifying their feelings and distress. Validating interventions also help to manage and treat core pathology by affirming the authenticity of the patient's feelings and countering self-invalidating ways of thinking that hinder self-development.

In many ways, validation is more a therapist attitude than a set of interventions. It is conveyed by how the therapist goes about the task of therapy showing nonjudgmental recognition and acceptance and an open, receptive, and accepting stance. Validation is achieved by not rushing the patient, by allowing adequate time to express affects and describe experiences, and by making an effort to search for meaning in the treatment narrative.

Motivation

Although motivation to change is essential if patients are going to seek help and to work productively on their problems, low motivation is common with personality disorder. For this reason, motivation cannot be a prerequisite for treatment, and therapists need to make extensive use of such techniques as motivational interviewing (Miller & Rollnick, 1991, 2002, 2013; Rosengren, 2009) to build a commitment to change. Hope and discontent are powerful motivators (Baumeister, 1994), so motivation is enhanced by expectations that treatment will be successful and by the person's discontent with the current state of his or her life.

When motivation is poor, the evidence suggests that the best course is to maintain a supportive stance while attempting to explore the consequences of maladaptive behavior. Although therapists are often tempted to react in more confrontational ways, this rarely works and usually has an adverse effects on the alliance. As Linehan, Davison, Lynch, and Sanderson (2006) noted, motivation is enhanced when the therapist deals with low motivation and therapeutic impasses in a supportive and flexible way and acknowledges that change is difficult.

Metacognition

Personality disorder involves impairments in a wide range of metacognitive processes (Bateman & Fonagy, 2004; Choi-Kain & Gunderson, 2008; Semerari, Carcione, Dimaggio, Nicolò, & Procacci, 2007) that hinder the emergence of a coherent self and the capacity to relate effectively to others. Smooth interpersonal exchange depends on an understanding of self and other and on being aware of, and able to reflect on, the mental states of both. Although a confusing array of overlapping constructs, such as mentalizing, metacognition, self-reflection, self-awareness, self-understanding, and so on, are used to conceptualize the processes involved, most therapies are concerned with increasing self-knowledge and self-reflective thinking. Self-knowledge is limited by tendencies to suppress or avoid distressing aspects of self-experience, leading to an impoverished and selective body of self-knowledge. Patients also have difficulties reflecting on this knowledge. Many are acutely aware of painful thoughts and feelings and are intensely self-focused but have difficulty thinking about the nature, origins, and consequences of their experiences.

Increasing self-knowledge and self-reflective capacity are crucial therapeutic tasks in IMT (see Bateman & Fonagy, Chapter 7, this volume, for a detailed description of the central role of mentalizing in the treatment of personality disorders). Within IMT, the work of therapy is conceptualized as engaging the patient in a collaborative description of his or her problems and psychopathology and the effect of these problems on his or her life and relationships (Livesley, 2003b). This process also includes encouraging patients to reflect on the nature of these problems and their consequences and to become increasingly curious about their own mental states. Self-knowledge is increased by helping patients to become more aware of their repetitive maladaptive patterns of behavior and experience, the factors that trigger these patterns, and how these patterns contribute to their problems. As a new understanding emerges and obstacles to self-awareness are overcome, the patient is drawn almost inevitably into contemplating both alternative perspectives on events and new ways of behaving.

The therapist's role is to guide the process by drawing attention to important issues, by asking for details when descriptions are too general and for clarification when things are unclear, and by incorporating more structured interventions as needed. The psychotherapy literature describes a wide variety of structured and unstructured methods that the therapist can draw on to match interventions with patient variables and the therapist's preferred mode of working. In the process of collaborative description, the therapist not only elicits descriptions of problems but also shapes the patient's understanding of these problems by the questions that are asked, by the material that is selected to reflect back to the patient for further description, and by summaries that reframe the patient's understanding. The result is a shared understanding that expands self-awareness, reframes patients' ideas about themselves, and reformulates problems so that they are less distressing. The process of collaborative description also enhances metacognitive processes. This idea is discussed by Dimaggio, Popolo, Carcione, and Salvatore (Chapter 8, this volume), who show how accessing autobiographical narratives helps to improve metacognitive functioning.

The goal of collaborative description is not a historical reconstruction of events but rather a detailed formulation of how the patient experiences, thinks about, and reacts to events in the present (Ryle, 1997). The process is a reconstruction in the sense that the person's knowledge about his or her life is extended; things outside awareness or dimly recognized enter awareness and in the process are changed and modified. It is also a creation in the sense that it generates new understandings that contribute to more adaptive behaviors and to the synthesis of a more integrated sense of self.

SPECIFIC TREATMENT MODULES AND PHASES OF CHANGE

The general modules are supplemented with specific interventions when the patient's mental state is sufficiently settled to allow him or her to use more specific interventions and when the alliance is satisfactory and the patient is motivated to change. Earlier we noted that the challenge in using an eclectic set of interventions drawn from therapies with different and even incompatible theoretical assumptions is to prevent therapy from becoming unfocused, as could occur when a combination of potentially conflicting interventions are used in rapid succession to address diverse problems. We attempt to circumvent this problem by organizing IMT around general treatment methods and selecting specific interventions according to the current phase of therapy. Confusion is also reduced by clearly differentiating an intervention from the theoretical assumptions on which it is based. Thus, for example, some DBT or schema-focused therapy (SFT) methods may be used without adopting all their underlying theories. However, the main way to limit confusion arising from technical eclecticism is to follow the phases-of change model, which assumes that treatment progresses through the five phases mentioned earlier. Although the general treatment modules are used throughout therapy, specific interventions differ substantially across phases. Consequently, the phases-of-change model offers a way to coordinate the use of specific interventions with a general progression from more structured to less structured methods.

Safety

Treatment of severe personality disorders, especially the emotionally dysregulated and dissocial forms, typically begins with a crisis characterized by emotional and behavioral instability and symptomatic distress, which may also involve regression, dissociation, and cognitive dysregulation with impaired thinking and quasi-psychotic symptoms. In these situations, the primarily goal is to ensure the *safety* of the patient and others. This is largely achieved through structure and support that is usually delivered through outpatient treatment or crisis intervention services or, occasionally, brief inpatient treatment. The assessment of suicidality and strategies for ensuring patient safety are discussed by Links and Bergmans (Chapter 9, this volume).

Containment

The safety phase quickly moves to containment, the goal of which is to contain and settle unstable emotions and impulses and restore behavioral control.

The safety and containment phases typically merge as components of crisis management, with the goals of returning the patient quickly to the precrisis level of functioning and laying the foundation for further treatment. Change is achieved through general mechanisms of support, empathy, and structure supplemented with medication as needed to treat specific symptoms of impulsivity, affective lability, or cognitive dysregulation (Soloff, 2000; see Silk & Friedel, Chapter 10, this volume).

Containment interventions are based on the understanding that patients in a crisis are primarily concerned with obtaining relief from distress and that relief comes from feeling understood (Joseph, 1983; Livesley, 2003b; Steiner, 1994; see also Links & Bergmans, Chapter 9, this volume). Thus the therapist's task is to acknowledge and align with the patient's distress, to endeavor to see things from the patient's perspective, and to reflect what the patient is experiencing without trying to change it. Containment interventions are used at any point in treatment when a crisis occurs or cognitive functioning is impaired by intense emotions or dissociative behavior.

Regulation and Modulation

Crisis resolution and the establishment of greater behavioral stability usually enhance the alliance and a greater commitment to change, which permit a gradual shift to the regulation and modulation phase. At this point in treatment, the general treatment modules that have been used almost exclusively to this point are supplemented with specific treatment modules to increase awareness of the nuances of emotional experiences and to promote more modulated emotional expression. The phase lends itself well to a transtheoretical modular approach that draws on interventions from a wide range of therapies, including DBT, cognitive therapy, MBT, SFT, acceptance-based therapies, and narrative therapies tailored to the needs of individual patients. These interventions are organized into modules designed to increase knowledge about normal and dysregulated emotions, to increase emotional awareness and acceptance, to build emotional self-regulation skills, and to enhance the capacity to process emotional experiences (see Livesley, Chapter 11, this volume, for further discussion of these modules).

Earlier descriptions of the regulation and modulation domain noted that impairments in emotional regulation involve either decreased emotional regulation or emotional constriction and inhibition. Although these patterns are treated with different specific intervention modules, there are some common elements, so that the same intervention modules may be used with most patients at the beginning of the control and modulation phase. Patients with both patterns benefit from psychoeducation about the functions and adaptive significance of emotions and from interventions to increase emotional awareness, acceptance, and tolerance, such as mindfulness (see Ottavi, Passarella, Pasinetti, Salvatore, & Dimaggio, Chapter 13, this volume, for a more detailed discussion of mindfulness tailored to treating personality disorder).

Steps to increase emotion awareness may be approached using structured exercises and homework assignments. However, we find that it is often more effective with severe personality disorder to introduce these interventions during sessions so that the therapeutic relationship and containment interventions may be used to modulate any ensuring distress.

Gradually, the treatment pathways for patients with emotional dysregulation and those with emotional constriction begin to diverge. With the latter group, progress tends to be slow, and considerable time needs to be spent on encouraging emotional expression, with a heavy focus on the interpersonal aspects of emotional expression and building the treatment relationship. Strategies for treating these problems are discussed by Lynch, Hempel, and Clark (Chapter 15, this volume).

The treatment of patients with emotional dysregulation in this phase continues with extensive use of cognitive-behavioral methods based on accumulating evidence of their effectiveness in reducing deliberate self-injury and building emotional control (Blum et al., 2008; Davidson, 2008; Evans et al., 1999; Linehan, Armstrong, Suarez, Allmon & Heard 1991; Schmidt & Davidson, 2004). Treatment is organized around the idea that deliberate self-harm and other crisis behavior are the endpoint of a sequence of events that begins with an interpersonal situation that triggers maladaptive cognitive–emotional personality schemas, especially those involving abandonment and rejection, that activate an escalating dysphoric state, a model that is consistent with the assumptions of both DBT (Linehan, 1993) and TFP (Clarkin et al., Yeomans & Kernberg, 2006; Swenson, 1989). Treatment begins by discussing this sequence with the patient, which helps the patient to begin to understand the links between problem behaviors, situational factors, emotional reactions, and associated cognitions, a process that is critical to effective outcomes (Critchfield & Benjamin, 2006). This work also often has a settling effect because it allows the patient to make sense of events and actions that previously seemed inexplicable.

As the sequence of events leading to crisis and self-harm is explored, the idea of delaying self-harm is introduced with the initial goal of reducing the frequency of these behaviors rather than eliminating them—an unrealistic goal early in treatment (see Links & Bergmans, Chapter 9, and Livesley, Chapter 11, this volume). Setting modest goals increases the probability of an early success, which is useful in building the alliance and the commitment to change. Simple behavioral interventions such as distraction, self-soothing, and response prevention are often useful. Medication may also help to reduce emotional reactivity and facilitate therapy (see Silk & Friedel, Chapter 10, this volume). At the same time, a psychoeducational element is introduced to explain that self-harm is often a self-regulation strategy to reduce distress. This is a validating explanation that helps to reduce self-criticism and encourages the patient to contemplate alternative ways to handle distress. This sets the stage for introducing cognitive-behavioral interventions to increase emotional control. It should be noted that, although the behavioral sequence has been discussed in terms of self-harming behavior, the same strategy also applies to other behaviors, such as aggression and violence (see Wong, Chapter 16, this volume, for a discussion of the treatment of violence in the context of psychopathy).

In tandem with these interventions, patients are encouraged to use self-soothing and distraction at the first signs of distress. Simple relaxation methods may be introduced as ways to self-manage emotions, and attention control is increased by teaching the patient how to divert attention from distressing experiences rather than ruminating about them. Specific cognitive interventions are also used to help the patient to change maladaptive ways of thinking that escalate distress, such as rumination, catastrophizing, and self-invalidation. Strategies for treating maladaptive ways of thinking about and processing emotions are discussed by Leahy (Chapter 12, this volume). It should also be noted that, although the acquisition of emotion regulation skills is part of the process, it is not considered sufficient; it is also important to improve emotion processing capacity and to understand the interpersonal significance of emotional experiences. The importance of improving emotional processing and ways to facilitate it are discussed by Livesley (Chapter 11, this volume).

Two other interventions are also useful during this phase. First, patients often benefit from learning more effective ways to seek help when a crisis looms. Most patients only seek help after harming themselves or "acting out" and do so in an angry and demanding manner that alienates those they turn to for help. Second, many crises can be averted if patients learn to examine interpersonal situations more carefully and avoid personalizing situations so readily. For example, a patient may assume that a friend's reluctance to meet is an indication that the friend does not really like him or her rather than recognizing that people have their own lives and may have prior commitments. Encouraging patients to question their interpretation of events often helps to restructure experiences and to decrease maladaptive perceptions that trigger crises and "acting out." Work on these issues gradually moves treatment to the next phase—the exploration and change of maladaptive interpersonal schemas and behaviors. The duration of the control and modulation phase varies considerably across different forms of disorder and cases. With more reactive conditions involving labile emotions and/or impulsivity, the phase is likely to be prolonged. Indeed, with such individuals, treatment may largely be confined to this phase.

Exploration and Change

This phase of treatment focuses primarily on the interpersonal domain, with particular attention to changing the cognitive–emotional schemas associated with self-harm and violence, dysfunctional interpersonal patterns, maladaptive traits such as submissiveness, social avoidance, and callousness, maladaptive cognitive styles such as catastrophic thinking and self-invalidation, and the interpersonal consequences of trauma. Work on these problems invariably involves dealing with emotionally charged memories associated with psychosocial adversity. This is the reason that more extensive work on these issues is deferred until the patient has acquired the capacity to handle distress without it disrupting cognitive functioning.

Treatment continues to make extensive use of cognitive interventions to restructure maladaptive schemas based on evidence of the effectiveness of these interventions in treating BPD (Giesen-Bloo et al., 2006). However, effective treatment of this domain also requires incorporation of methods from other schools of therapy, especially psychodynamic and interpersonal therapy. Psychodynamic techniques become increasingly useful in treating avoidance behavior and in increasing awareness of maladaptive interpersonal patterns. The psychodynamic focus on the patient–therapist relationship helps to identify broad patterns of thinking and relating. This can then be followed with behavioral analyses of these patterns using cognitive-behavioral methods to clarify the specific ways these patterns are expressed and the environmental contingencies that evoke and maintain them. Psychodynamic interventions also take on greater importance because the treatment relationship becomes a major vehicle for changing core interpersonal schemas involving distrust, rejection, abandonment, self-derogation, and shame. Examination of the activation of these schemas in the here and now of therapy provides opportunities to make synergistic use of cognitive and psychodynamic interventions to explore triggering factors, the feelings associated with schema activation, and the way schemas shape interpersonal behavior. Interpersonal methods are particularly useful in changing core schemas (Young, Klosko, & Weishaar, 2003) because patients with severe personality disorder often have difficulty using standard cognitive interventions (Davidson, 2008; Layden, Newman, Freeman, & Morse, 1993).

Attention also has to be given to changing the core interpersonal patterns that characterize the different forms of personality disorder. This usually requires the use of methods drawn from different forms of interpersonal therapy. Cain and Pincus (Chapter 14, this volume) discuss effective interpersonal techniques based on the concept of interpersonal signature.

Cognitive restructuring is also useful in modulating the expression of maladaptive traits. Although traits are highly heritable, change is possible. However, it may be more effective to focus on reducing the frequency and intensity of trait expression by modifying associated schemas than to attempt more radical changes in trait structure. For example, reckless and sensation-seeking behaviors may be modulated by modifying beliefs about personal invulnerability, or emotional traits such as anxiousness may be modulated with a combination of a restructuring of beliefs about the threatening nature of the world and personal competency in coping with threats and emotion-regulating skills. With other traits, it may be more effective to help the patient to learn more adaptive ways to express them. For example, many patients with borderline and antisocial personalities are highly sensation seeking, which contributes to crises and interpersonal conflicts due to their need for excitement. These individuals can often be helped to find more adaptive ways to meet the need for stimulation.

Integration and Synthesis

The goal of the final phase of treatment is to construct a more adaptive sense of self or identity, a phase of treatment that is not reached by many patients. The transition from the previous phase is usually imperceptible. Self- and interpersonal pathology are inextricably intertwined; both emerge from the same interactional matrix. Exploration and resolution of interpersonal patterns inevitably incorporate discussion of important aspects of the self, and gradually the therapeutic focus increasingly deals with self problems and the development of a worthwhile life and hence a more adaptive sense of self and one's relationship with the interpersonal world.

We know considerably less about the most effective methods to promote an adaptive self-structure and sense of identity than we do about treating other aspects of personality pathology. The achievement of a sense of self probably does not involve only changing maladaptive and conflicted ways of being but also synthesizing a new and more coherent self-structure, more integrated representations of others, and development of the capacity for self-directedness. Such changes usually require longer-term treatment. Although there is little empirical research to guide intervention strategies, the nature of self-pathology points to the importance of general therapeutic strategies in providing a stable experience of the self in relationship with the therapist, which challenges core schemas and promotes self-understanding by providing consistent and veridical feedback. In addition, some the more specific strategies of self-psychology, constructionist therapies, and cognitive analytic therapy (Ryle, 1997) may also assist in constructing a more adaptive self-narrative. Three chapters in this volume offer differing perspectives on this neglected but important phase of treatment. In Chapter 17, Dimaggio, Popolo, Carcione, Salvatore, and Stiles discuss ways to extend the self-narratives that are important in understanding oneself in an interpersonal context. Clarkin, Yeomans, De Panfilis, and Levy (Chapter 18) offer ideas for incorporating psychoanalytical strategies for constructing an adaptive self-structure within an integrated approach. In Chapter 19, Salvatore, Popolo, and Dimaggio consider ways to integrate the different self-states that are a common feature of disordered personality.

An important step in promoting more adaptive self- and more integrated personality functioning is to help the patient to construct a personal niche that allows expression of personal aspirations, talents, interests, and traits while also helping the patient to avoid situations that activate vulnerabilities and conflicts. Essentially, it involves helping patients to "get a life" for themselves that is more adaptive than the life of a psychiatric patient or an offender. Although systematic work on this goal occurs toward the end of therapy, work on "getting a life" begins much earlier. Therapists always need to keep an eye on this objective and encourage the search for more adaptive relationships and ways of living throughout treatment. However, the construction of a more adaptive sense of identity or life script is more largely the achievement of the latter phases of therapy. This is an important part of comprehensive treatment: Long-term studies of patients without treatment suggest that success in finding an adaptive niche that created security and a sense of identity was linked to good outcomes (Paris, 2003).

HIERARCHY OF TREATMENT FOCI

Several times in this chapter we have alluded to the problem of how to coordinate the delivery of a complex array of interventions and how we consider this a major obstacle to the use of an integrated approach. In this section we discuss this issue in more detail. Later in the book we present an actual treatment case (Clarkin, Livesley, & Dimaggio, Chapter 20) to illustrate how this problem may be handled. The reader may wish to peruse this chapter before reading chapters on specific treatment methods to get an overview of how an integration-oriented therapist works with the patient to focus sequentially on areas of safety and change.

We argue that the logical sequence of change should proceed from patient safety to containment of disruptive emotions to interpersonal functioning and finally to building self-functioning that is satisfying and provides a sense of commitment and accomplishment for the individual. There are some obvious and not-so-obvious reasons for this hierarchy of intervention. Safety of the patient and those individuals around the patient is of obvious concern. This would be especially relevant with patients with chronic suicidal and/or self-destructive behavior. There are other not-so-obvious behaviors that are of safety concern, such as patients who are HIV-positive who endanger their sexual partners with minimal conscious concern. When safety concerns are met with appropriate treatment, or in the absence of such concerns, the therapist can turn to containment of symptoms, intense emotions, and impaired cognitive functioning and provide structure and consistent support. Having achieved some progress in containment, the therapist and patient can proceed to areas that are in some ways more complex and slower to change. This involves examining interpersonal functioning and the patient's self-direction and personal goals and values and helping the patient to integrate these self-conceptions by finding a satisfying niche in terms of work and intimate relations. We suggested that this sequence imposes some structure on the treatment process and begins to narrow the range of interventions to those appropriate to the phase of therapy. This is achieved by linking domains to intervention strategies.

Besides this general structure, therapists also need guides to help them decide when to change from one form of intervention to another, when to shift the therapeutic focus to a new problem, and when to move from one phase of treatment to the next phase.

Incorporating Specific Interventions

The first and probably the most straightforward transition in IMT is the decision about when to add specific interventions to the framework established by the general modules. Previously, we recommended that specific interventions be used only when the therapeutic conditions that the general modules are designed to promote have been achieved and the patient is not in a highly symptomatic or dysregulated state. Essentially, this means specific interventions are used only when the alliance and treatment bond are sufficiently robust to withstand the additional stress created by a more direct focus on change and the patient is sufficiently settled and motivated to make use of specific interventions.

With patients with more dysregulation, treatment often begins with the patient in a decompensated state so that therapy is initially concerned with ensuring safety, containing distress and reactivity, and engaging the patient in treatment. This usually involves using generic interventions to provide support and containment. The only specific intervention used at this time is medication to begin treating symptoms. As the distress settles and a connection is made with the patient, opportunities arise to begin using more specific interventions. The transition is usually smooth because appropriate interventions are relatively straightforward and highly structured, such as distraction to reduce emotional dyscontrol and deliberate self-harm, initial attempts to identify and label emotions, and discussion of practical ways to organize and schedule the patient's day and manage distress. Although these treatment methods hardly qualify as specific interventions, they pave the way for introducing skill-building and related modules to increase emotional control and reduce deliberate self-harm (see Livesley, Chapter 11, this volume). These methods are added as rapport deepens and, equally importantly, the patient's trust in treatment and in the therapist builds. With patients with more emotional constriction, the process is similar except that considerably more time is given to building the alliance in a nonintrusive way. With all cases, additional interventions are used only when there is a good alliance and a motivated patient. Because both the alliance and motivation for change fluctuate during therapy, this general rule operates throughout treatment.

Managing Transitions across Phases of Treatment

In contrast to the relatively straightforward decision of when to use specific interventions, the decision to move to the next phase of therapy requires considerably more clinical judgment. Within the phases-of-change model we have proposed, the change between *safety* and *containment* phases is usually seamless: Both are facets of crisis management. Also as noted, the transition from containment to the *regulation and modulation* phase is best managed by gradually incorporating cognitive-behavioral interventions as rapport builds. This development ushers in a relatively long phase focusing on building and modulating self-regulation skills and processes in patients with either emotional dysregulation or emotional constriction.

With patients with emotional dysregulation, the regulation and modulation phase of treatment nicely illustrates the benefits of a unified modular approach that allows deployment of a variety of specific interventions to develop the skills and processes needed for effective self-management of emotions. As described by Livesley (Chapter 11, this volume), improved emotion management involves the development of three basic capacities: (1) abilities linked to awareness and ability to identify the nuances of emotional experience coupled with the capacity to accept and tolerate emotions; (2) the use of emotion management skills; and (3) the ability to process emotions in terms of their interpersonal origins and consequences. Most therapies include interventions that address facets of these capacities, but few cover all aspects thoroughly. Integrated treatment allows flexible use of all relevant interventions as required to treat the problems of individual patients. Cognitive-behavioral strategies are likely to predominate. However, these are drawn from different forms of cognitive therapy, including standard Beckian therapy, and developments such as emotional schema therapy (see Leahy, Chapter 12, this volume), acceptance and commitment therapies, and more transtheoretical methods such as mindfulness (see Ottavi et al., Chapter 13, this volume). The development of enhanced emotion processing capacities will also require systematic application of more generic interventions concerned with enhancing self-reflection and metacognitive capacities related to emotion processing (see Bateman & Fonagy, Chapter 7, and Dimaggio et al., Chapter 8, this volume). The only other specific interventions used are likely to be psychodynamic strategies to address aspects of suppression of emotions and avoidance of emotional situations.

The most complex decision for the therapist involves when to progress from the control and regulation phase to exploration and change. This is a more complex transition because the primary focus of therapy changes from enhancing self-regulation of emotions and impulses to exploring and changing the maladaptive interpersonal schemas and patterns that underlie symptoms and emotional distress. This process requires changing from an essentially emotion-containment approach to a more emotion-arousing one, with the systematic exploration of thoughts and memories associated with adverse and traumatic experiences. There are no fundamental guidelines to help the therapist through this transition. It is largely a matter of clinical judgment. However, there are some factors that we have found helpful.

Transitions should be gradual rather than abrupt, and there is usually considerable movement back and forth across phases. When moving to a new phase, the problems and issues raised by the patient do not necessarily change. Instead, the therapist gradually responds to the therapeutic narrative differently while carefully gauging the patient's ability to manage emotional arousal. Throughout therapy, the narrative usually involves accounts of episodes and events that cause concern. Initially, these episodes are discussed in ways that build the alliance and contain distress. These discussions largely involve listening, reflecting, and seeking clarification. During the control and regulation phase, the same episode may be used to build emotional control by exploring the episode to establish what happened, to identify the feelings involved, to establish emotional triggers and patient responses to the event, and so on. Other elements of the episode are only explored to the degree needed to validate the significance of the episode and the feeling evoked before working with the episode to build emotion-regulation capacities. In the exploration and change phase, the same episode would be explored in more detail in terms of the interpersonal schemas activated, the interpersonal patterns involved, the associated affects, and so on. Thus the transition from regulation to exploration is largely a matter of the depth to which episodes are explored.

These ideas provide a context for considering the factors therapists should weigh when considering whether to proceed with more active exploration of psychopathology, including adverse and traumatic events and their long-term consequences. The important issue is whether the patient has developed the capacity to self-manage the levels of emotional arousal that are likely to accompany detailed exploration of adversity and traumas. The indicators of this capacity are a significant decrease in crises, including deliberate self-harm, increased emotion tolerance, consistent use of emotion-regulating skills inside and outside therapy, and the capacity to process emotional events as demonstrated by recognition of triggering events and the occurrence of more adaptive responses to emotional arousal.

An additional consideration is the quality of the alliance. Progression through the regulation and control phase is usually accompanied by greater trust in the therapist, manifested by a deepening bond and greater self-revelation. As this occurs, the patient becomes progressively more relaxed during sessions and less cautious—changes that are often accompanied by more humor that is appropriate to the context. Doubts about the therapist's availability and responsiveness also decrease, along with concerns about the therapist terminating therapy. Greater use is made of the therapist's comments both within and outside sessions, which usually reflects increased motivation for change.

As exploration of potentially distressing material deepens, the therapist needs to continue monitoring the patient's level of emotional arousal. If this increases to the point of impairing information processing, further exploration of emotionally arousing material is deferred and containment interventions are used to reestablish emotional control, as described earlier (see also Links & Bergmans, Chapter 9). These interventions simply involve recognizing the distress, providing support, and reflecting back the therapist's understanding of the patient's feelings. When these events occur (and in most therapies they do), it is important not to see the distress and confusion simply as a defense to avoid dealing with traumatic material that needs to be interpreted but rather as a manifestation of an underlying vulnerability. Hence, little is gained from interpreting these feelings or continuing with their exploration until cognitive functions are restored.

The final transition from the exploration and change phase to the integration and synthesis phase rarely presents problems. Many therapies do not reach this phase. In those that do, exploration of salient interpersonal problems often incorporates a self- or identity component so that the distinction is largely a difference in emphasis as concern progressively focuses on helping the patient to explore the implications of work on interpersonal difficulties for understanding the self.

Managing Changes between Specific Interventions

Often the most difficult decision for the therapist using IMT is when to adopt a new specific intervention. Rapid changes are confusing to patients, and as a general principle such changes should be kept to a minimum, and any change should be consistent with the phase of treatment and issues that are the focus of attention during a given session. Confusion is also minimized if the new intervention targets the same problem. A feature of IMT is the synergistic use of different interventions to treat a given problem. This often occurs early in treatment, when several interventions may be proposed to help the patient to reduce deliberate self-harming behavior. Under these circumstances, the therapist should explain to the patient that change often results not from a single intervention but rather from the accumulative effects of different methods, each having a small effect. For example, deliberate self-harming behavior may not respond to a single intervention but rather may improve when the patient uses several strategies such as distraction, self-soothing, and relaxation.

The most disruptive and confusing changes are abrupt transitions that use radically different interventions to target a new problem—for example, changing from using skill building to detailed exploration of trauma in response to the patient's suddenly describing a traumatic event. When the patient suddenly raises an important and painful issue, especially early in treatment, the therapist needs to listen carefully, validate the patient's concerns, and attempt to use the occurrence to address the problems that are being managed at that time. If the patient insists on dealing with such matters before the therapist thinks the patient is ready, it is best to acknowledge that the issue is important and that it has to be dealt with at some point, but then ask whether it would be possible to defer dealing with the issue in depth until the patient feels stable enough to handle the pain involved. If there is a good alliance, patients are usually content to defer to the therapist's suggestions.

CONCLUDING COMMENTS

The framework offered for thinking about and organizing integrated modular treatment is intended to be sufficiently structured to provide the consistent approach needed for effective outcomes but also sufficiently flexible that therapists may tailor treatment to their specific style, patient needs, treatment setting, and therapeutic modality. Consequently, the principles of IMT are relevant to short-term crisis intervention lasting at most a few months, to medium-term treatment lasting perhaps a year or so that is primarily concerned with increasing emotion and impulse regulation and decreasing self-harming behavior, and to long-term treatment lasting several years that is intended to change interpersonal patterns and promote more integrated personality functioning. The proposed framework is also intended to be sufficiently flexible to allow it to be modified to accommodate empirical and conceptual advances. In this sense, the framework is simply an interim position until a truly integrative model can be constructed based on a comprehensive, evidence-based theory of personality disorder.

REFERENCES

American Psychiatric Association. (2013). *Diagnostic and statistical manual of mental disorders* (5th ed.). Arlington, VA: Author.

Angus, L., & McLeod, J. (Eds.). (2004). *The handbook of narrative and psychotherapy: Practice, theory and research.* Thousand Oaks, CA: Sage.

Barlow, D. H., Farchione, T. J., Fairholme, C. P., Ellard, K. K., Boieseau, C. L., Allan, L. B., et al. (2011). *Unified protocol for transdiagnostic treatment of emotional disorders.* Oxford, UK: Oxford University Press.

Bateman, A., & Fonagy, P. (2004). *Psychotherapy for borderline personality disorder.* Oxford, UK: Oxford University Press

Baumeister, R. F. (1994). The crystallization of discontent in the process of major life change. In T. F. Heatherton & J. L. Weinberger (Eds.), *Can personality change?* (pp. 281–297). Washington, DC: American Psychological Association.

Beck, A. T., Freeman, A., Davis, D. D., & Associates. (2004). *Cognitive therapy of personality disorders.* New York: Guilford Press.

Benjamin, L. S. (1993). *Interpersonal diagnosis and treatment of personality disorders.* New York: Guilford Press.

Benjamin, L. S. (2003). *Interpersonal reconstructive therapy: An integrative, personality-based treatment for complex cases.* New York: Guilford Press.

Blum, N., St. John, D., Pfohl, B., Stuart, S., McCormick, B., Allen, J., et al. (2008). Systems training for emotional predictability and problem solving (STEPPS) for outpatients with borderline personality disorder: A randomized controlled trial and 1-year follow-up. *American Journal of Psychiatry, 165*, 468–478.

Bowlby, J. (1980). *Loss.* London: Hogarth Press.

Castonguay, L. G., & Beutler, L. E. (2006a). Common and unique principles of therapeutic change: What do we know and what do we need to know? In L. G. Castonguay & L. E. Beutler (Eds.), *Principles of therapeutic change that work* (pp. 353–369). New York: Oxford University Press.

Castonguay, L. G., & Beutler, L. E. (Eds.). (2006b). *Principles of therapeutic change that work.* New York: Oxford University Press.

Cervone, D. (2005). The architecture of personality. *Psychological Review, 111*, 183–204.

Choi-Kain, L. W., & Gunderson, J. G. (2008). Mentalization: Ontogeny, assessment and application in the treatment of borderline personality disorder. *American Journal of Psychiatry, 165*, 1127–1135.

Clarkin, J. F., Yeomans, F. E., & Kernberg, O. (2006). *Psychotherapy for borderline personality: Focusing on object relations.* Washington, DC: American Psychiatric Publishing.

Crawford, M. J., Koldobsky, N., Mulder, R., & Tyrer, P. (2011). Classifying personality disorder according to severity. *Journal of Personality Disorders, 25,* 321–330.

Critchfield, K. L., & Benjamin, L. S. (2006). Integration of therapeutic factors in treating personality disorders. In L. G. Castonguay & L. E. Beutler (Eds.), *Principles of therapeutic change that work* (pp. 253–271). New York: Oxford University Press.

Davidson, K. (2008). *Cognitive therapy for personality disorders* (2nd ed.). New York: Routledge.

Dimaggio, G., Semerari, A., Carcione, A., Nicolò, G., & Procacci, M. (2007). *Psychotherapy of personality disorders: Metacognition, states of mind, and interpersonal cycles.* London: Routledge.

Evans, K., Tyrer, P., Catalan, J., Schmidt, U., Davidson, K., Tata, P., et al. (1999). Manual-assisted cognitive-behavioral therapy (MACT): A randomized controlled trial of a brief intervention with bibliotherapy in the treatment of recurrent deliberate self-harm. *Psychological Medicine, 29,* 19–25.

Fonagy, P., Gergely, G., Jurist, E. L., & Target, M. (2002). *Affect regulation, mentalization, and the development of the self.* New York: Other Press.

Giesen-Bloo, J., van Dyck, R., Spinhoven, P., van Tilberg, W., Dirksen, C., van Asselt, T., et al. (2006). Outpatient psychotherapy for borderline personality disorder: Randomized trial of schema-focused therapy vs. transference-focused therapy. *Archives of General Psychiatry, 63,* 649–658.

Gold, J. R. (1990a). Culture, history, and psychotherapy integration. *Journal of Integrative and Eclectic Psychotherapy, 9,* 41–48.

Gold, J. R. (1990b). The integration of psychoanalytic, interpersonal, and cognitive approaches in the psychotherapy of borderline and narcissistic disorders. *Journal of Integrative and Eclectic Psychotherapy, 9,* 49–68.

Gold, J. R. (1996). *Key concepts in psychotherapy integration.* New York: Plenum Press.

Gray, J. A. (1987). *The psychology of fear and stress.* Cambridge, UK: Cambridge University Press.

Hermans, H. J. M., & Dimaggio, G. (Eds.). (2004). *The dialogical self in psychotherapy.* London: Brunner/Routledge.

Horowitz, M. J. (1998). *Cognitive psychodynamics: From conflict to character.* New York: Wiley.

Joseph, B. (1983). On understanding and not understanding: Some technical issues. *International Journal of Psychoanalysis, 64,* 291–298.

Kernberg, O. F. (1984). *Severe personality disorders.* New Haven, CT: Yale University Press.

Kohut, H. (1971). *The analysis of the self.* New York: International Universities Press.

Lambert, M. J. (1992). Psychotherapy outcome research: Implications for integrative and eclectical therapists. In J. C. Norcross & M. R. Goldfried (Eds.), *Handbook of psychotherapy integration* (pp. 94–129). New York: Basic Books.

Lambert, M. J., & Bergen, A. E. (1994). The effectiveness of psychotherapy. In A. E. Bergin & S. L. Garfield (Eds.), *Handbook of psychotherapy and behavior change* (4th ed., pp. 143–189). New York: Wiley.

Layden, M. A., Newman, C. F., Freeman, A., & Morse, S. B. (1993). *Cognitive therapy of borderline personality disorder.* Needham Heights, MA: Allyn & Bacon.

Linehan, M. M. (1993). *Cognitive-behavioral treatment of borderline personality disorder.* New York: Guilford Press.

Linehan, M. M., Armstrong, H. E., Suarez, A., Allmon, D., & Heard, H. (1991). Cognitive-behavioral treatment of chronically parasuicidal borderline patients. *Archives of General Psychiatry, 48*, 1060–1064.

Linehan, M. M., Davison, G. C., Lynch, T. R., & Sanderson, C. (2006). Techniques factors in treating personality disorders. In L. G. Castonguay & L. E. Beutler (Eds.), *Principles of therapeutic change that work* (pp. 239–252). New York: Oxford University Press.

Livesley, W. J. (2003a). Diagnostic dilemmas in the classification of personality disorder. In K. Phillips, M. First, & H. A. Pincus (Eds.), *Advancing DSM: Dilemmas in psychiatric diagnosis* (pp. 153–189). Washington, DC: American Psychiatric Publishing.

Livesley, W. J. (2003b). *Practical management of personality disorder.* New York: Guilford Press.

Livesley, W. J. (2008a). Integrated therapy for complex cases of personality disorder. *Journal of Clinical Psychology, 64*, 207–221.

Livesley, W. J. (2008b). Toward a genetically informed model of borderline personality disorder. *Journal of Personality Disorders, 22*, 42–71.

Livesley, W. J., & Jang, K. L. (2008). The behavioral genetics of personality disorders. *Annual Review of Clinical Psychology, 4*, 247–274.

Luborsky, L. (1984). *Principles of psychoanalytic psychotherapy.* New York: Basic Books.

Miller, W. R., & Rollnick, S. (1991). *Motivational interviewing: Preparing people to change addictive behavior.* New York: Guilford Press.

Miller, W. R., & Rollnick, S. (2013). *Motivational interviewing* (3rd ed.): *Helping people change.* New York: Guilford Press.

Mischel, W. (2004). Toward an integrative science of the person. *Annual Review of Psychology, 55*, 1–22.

Mischel, W., & Shoda, Y. (1995). A cognitive-affective system theory of personality: Reconceptualizing situations, dispositions, dynamics, and invariance in personality structure. *Psychological Review, 102*, 246–268.

Morf, C. C., & Mischel, W. (2012). Self as a psycho-social dynamic processing system: Toward a converging science of selfhood. In M. R. Leary & J. P. Tangney (Eds.), *Handbook of self and identity* (2nd ed., pp. 21–49). New York: Guilford Press.

Neimeyer, R. A. (2000). Narrative disruptions in the construction of the self. In R. A. Neimeyer & J. D. Raskin (Eds.), *Constructions of disorder* (pp. 207–241). Washington, DC: APA Press.

Paris, J. (2003). *Personality disorders over time.* Washington, DC: American Psychiatric Press.

Rosengren, D. B. (2009). *Building motivational interviewing skills: A practitioner workbook.* New York: Guilford Press.

Rutter, M. (1987). Temperament, personality, and personality disorder. *British Journal of Psychiatry, 150*, 443–458.

Ryle, A. (1997). *Cognitive analytic therapy and borderline personality disorder.* Chichester, UK: Wiley.

Safran, J. D., Muran, J. C., & Samstag, L. W. (1994). Resolving therapeutic alliance ruptures: A task analytic investigation. In A. O. Horvath & L. S. Greenberg

(Eds.), *The working alliance: Theory, research, and practice* (pp. 225–255). New York: Wiley.

Safran, J. D., Muran, J. C., Samstag, L. W., & Stevens, C. (2002). Repairing alliance ruptures. In J. C. Norcross (Ed.), *Psychotherapy relationships that work: Therapist contributions and responsiveness to patients* (pp. 235–254). New York: Oxford University Press.

Schmidt, U., & Davidson, K. (2004). *Life after self-harm.* Hove, UK: Brunner-Routledge.

Semerari, A., Carcione, A., Dimaggio, G., Nicolò, G., & Procacci, M. (2007). Understanding minds, different functions and different disorders?: The contribution of psychotherapeutic research. *Psychotherapy Research, 17,* 106–119.

Soloff, P. H. (2000). Psychopharmacology of borderline personality disorder. *Psychiatric Clinics of North America, 23,* 169–190.

Steiner, J. (1994). Patient-centered and analyst-centered interpretations: Some implications of containment and countertransference. *Psychoanalytic Quarterly, 14,* 406–422.

Swenson, C. (1989). Kernberg and Linehan: Two approaches to the borderline patient. *Journal of Personality Disorders, 3,* 26–35.

Tickle, J. J., Heatherton, T. F., & Wittenberg, L. G. (2001). Can personality change? In W. J. Livesley (Ed.), *Handbook of personality disorders: Theory, research, and treatment* (pp. 242–258). New York: Guilford Press.

Toulmin. S. (1978). Self-knowledge and knowledge of the "self." In T. Mischel (Ed.), *The self: Psychological and philosophical issues* (pp. 291–317). Oxford, UK: Oxford University Press.

Tyrer, P., Crawford, M., Mulder, R., Blashfield, R., Farnam, A., Fossati, A., et al. (2011). The rationale for the reclassification of personality disorder in the 11th revision of the International Classification of Diseases (ICD-11). *Journal of Personality and Mental Health, 5,* 246–259.

Wachtel, P. L. (1991). From eclecticism to synthesis: Toward a more seamless psychotherapeutic integration. *Journal of Psychotherapy Integration, 1,* 43–54.

Weisz, J. R., Chorpita, B. F., Palinkas, L. A., Schoenwald, S. K., Miranda, J., Bearman, S. K., et al. (2012). Testing standard and modular designs for psychotherapy treating depression, anxiety, and conduct problems in youth: A randomized effectiveness trial. *Archives of General Psychiatry, 69,* 274–282.

Widiger, T., & Simonsen, E. (2005). Alternative dimensional models of personality disorder: Finding a common ground. *Journal of Personality Disorders, 19,* 110–130.

Young, J. E., Klosko, J. S., & Weishaar, M. E. (2003). *Schema therapy: A practitioner's guide.* New York: Guilford Press.

part two

ASSESSMENT, TREATMENT PLANNING, AND THE TREATMENT CONTRACT

chapter 3

Diagnosis and Assessment

W. John Livesley and John F. Clarkin

Assessment and treatment are closely intertwined in integrated modular treatment (IMT). Diagnostic assessment provides not only the information needed to construct a formulation and plan treatment but also an opportunity to begin shaping the treatment alliance, building a commitment to change, and encouraging self-appraisal and self-reflection. The basic principle of integration—that treatment involves a combination of methods based on common change mechanisms and specific interventions tailored to individuals' problems—requires systematic evaluation of the diverse components of personality disorder. Assessment limited to specific categorical diagnoses such as borderline or antisocial personality disorder are usually considered sufficient, with the assumption that current diagnoses identify sufficiently homogeneous conditions to justify using a standardized protocol. Unfortunately, the assumption conflicts with the protean form and content of personality pathology that encompass most aspects of personality, creating enormous heterogeneity, even among those with the same categorical diagnosis. Responding to this heterogeneity with appropriate levels of treatment intensity and interventions requires a thorough evaluation of all aspects of personality disorder; it is not sufficient to rely exclusively on a categorical diagnosis. Consequently, we begin discussing assessment by examining sources of heterogeneity and their implications.

HETEROGENEITY OF PERSONALITY DISORDER

A major cause of heterogeneity is the convention that diagnosis requires the presence of a specified number of criteria from a larger set, which results in some individuals with the same diagnosis having few features in common. Nevertheless, diagnostic practice and contemporary treatments consider all individuals meeting a diagnostic threshold to be the same. Unfortunately, this is clearly not the case. For example, patients meeting criteria for borderline personality disorder (BPD) with high levels of cognitive dysregulation that cause cognitive processes to become disorganized when stressed need to be managed differently from patients without this feature; emotional arousal needs to be managed to prevent emotions overwhelming cognitive functions. The tendency to assume similarity among all individuals with the same diagnosis is also challenged by evidence that severity predicts outcome better than categorical diagnoses (Crawford, Koldobsky, Mulder, & Tyrer, 2011). Hence, both DSM-5 and proposals for the *International Classification of Diseases* (ICD-11) (Tyrer et al., 2011) incorporate a measure of severity. Heterogeneity also arises because the trait constellations delineating categorical disorders occur in the context of other personality traits that also influence treatment. For example, some patients with DSM-IV BPD also have elevated traits such as sensation seeking and recklessness that are more commonly associated with antisocial personality disorder. The need for stimulation and excitement associated with these traits contribute to the crises and maladaptive lifestyles often associated with borderline pathology. The management of such patients is likely to differ from that of other patients with BPD who are more socially avoidant. This suggests the need to assess all traits, not just the narrow range described by each DSM-IV or DSM-5 diagnosis.

Extensive *between-individual heterogeneity* is complemented by extensive *within-individual heterogeneity* that occurs because pathology involves all aspects of personality, leading to diverse problems, including symptoms, dysregulation of emotions and impulses, interpersonal problems, and self-identity pathology. Evaluation of these domains is important because the evidence suggests that outcome is domain specific (Piper & Joyce, 2001); interventions that work for one set of problems do not necessarily work for another. This suggests that interventions need to be selected according to the domain being treated rather than by a global categorical diagnosis. For this reason, we advocate decomposing global diagnoses such as antisocial and borderline personality disorders into four domains of functionally related impairments: symptoms, regulation and modulation, interpersonal, and self or identity. The value of this approach is that it systematically links assessment to treatment goals and methods, something that is not possible with categorical diagnosis.

Our examination of heterogeneity leads us to propose an assessment process that establishes (1) the presence of personality disorder and level of severity, (2) individual differences in clinically significant personality dimensions, and (3) impairment across domains of personality functioning. Before considering the assessment of these features, we examine other proposals for assessing personality disorder to place our recommendations in a broader context.

REVIEW OF OTHER RECOMMENDATIONS

Perhaps surprisingly, the clinical literature contains few systematic recommendations for assessing individuals with potential personality disorder. Recommendations also vary widely. A common distinction is whether a specific DSM-IV/DSM-5 or ICD-10 diagnosis is considered sufficient to implement treatment. Within those approaches that advocate more extensive assessment, there is considerable divergence of opinion on what additional information is needed and, indeed, whether categorical diagnosis is important. We began our overview by considering the recommendations in manuals describing empirically supported treatments, although unfortunately most deal with BPD.

Linehan's (1993) account of dialectical behavior therapy (DBT) does not formally discuss assessment. However, different definitions of BPD are discussed, which suggests that categorical diagnosis is the only formal assessment. Nevertheless, DBT incorporates the idea that behavioral analysis is an ongoing part of treatment. DBT's reliance on diagnosis contrasts with the more detailed assessment recommended by other cognitive therapies. Young, Klosko, and Weishaar (2003), in their manual for schema-focused therapy, emphasize a case formulation approach based on a broad assessment strategy covering dysfunctional life patterns, early maladaptive schemas and their origins, coping styles and responses, and temperament that makes little reference to formal diagnosis. Davidson (2008) recommends a similar approach in her account of cognitive therapy for personality disorders. With these purely cognitive therapies, assessment is designed to provide the information needed to construct a road map that allows treatment to be tailored to the individual within the parameters of the cognitive model.

Clarkin, Yeomans, and Kernberg's (2006) manualization of transference-focused psychotherapy (TFP) recommends a two-level strategy that goes beyond categorical diagnosis to assess symptoms and level of structural organization. The former involves evaluating DSM-IV personality disorder criteria, which may involve using structured interviews. They also discuss the importance of differentiating among major depression, characterological depression, and BPD. The latter assessment involves a structural interview to assess Kernberg's concept of borderline personality organization. Interestingly, much of the assessment chapter is devoted to a case illustration of the structural interview reflecting the authors' emphasis on clinical assessment. Three features of this approach are directly relevant to assessment for integrated treatment. First, Clarkin and colleagues note the limitations of categorical diagnosis while emphasizing the importance of careful differential diagnosis. Second, as with the cognitive therapies, detailed case formulation is used to accommodate both patient heterogeneity and the unique features of each case. Finally, they adopt a clinical assessment approach—a recommendation that we follow.

The manual for mentalizing-based therapy (MBT; Bateman & Fonagy, 2004), like that for DBT, does not include a systematic discussion of diagnosis. A short section indicates that the Structured Clinical Interview for DSM-IV Axis I and Axis II Personality Disorders (SCID-I, SCID-II) and the Diagnostic Interview for Borderlines (DIB) are used to establish diagnosis prior to treatment. A subsequent volume (Bateman & Fonagy, 2006), however, discusses assessment of mentalizing and the interpersonal relationships largely using clinical methods and indicators such as chaotic lifestyle, unstable housing, suicide risk, substance abuse, and problems with impulse control, features that we refer to as *severity indicators*.

Other experts generally recommend a broad assessment strategy. Widiger and Lowe (2012), for example, provided a comprehensive review of the instruments and empirical research on assessment related to treatment planning. They acknowledged that clinicians do not typically use structured interviews (e.g., SCID-II, International Personality Disorder Examination [IPDE]) and recommended a combination of patient self-report measures, clinical interview, and selected components of semistructured interviews (based on the patient's individual domains of difficulty). Beutler and Groth-Marnat (2003) also recommend going beyond an emphasis on diagnosis. They advocate using a diagnosis evaluation and additional information to shape a treatment formulation, although they focus less on official diagnoses and more on dimensions of personality functioning that are empirically related to treatment foci and outcome. The approach matches empirically derived patient variables to treatment planning decisions (Beutler, Clarkin, & Bongar, 2000). This is a useful feature that is closely related to our recommendations. Currently, diagnostic assessment is poorly related to treatment decisions, including the selection of interventions. This is an unfortunate disconnection given that diagnosis is primarily designed to help clinicians make informed decisions. Beutler and colleagues (2000) focus on the following patient variables: (1) functional impairment in social and intimate relationships, (2) level of social support, (3) problem complexity (chronicity and comorbidity issues), (4) characteristic ways of coping, and (5) acceptance or resistance to outside influences. Assessment utilizes an organized clinical interview and selected self-report instruments to measure these characteristics.

Although this brief overview of recommendations for assessing personality disorders reveals little consensus, several themes emerged that are helpful in establishing assessment parameters for IMT. First, most recommendations downplay the importance of official diagnoses in favor of a more broadly based evaluation of critical patient variables that includes a personality profile. This concurs with our conclusions derived from a consideration of the heterogeneity of personality pathology. It is also consistent with the way therapy is conducted: Interventions tend to focus on relatively specific features of personality pathology such as emotional lability and aggressivity rather than global diagnoses (Leising & Zimmermann, 2011; Sanderson & Clarkin, 2013). A second theme is the focus on patient variables related to treatment decisions—what we have referred to as *domains of impairment*. Third, emphasis is placed on clinical assessment supplemented with structured assessment methods. Fourth, assessment is closely tied to case formulation that shapes the treatment process (see Links, Mercer, & Novick, Chapter 5, this volume).

RECOMMENDATIONS FOR ASSESSMENT

A major assessment decision concerns what aspects of dysfunction to focus on. This is precisely where choices must be made because the advocates of the various treatments for the personality disorders emphasize different impairments. DBT emphasizes assessment of suicidality and emotional dysregulation. MBT emphasizes deficits in mentalization. TFP emphasizes intervention with mental representations of self, others, and related relationship disruptions and difficulties. Unfortunately, although the empirically supported treatments focus on different domains of dysfunction, there is little evidence that the treatments are specific to the domains of dysfunction they emphasize. Hence they offer limited guidance in identifying critical assessment variables. For this reason, we recommend an assessment strategy based on our analysis of heterogeneity of personality and the recommendations of others to match patients to the most appropriate level of treatment intensity and combination of treatment methods. Besides obtaining a thorough personal history and evaluation of mental state, including any comorbid symptom constellations (e.g., depression, anxiety), this requires evaluation of three sets of personality variables: (1) a diagnosis of personality disorder, including severity; (2) clinically relevant individual differences in personality traits; and (3) impairments in four domains of personality functioning, namely, symptoms, regulation and modulation mechanisms, interpersonal, and self/identity. This information is used to construct a case formulation and treatment plan derived logically from the formulation that (1) links evaluation of severity and domains of impairment to treatment intensity, therapeutic pathways, and intervention strategies and (2) includes practical decisions about frequency of treatment, treatment setting, likelihood of crises, and so forth. Although this appears to require a complex assessment, we do not believe that this is the case. We also suggest that this type of assessment occurs implicitly with all treatments because clinicians need to isolate specific features in order to identify effective interventions.

This alternative to categorical diagnosis is consistent with emerging trends in diagnostic classification. The ascent of dimensional classification has prompted suggestions for a two-component classification consisting of definitions of general personality disorder and severity and a system to describe clinically significant individual differences in personality (Cloninger, 2000; Leising & Zimmerman, 2011; Livesley, 1998, 2003). Before discussing the three-component assessment of personality disorder, we briefly consider the relative merits of clinical and structured assessment.

A major decision for the clinical assessor is whether to use a free-flowing clinical interview or a semistructured interview with set areas of inquiry. The former is the time-honored approach (MacKinnon, Michels, & Buckley, 2009) that has the advantage of favoring the freedom of a talented and experienced clinician. The latter provides an assurance of standard coverage of crucial areas and allows clinicians to compare their assessments with those of others. On balance, we recommend using the clinical interview as the primary assessment tool for routine clinical practice because it allows the clinician to elicit information in ways that foster the alliance and engage patients in treatment. This is important because many patients drop out either during assessment or between assessment and therapy, even under the carefully constructed conditions of a randomized clinical trial (Giesen-Bloo et al., 2006), which suggests that assessors should not lose sight of the process of the interview and rapport in the quest for information.

Another decision is whether to supplement the interview with ancillary measures such as questionnaires and/or more extensive assessment instruments. Whereas self-report questionnaires and, in fact, a whole battery of psychological and neurocognitive tests can be used to evaluate the patient (Clarkin, Howieson, & McClough, 2008), efficiency and limited resources in many mental health systems lead clinicians to use the interview as the most efficient way to approach diagnostic assessment and treatment planning.

Every clinician develops his or her own preferred approach to the initial assessment interview, and it is not our intent to discuss in detail how the initial evaluation should be structured. However, our assumption is that the interview will cover (1) current symptoms and problems and reasons for seeking help, including a recent history of symptoms and problems and their onset; (2) personal history that includes information about the nuclear family and early development, reactions to major developmental transitions such as early school experiences, adolescence, sexuality, peer relationships, experiences of abuse, trauma and other forms of adversity, and important memories; and (3) examination of mental state.

In collecting this information, a pertinent decision required of the assessor is the balance between a focus on present functioning as opposed to developmental history. Within the dictates of time, we recommend a thorough evaluation of the patient's present functioning with relatively less attention to the past. Information about past difficulties in development, traumatic experiences, and the history of current ways of relating to others is most relevant. When time constraints are not a problem, it is always valuable to have detailed developmental and life history information.

ASSESSING PERSONALITY DISORDER AND SEVERITY

This section covers various issues related to the diagnosis of personality disorder and assessment of severity. We begin by examining definitions of personality disorder to identify a clinically useful approach. This is followed by a consideration of the meaning and assessment of severity. The section concludes with a discussion of how disorder and severity can be assessed simultaneously in the clinical interview.

The first clinical decision is whether the patient has personality disorder or not. Although this decision is usually considered categorical, it is essentially dimensional: To what extent, to what degree does a patient show stigmata of personality pathology? There is a wide range of personality difficulties to consider here. Does a successful man with narcissistic traits whose spouse experiences him as distant and not interested in her meet criteria for personality disorder or not? One could sensibly ask: Does it really matter? There are marital conflicts that have brought the couple to treatment to alleviate the interpersonal difficulties. In contrast, consider the patient who has multiple symptoms (anxiety, depression, angry outbursts, wrist cutting, and creation of conflict in relationships) who meets the severity criteria for self- and other relations and severe trait disturbances that clearly place her in the realm of personality disorder. These examples illustrate the distinction between personality dysfunction and disorder. Although this distinction may not be important in initiating treatment, it has implications for how treatment is conducted—severity is the main factor determining treatment intensity and intervention strategy.

Definition of Personality Disorder

Although there is currently little consensus on how to define personality disorder, some approaches are clearly less useful than others, and some trends are emerging that provide the outline of a practical clinical definition. DSM-III's (American Psychiatric Association, 1980) definition of personality disorder as maladaptive traits initially leads to simple definitions based on having an extreme level of traits that are expressed in rigid or maladaptive ways (Cloninger, 2000; Eysenck, 1987; Kiesler, 1986; Leary, 1957; Wiggins & Pincus, 1989). The idea has not proved useful because an extreme level of trait does not necessarily imply disordered functioning (Parker & Barrett, 2000; Verheul et al., 2008). Moreover, terms such as *maladaptive* and *inflexible* are too vague and poorly defined (Wakefield, 2008) for reliable assessment. Definitions based solely on traits also fail to recognize that personality includes other features besides traits, such as motives, roles, goals, strategies, values, representations of self and others, and life narratives (McAdams, 1994; McAdams & Pals, 2006). Equally important, they neglect the integrating and organizing aspects of personality (Allport, 1961; Cervone & Shoda, 1999; McAdams, 1994; Rutter, 1987). As Millon noted, personality "is not a potpourri of unrelated traits and miscellaneous behaviors but a tightly knit organization of stable structures (e.g., internalized memories and self-images) and coordinated functions (e.g., unconscious mechanisms and cognitive processes)" (1996, p. 13). Similarly, Mischel and Shoda (1995) noted that the "personality system functions literally as a whole—a unique network of organized interconnections among cognitions and affects, not a set of separate, independent discrete variables, forces, factors, or tendencies. The challenge becomes to understand the psychological meaning of the organization of the relationships within the person" (pp. 258–259). This aspect of personality is directly applicable to defining personality disorder because the essential feature of disorder is an enduring disturbance of the organizational and integrative aspects of personality (Livesley, 2003; Livesley & Jang, 2000; Rutter, 1987; Wakefield, 2008).

As background to this issue, we note how the unfortunate divide between the study of normal and disordered personality has hindered the development of a definition of personality disorder by preventing the study of personality disorder from benefiting from the evolution of an understanding of the self and personality in psychology, especially the development in social-cognitive approaches. These emphasized the functional and adaptive aspects of the self (self-regulation, self-direction, and self-defense) and concepts of identity and object relations leading to the recognition of the self as a causal agent with growing emphasis on emotion as a motivating force (Carver, 2011; Carver & Scheier, 1998; Mischel & Morf, 2003; Sheldon & Elliot, 1999), ideas that have obvious implications for conceptualizing the functional disturbances in self and interpersonal relationships. In the next section, we draw on ideas about the organizational component of personality and the cognitive and motivational aspects of the self to formulate a working definition of personality disorder to guide assessment.

Personality Disorder as Adaptive Impairment

Defining personality disorder as an impairment in the organization and integration of personality immediately raises the question of what indicators are clinically useful in evaluating such a generalized impairment. Clinicians have traditionally focused on two general indicators: chronic interpersonal problems and an impaired sense of self or identity. General and interpersonal psychiatry consider impaired interpersonal functioning to be the core feature of personality disorder (Hopwood, Wright, Ansell, & Pincus, 2013; Pincus & Hopwood, 2012; Rutter, 1987; Vaillant & Perry, 1980). Rutter (1987), for example, defined personality disorder as "characterized by a persistent, pervasive abnormality in social relationships and social functioning generally" (p. 454). In contrast, the psychoanalytical literature has focused on self-pathology as illustrated by Kohut's (1971) description of the lack of a cohesive self-structure in narcissistic conditions and Kernberg's (1984) concept of identity diffusion (disorganized representations of self and others) in borderline personality organization. Interestingly, this clinical tradition is consistent with cognitive models of the self as a cohesive structure of self-schemas.

The conception of personality disorder emerging from clinical practice is also consistent with ideas about the adaptive origins of personality. Personality structures presumably evolved because they aided fitness in our remote ancestors. The gradual emergence of community living over the last 2 million years created the need for mechanisms to manage the problems created by social living. To function effectively in the small social groups that were the context in which many personality structures and mechanisms evolved required the development of a sense of self or identity that defined one's place in the group, the capacity for attachment and intimacy, and the ability to function in an altruistic and prosocial way. Combining this understanding of the adaptive functions of personality with clinical conceptions of personality disorder suggests the working definition that disorder involves at least one of the following: (1) an impaired sense of self and identity, (2) a seriously impaired capacity for intimacy and attachment, and/or (3) a poorly developed capacity for prosocial, altruistic, and cooperative behavior (Livesley, 1998, 2003).

The definition of personality disorder in DSM-5 (Section III) drew on this conception. To be useful clinically, the different components need to be defined explicitly. The DSM-5 proposal attempted to do this by defining self-pathology in terms of identity and self-directedness and interpersonal pathology as problems with intimacy and empathy. Unfortunately, the proposed descriptions of both self- and interpersonal pathology are too confusing and ambiguous for reliable clinical assessment. Also, the proposal fails to capture the basic idea that identity defines one's sense of self and one's place in the social contexts in which one lives. And the suggestion that identity involves "experience of oneself as unique" may lead to identity being equated with narcissistic tendencies. It is also culturally bound, seeming to be more applicable to Western cultures than to cultures that emphasize connectedness to other persons (Mulder, 2012). Equally problematic is the description of self-directedness that confuses the motivational aspect of the self with the unrelated concept of prosocial behavior and the metacognitive process of self-reflection. Given these problems, we suggest an alternative scheme.

Clinical Definition of Personality Disorder

The alternative approach that we propose defines self-pathology in terms of cognitive and motivational impairments (Livesley, 2003). The cognitive component is described as problems with the *differentiation* and *integration* of the person's knowledge of the self. Knowledge about the self accumulates during development through interaction with the social environment. As self-knowledge accumulates, the self takes structure. Poor differentiation of the self is manifested as an impoverished set of self-schemas, lack of clarity or certainty about personal attributes, a sense of inner emptiness, and poor interpersonal boundaries. In parallel with the process of differentiation is an integrative process that combines items of self-knowledge or self-schemas into different images of the self, resulting ultimately in an autobiographical sense of self that organizes diverse aspects of self-knowledge into an overarching self-narrative. The interconnections created within self-knowledge form the basis for the subjective sense of personal unity, continuity, and coherence that characterizes an adaptive self-system (Harter, 2012; Toulmin, 1978). Problems of integration include lack of a sense of historicity or continuity in one's experience of the self, fragmentary self-representations, and disconnected self-states (Kernberg, 1984; Livesley, 2003).

The second component of the self is motivational: Meaningful goals contribute to the coherence of the self. Goals integrate by drawing together different aspects of personality by linking needs and wishes with the abilities and skills needed to attain them. It is this striving toward a goal that integrates, not its attainment (Allport, 1961). As Read, Jones, and Miller (1990) noted, "behavioral organization becomes understandable in terms of the individual's goals, plans, resources, and beliefs" (p. 1060). Striving to attain goals contributes to a sense of personal autonomy and agency that gives meaning, direction, and purpose to life (Carver, 2011; Carver & Scheier, 1998; Shapiro, 1981).

The interpersonal component of personality disorder is more straightforward. It involves impaired capacity for (1) intimacy, attachment, and affiliative relationships and (2) prosocial and cooperative behavior. In evolutionary terms, these may be considered impaired functioning in kinship and societal relationships, respectively. Before considering ways to assess these impairments, we need to consider briefly the literature on the related problem severity of personality disorder.

Definition of Severity

Despite growing recognition that severity is central to treatment planning, the assessment of severity remains a subject of confusion. Several proposals have been advanced, and we review a few here. However, it is useful to keep in mind that although researchers are looking for the optimal way to arrive at a summary score for severity, such a rating may not be particularly useful to the clinician; it may be more useful to identify areas of deficit indicative of severity than are likely to modify the treatment response.

Parker was among the first to highlight the significance of severity and the problem of confounding severity and personality category (see Parker & Barrett, 2000). Parker and colleagues (2004) recommended a general rating based on failures in cooperating and coping with the interpersonal world. Bornstein (1998) also recommended a severity rating of global personality pathology but focused on the dysfunction suffered by the individual patient. He noted areas of dysfunction, such as distorted cognition, inappropriate affectivity, impaired interpersonal functioning, and impulse control problems. Widiger and colleagues (2002) recommended using the Global Assessment of Functioning (GAF) score. Tyrer and Johnson (1996) viewed severity as the extent of comorbidity—the sum of all criteria observed across all personality disorders.

In a reanalysis of a longitudinal study, Hopwood and colleagues (2011) found that generalized severity was the most predictive of current and future dysfunction but that personality style indicated specific areas of difficulty. Based on their findings, this group recommended a three-part assessment: (1) global rating of severity (sum of all personality disorder criteria as proposed by Tyrer & Johnson, 1996), (2) ratings of stylistic elements of personality disorder (captured as factors representing peculiarity, withdrawal, fearfulness, instability, and deliberateness), and (3) a rating of normative traits.

Although there is little agreement, a common approach is to base a rating of severity on the amount of personality pathology present as indexed by either the number of DSM-IV/DSM-5 personality disorders or total number of diagnostic criteria. Thus a case that meets criteria for a single disorder is considered less severe than a case that meets criteria for two or more disorders, and a case manifesting 15 diagnostic criteria is considered more severe than one showing 10 criteria. Although there is evidence supporting this assumption (Dimaggio et al., 2013), the method equates severity with breadth of pathology (the number of criteria present) and not with degree of impairment. Thus it is conceivable for a patient to manifest a wide range of criteria that are all relatively mild.

In the absence of an agreed measure of severity, we propose using a clinical evaluation based on the degree of impairment in the core features of personality disorder, thereby combining the diagnosis of personality disorder with assessment of severity. Although severity is a graded construct, we suggest that until a generally accepted rating scale is available, it is sufficient for most clinical purposes to recognize two levels of severity: personality disorder and severe personality disorder. Table 3.1 describes differences in severity for each defining feature of general personality disorder. We recommend using these descriptions to make a global determination of severity.

When making this assessment, it is important to distinguish severity of pathology from intensity of distress. Some forms of personality disorder may show little distress even though there is severe impairment in personality functioning—for example, patients with high levels of social avoidance (DSM-IV/DSM-5 schizoid personality disorder)—whereas with some of the more emotionally unstable disorders, extreme levels of distress may occur with relatively low severity.

Clinical Assessment of Personality Disorder and Severity

Although evaluation of self- and interpersonal pathology based on the preceding conceptualization may appear a daunting and highly subjective task, this is not the case. The definitions of self- and interpersonal pathology shown in Table 3.1 are sufficiently precise to construct reliable self-report scales that differentiate personality disorder from other mental disorders (Berghuis, Kamphuis, Verheul, Larstone, & Livesley, 2012; Hentschel & Livesley, 2013a, 2013b), and these definitions are easily applied in clinical assessment.

TABLE 3.1. Definition of Personality Disorder and Levels of Severity

Personality disorder is characterized by an impaired self/identity and/or by chronic interpersonal dysfunction that differs markedly from the expectations of the individual's culture.

Self-pathology

Impaired self/identity as manifested by at least one of the following: (1) poor differentiation, (2) fragmented self-concept, and/or (3) low self-directedness.

Differentiation

Poorly developed self-structure with limited development of self-schemas and impaired interpersonal boundaries.

Personality disorder: Self-description is limited to a few relatively concrete qualities with a lack of clarity and certainty about personal qualities, feelings, and wants, leading to a poorly developed sense of identity; wants and emotions do not feel real or authentic—for example, questions whether emotions are real or genuine; relies extensively on others to confirm the appropriateness of thoughts and experiences and to help decide how he or she feels; interpersonal boundaries are present but poorly developed; feels empty or "hollow."

Severe personality disorder: Severely impoverished self-concept—difficulty describing personal qualities and attributes; lacks a sense of identity; minimal interpersonal boundaries leading to enmeshed relationships and the "sense of losing oneself" when with others, which may lead to dissociation; assumes that personal experiences and those of others are identical.

Integration

Self-structure is poorly integrated, leading to a fragmented and unstable sense of self and a limited sense of personal unity and continuity.

Personality disorder: Experiences shifting and poorly integrated or unrelated self-states but is able to recall experiences in other self-states than the current state; sense of self varies substantially across situations; feels a sense of discontinuity between the self presented to the world and the "real" self.

Severe personality disorder: Integration is minimal; self-experience consists of a series of discrete disconnected experiences and distinct self-state with little recall experiences across different self-states.

Self-directedness

Difficulty setting and attaining satisfying personal goals.

Personality disorder: Low motivation leading to difficulty establishing realistic goals; unable to sustain work on achieving long-term goals; limited sense of personal autonomy and agency.

Severe personality disorder: Lacks the ability to establish lasting long-term goals; lacks direction and purpose; passive and lacks motivation; lacks a sense of agency and autonomy.

Interpersonal pathology

Chronically impaired interpersonal functioning as manifested by either by impaired capacity for intimacy and attachment and/or socialization.

Intimacy and attachment

Impaired capacity for close relationships.

(*continued*)

TABLE 3.1. *(continued)*

Personality disorder: Exhibits one or more of the following difficulties: (1) impaired capacity for intimacy due to personality traits (e.g., narcissism, insecure attachment, compulsivity), although may be able to tolerate more distant social relationships; (2) unstable and conflicted relationships; (3) difficulty tolerating the autonomy and individuality of others; (4) attachment problems involving either difficulty establishing adult patterns of attachment or inability to function as a responsible attachment figure.

Severe personality disorder: Severely impaired capacity to relate to others, involving either difficulty differentiating self and other (symbiotic relationships) or avoidance of relationships.

Prosocial behavior

Impaired socialization as evidenced by severely impaired prosocial behavior and/or moral development.

Personality disorder: Impaired respect for culturally typical moral behavior; impairment in altruistic behavior.

Severe personality disorder: Lacks the capacity for culturally typical moral behavior; devoid of altruism.

Establishing the presence or absence of disorder need not be a lengthy process that requires assessing all facets of self-pathology. Rather, we suggest that clinicians become familiar with the concepts and use the definitions as a prototype to evaluate the degree to which the patient matches the description. Most clinical interviews provide sufficient information to make a reliable evaluation. For example, patients may mention uncertainty about who they are or what they think or feel, losing themselves in other people, or not knowing what they want from life. Such statements respectively hint at poor differentiation of the self, uncertainty about personal qualities, boundary problems, and low self-directedness that can readily be pursued to establish a diagnosis of personality disorder. This information can then be supplemented with a few specific questions to explore different facets of the definition.

Clinical Assessment of Self-Pathology

We find it helpful to begin assessing these problems by eliciting a self-description: "Perhaps we could now talk about how you see yourself. What sort of person do you think you are? How would you describe yourself?" This question usually produces important diagnostic information relatively quickly. Having posed the question, the interviewer observes how the patient responds.

Those with a poorly differentiated self often struggle with the task and comment about being unsure about who they are. Others provide a brief description consisting of a few general or concrete attributes. For example, "I am not sure what to say. I am a nice person, I like dancing, and I am very attached to my dog. . . . I do not know what else to say." A few probing questions to elicit more information usually reveals the extent of differentiation problems. Poor differentiation is often accompanied by feelings of "inner emptiness" that is easily assessed by asking: "Do you feel as if there is nothing inside, as if you are empty and hollow inside?" Information on interpersonal boundaries is especially important because the distinction between self and others is a prerequisite for the emergence of the self. Useful questions to explore boundary problems are: "Do you ever feel very vulnerable and exposed because it feels as if nothing separates you from other people?" "Do you ever confuse other people's ideas with your own?" "Do ever worry that you will lose the sense of who you really are or lose yourself in others?"

The differences between personality disorder and severe personality disorder are reflected in the degree of differentiation. Lower severity typically produces a self-description limited to a few concrete qualities and some uncertainty about personal qualities. With severe disorder, the self-concept is severely impoverished, leading to difficulty describing personal qualities and attributes. Instead, the self is defined very much by the moment and the expectations of others. There are also differences in boundaries: With increasing severity, interpersonal boundaries become almost nonexistent, leading to enmeshed relationships and a sense of losing oneself by merging with others.

Patients with integration problems may respond to the request for a self-description by commenting that it is difficult to describe themselves because their ideas about themselves change frequently. For example, patients may note that "It is hard to say . . . my feelings about myself change all the time"; "Sometimes it feels as if there are lots of different me's." Such statements suggest discontinuity in experiences of the self that can be assessed further by asking such questions as: "Does your sense of who you are change a lot from day to day?" "Do you have contradictory feelings about yourself and who you are?" and "Do you ever get the feeling that you are several different people?"

The preceding responses are typical of patients with emotional dysregulation problems as associated with DSM-IV/DSM-5 BPD. In more schizoid or socially withdrawn individuals, problems with integration may take the form of feeling that the self presented to the world is a facade and that the "real" self is hidden inside and never exposed to others. Differences in severity are less marked than in the case of differentiation problems. A major differentiating feature is that with severe pathology there is greater disjunction between self-states such that experiences when in one state are poorly recalled in another state. For example, one patient with severe disorder showed several self-states, including a more settled optimistic state and a state of intense agitation associated with almost painful feelings of inner emptiness that he found terrifying, a state that was largely characterized by a combination of intense anger and neediness. When experiencing the state of inner emptiness, he found it difficult to recall and even imagine that he ever felt any different, even though he had been in a more settled state only a few hours previously. This inability to recall that he had felt different increased his distress because the despair felt timeless, as if it had always existed and always would.

Low self-directedness, the motivational component of the self, has several components: low self-efficacy—a sense of being unable to control oneself and one's destiny—a lack of meaning and purpose to life, and difficulty setting and attaining long-term goals. All components can usually be evaluated when taking a personal history because it often becomes apparent whether the individual has lived a life imbued with purpose with clearly defined goals or whether life has been less purposeful. This initial assessment can then be followed up with a few questions, such as: "Do you feel as if you are not in control of your own life, as if there is nothing that you can do to change your life?" "Does it feel as if your life has meaning? Does it seem as if nothing that you do has much purpose?" "Do you have difficulty deciding what you want to achieve in life and in setting goals?" Patients with less severe pathology often set goals, but their goals often change rapidly due to uncertainty about self-attributes, including goals, and they have difficulty sustaining the effort to achieve longer-term objectives. With increasing pathology there is almost total lack of goal setting that is associated with low motivation and a pervasive sense of passivity.

Clinical Assessment of Interpersonal Pathology

Information on interpersonal functioning is readily elicited in a clinical interview. Standard questions about relationships with significant others, childhood peer relationships, and adult relationships, including romantic relationships, usually provide sufficient information to evaluate the ability to establish meaningful relationships and the capacity to sustain attachment and intimacy. Exploration of current circumstances adds additional information about the extent and quality of relationships, number of friends, and stability of relationships that is readily translated into a clinical evaluation of the intimacy and affiliative component of interpersonal pathology. Just as the assessor asks the patient to describe him- or herself, he or she can also ask the patient to describe a significant other to evaluate the depth (differentiation) and degree of integration of the representation of that person. Patients with less severe disorder can often form relationships but have difficulty with sustained intimacy and attachment, which may or may not be associated with unstable and conflicted relationships. Greater severity is associated with a substantially impaired capacity to relate to others involving either difficulty differentiating between self and other, leading to symbiotic relationships, or almost total avoidance of relationships.

A comprehensive clinical interview also reveals information about impaired socialization that leads to problems with prosocial and moral behavior and that can clarified with a few questions about whether the patient likes working with others or has problems with cooperation, whether he or she would ever "sacrifice yourself to help others," or whether he or she "makes sure that you get what you want regardless of the consequences for others."

Greater severity is associated with an absence of concern for others, disregard for culturally typical moral behavior, and an absence of altruism.

ASSESSING TRAIT CONSTELLATIONS AND PRIMARY TRAITS

The second part of the assessment of personality disorder is to evaluate individual differences in clinically important personality characteristics. An understanding of the individual's salient personality characteristics is needed to establish treatment pathways and identify suitable intervention strategies (see Links, Mercer, & Novick, Chapter 5, this volume). Although categorical diagnoses have traditionally been used prior to treatment, we advocate dimensional classification because of the well-established limitations of categorical diagnoses, extensive evidence supporting dimensional diagnosis, and direct links between traits such as emotional lability and impulsivity and treatment methods. Despite the evidence, however, there is considerable resistance to using dimensional assessment. For this reason, we briefly consider its advantages before discussing practical ways to assess clinically important traits.

Advantages of Dimensional Assessment

Dimensional models are more consistent with the evidence than category models (Trull & Durrett, 2005). The multiple shortcomings of categorical diagnoses include extensive diagnostic overlap, limited structural validity, and poor coverage. Because nearly 40% of patients with personality disorders cannot be adequately diagnosed using DSM-IV (Westen & Arkowitz-Westen, 1998), personality disorder—not otherwise specified is often the most common diagnosis in clinical practice (Verheul & Widiger, 2004), a significant limitation for treatment purposes. Also, as noted earlier, the extensive heterogeneity among patients with the same categorical diagnosis severely limits the value of these diagnoses in treatment planning. Dimensional models account for heterogeneity better and provide a comprehensive assessment of both adaptive and maladaptive features. The comprehensiveness of dimensional models also means that they can accommodate important forms of personality pathology not recognized by the DSM system, such as sadistic and oppositional traits.

Trait assessment is also more closely linked to intervention strategies because most interventions target specific traits or symptom clusters rather than global diagnoses (Leising & Zimmerman, 2011; Livesley, 2003; Sanderson & Clarkin, 2013). This is clearly illustrated by the use of medication with BPD to target specific symptom clusters such as cognitive dysregulation, emotional lability, and impulsivity (Soloff, 2000). Likewise, psychotherapeutic interventions focus on specific behaviors, such as deliberate self-harm, and specific traits, such as emotional dysregulation, aggression, and abandonment anxiety. Overall, the typical level of clinical intervention is with specific primary traits or their component behaviors (Leising & Zimmermann, 2011).

Dimensional Models

The decision to use dimensional assessment raises the question of which model to use. Although this appears a difficult problem due to multiple competing models, there are only two main choices: whether to use a model of normal personality or a specific model of personality disorder. Alternative ways to classify personality disorders based on models of normal personality include Eysenck's three-dimensional model (1987; Eysenck & Eysenck, 1985), the five-factor approach (Costa & Widiger, 1994; Widiger, Trull, Clarkin, Sanderson, & Costa, 1994), Cloninger's biologically based model (1987; Svrakic, Whitehead, Przybeck, & Cloninger, 1993), and the interpersonal circumplex (Kiesler, 1982; Wiggins, 1982). However, our preference is to use a clinically based model that incorporates traditional clinical concepts (Clark, 1990; Livesley, Jackson, & Schroeder, 1992; Livesley & Jang, 2000) because there is a reasonable consensus that four broad factors provide an adequate representation of the trait structure of personality disorder (Mulder, Newton-Howes, Crawford, & Tyrer, 2011; Widiger & Simonsen, 2005). Table 3.2 lists the primary traits associated with each higher-order factor.

Clinical Assessment of Traits

Dimensional assessment readily lends itself to structured measures. Two questionnaires are available that were specifically designed to evaluate personality disorder: the Schedule for Nonadaptive and Adaptive Personality (SNAP; Clark, 1993) and the Dimensional Assessment of Personality Pathology—Basic Questionnaire (DAPP-BQ; Livesley & Jackson, 2009). Both were developed using a "bottom-up" strategy that began with a representative pool of descriptive terms and then gradually built a final structure based on the empirical structure identified in the original pool. With the SNAP, the original descriptors were personality terms used in DSM-III, whereas the DAPP-BQ relied on terms identified through a broad literature search. Nevertheless, the final structure of the two measures is remarkably similar (Clark & Livesley, 1994; Harkness, 1992).

A practical alternative to a questionnaire is to assess traits during the clinical interview. The most comprehensive way is to assess all primary traits shown in Table 3.2 using information obtained from the interview, supplemented as needed with questions based on the definitions of each trait to establish whether it is present to a clinically significant degree. Table 3.3 provides detailed definitions of each trait based in part on Livesley and Jackson (2009). A more parsimonious approach is to assess only the most salient traits in each cluster using interview information and clarifying questions (Livesley, 1998). These traits are shown in bold in Table 3.2. The most salient traits are those with the highest loadings in the analyses used to establish the structure (Livesley & Jackson, 2010; Livesley, Jang, & Vernon, 1998). If these screening traits are considered clinically significant—that is, if they are associated with

TABLE 3.2. Trait Constellations and Primary Traits

Secondary domain	Primary trait
Emotional dysregulation	**Anxiousness**
	Emotional lability:
	Emotional reactivity
	Emotional intensity
	Pessimistic anhedonia
	Submissiveness
	Insecure attachment
	Cognitive dysregulation
	Need for approval
	Social apprehensiveness
	Oppositional
	Self-harming acts
	Self-harming ideas
Dissocial	**Callousness**
	Lack of empathy/remorselessness
	Exploitativeness
	Egocentrism
	Sadism
	Hostile dominance
	Conduct problems
	Impulsivity
	Sensation seeking
	Narcissism
	Suspiciousness
Social Avoidance	**Low affiliation**
	Restricted emotional expression
	Avoidant attachment
	Self-containment
	Inhibited sexuality
	Attachment need
Compulsivity	**Orderliness**
	Conscientiousness

Note. The most salient traits for each factor are shown in **bold**.

impaired social and/or occupational functioning—then the remaining traits defining the cluster can be assessed to provide a detailed picture of the constellation. With this strategy, traits can be assessed relatively quickly, at least for clinical purposes. For example, the emotional-dependency cluster can be assessed based on four traits: emotional lability, anxiousness, insecure attachment, and submissive-dependency. The underlying conflict between neediness and fear of rejection can be assessed at the same time by inquiring about attachment needs. The diagnostic process would extend to the salient traits of the dissocial (antisocial/psychopathic), social avoidance (schizoid/avoidant), and compulsivity constellations. In many cases, this information is sufficient

TABLE 3.3. Primary Traits of Personality Disorder

Primary trait	Definition
Anxiousness	Readily feels fearful, worried, tense, and threatened; lifelong sense of tension and feeling "on the edge"; broods about unpleasant experiences, unable to divert attention from painful thoughts; unable to make decisions due to fear of making a mistake; pervasive sense of guilt.
Attachment need	Strong need for attachment relationships; distressed by lack of intimacy.
Avoidant attachment	Avoids attachment relationships; fearful of attachments; does not seek out others when stressed or distressed; shows little reaction to separations or reunions.
Cognitive dysregulation	Thoughts tend to become disorganized when stressed; may experience brief stress psychosis; tends to experience feelings of depersonalization or derealization and show dissociative behavior; often manifests schizotypal cognition (e.g., mild paranoid thoughts, illusions, and pseudohallucinations).
Conduct problems	Violates social norms and laws; violent; resorts to threats and intimidation; often has a history of juvenile antisocial behavior; tends to engage in substance misuse; routinely prevaricates and rationalizes actions; deliberately flouts authority.
Conscientiousness	Strong sense of duty and obligation; completes all tasks thoroughly and meticulously.
Egocentrism	Preoccupied with self; perceptions dominated by own point of view, interests, and concerns; defines and pursues own needs without regard for those of others; believes he or she knows what is best for others.
Emotional intensity	Feels and expresses emotions intensely; overreacts emotionally; exaggerates emotional significance of events.
Emotional reactivity	Experiences frequent and unpredictable emotional changes; moody; irritable with low threshold for annoyance; impatient; intense, frequent, and easily aroused anger; poor anger control.
Exploitativeness	Takes advantage of others for personal gain; charming and ingratiating when suits own purpose; believes that others are easily manipulated or conned; considers self to be adroit at taking advantage of others.
Hostile dominance	Antagonistic and unfriendly to others; verbally abusive; enjoys taking charge, assumes leadership roles, likes to influence others, frustrated when not in charge.
Impulsivity	Does things on the spur of the moment; many actions unplanned or without much thought about the consequences; fails to follow established plans; impulsivity overrules previous experiences and hence appears not to learn from experience.
Inhibited sexuality	Lacks interest in sexuality; derives little pleasure from sexual experiences; fearful of sexual relationships.

(*continued*)

TABLE 3.3. *(continued)*

Insecure attachment	Fears losing attachments; coping depends on presence of attachment figure; urgently seeks proximity with attachment figure when stressed; strongly protests separations; intolerant of aloneness; avoids being alone and plans adequate activities to avoid being alone.
Lack of empathy	Does not notice or respond to others' feelings or problems; has difficulty understanding others' feelings; lacks guilt about the effects of own actions; unable to express remorse.
Low affiliation	Seeks out situations that do not include other people; declines opportunities to socialize; does not initiate social contact.
Narcissism	Grandiose, exaggerates achievements and abilities, craves admiration; preoccupied with fantasies of unlimited success, power, brilliance, or beauty; feels and acts as if entitled; acts to be noticed; strong need for acceptance and approval.
Need for approval	Strong need for demonstrations of acceptance and approval; constantly seeks reassurance that he or she is a worthy person.
Oppositionality	Resists satisfactory performance of routine tasks and hence fails to meet others' requests and expectations; resents authority figures; lacks ambition, rarely takes the initiative; shows low levels of activity and fails to take control of own life; fails to get things done on time, "forgets" to do things; does not plan or organize ahead; passively resists cooperating with others.
Orderliness	Methodical and organized; concerned with cleanliness; concerned with details, time, punctuality, schedules, and rules.
Pessimistic anhedonia	Derives little pleasure from experiences or relationships; no sense of fun; pervasive feelings of hopelessness; negative expectations for the future; accentuates the negative, strongly adheres to negative beliefs.
Restricted emotional expression	Does not express emotions; appears unemotional; avoids emotional situations; shows little reaction to emotionally arousing situations.
Sadism	Cruel; humiliates and demeans others; fascinated by violence and torture; amused by/enjoys the suffering of others; considers others to be worthless; despises others; cynical.
Self-containment	Reluctant to share personal information; avoids inadvertent self-disclosure; fears personal information may be used against self; self-reliant and self-sufficient; prefers to cope independently, does not to seek help from others; fears having to rely on others.
Self-harming acts	Deliberate self-damaging acts (e.g., self-mutilation, drug overdoses).
Self-harming ideas	Frequent thoughts about suicide and hurting self; stress or distress readily activates thoughts of self-harm.
Sensation seeking	Craves excitement; needs variety; has difficulty tolerating the normal or routine; reckless, enjoys taking unnecessary risks and does not heed own limitations; denies the reality of personal danger.

(continued)

TABLE 3.3. *(continued)*

Social apprehensiveness	Fears hurt and rejection; poor social skills; uncertain about appropriate social behavior, awkward in social settings.
Submissiveness	Subservient and unassertive; subordinates self and own needs to those of others; passively follows the interests and desires of others; submits to abuse and intimidation to maintain relationships; seeks advice and reassurance about all courses of action; readily accepts others' suggestions and often appears gullible.
Suspiciousness	Mistrusts other people, hyperalert to signs of trickery or harm; searches for hidden meanings in events, questions others' loyalty, often feels persecuted.

for planning and initiating treatment. More detailed assessment can subsequently be incorporated into treatment.

DOMAINS OF PSYCHOPATHOLOGY

A distinguishing feature of IMT is an emphasis on decomposing personality pathology not only into traits but also into domains that are linked to specific intervention modules. Because personality pathology can be parsed into domains in various ways, we sought to base domains on descriptive concepts closely tied to the traditional subdivisions of personality, clinical descriptions of personality disorder, and the problems clinicians typically address in therapy. Four functional domains are specified:

1. *Symptoms:* a wide variety of symptoms are associated with personality disorders, including dysphoria, anxiety, deliberate self-harm, dissociative features, quasi-psychotic symptoms, aggression, rage, and violent behavior.
2. *Regulation and modulation:* Problems arising from impaired regulatory structures that inhibit behavioral responses and mediate action and metacognitive processes involved in modulating personality processes:
   a. Undercontrol of emotions and impulses: unstable emotions, frequent mood changes, impulsive behaviours, violence, and impulsive aggression
   b. Overcontrol of emotions and impulses resulting in constricted emotions and inhibited behavior.
3. *Interpersonal:* the range of problems covers inability to establish social relationships, problems with intimacy and attachment, conflicted interpersonal behaviors, unstable relationships, callousness, and disregard for the well-being and welfare of others.
4. *Self/identity:* problems with the contents and structure of self and identity, including difficulties with the regulation of self-esteem,

maladaptive self-schemas, unstable sense of self or identity, poorly developed self-system, and dysfunctional and biased perceptions of self in relation to others.

The trait system discussed previously is not independent of functional domains but rather cuts across domains. For example, traits such as anxiousness and emotional lability predispose to mood symptoms, interpersonal problems, and self-pathology, and cognitive dysregulation predisposes to impaired thinking when stressed and the development of quasi-psychotic symptoms, such as illusions and pseudohallucinations. Interpersonal traits such as callousness, insecure attachment, and social avoidance play an important role in the development of interpersonal problems.

Because domain assessment identifies impairments that form treatment targets, it helps to map the broad directions of therapy. It also helps to structure discussions with patients about the personal concerns that they want to address in treatment, which is part of working with the patient to establish the collaborative goals that will be the focus of therapeutic work. Table 3.4 describes the relationships between domains, goals, and assessment and illustrates typical problems associated with each domain. This list is not intended to provide an exhaustive account of each problem domain but rather to illustrate the range of issues to consider in each domain. We suggest that these guidelines be used as the basis for a systematic assessment of each domain. At some point toward the end of the assessment process, it is useful to conduct a systematic evaluation of each domain, rather like the systematic review that is part of a mental state examination. This information obtained during the clinical interview will include details of impairments across domains so that completion of a domain assessment need not be time-consuming. It is a useful way to conclude the assessment because it paves the way for a discussion of the formulation and treatment options, as discussed by Clarkin and Livesley (Chapter 4, this volume).

THE TREATMENT ALLIANCE DURING THE ASSESSMENT PROCESS

Earlier, we suggested that assessment should also be used to foster engagement because of the association between the quality of the alliance and early dropout. This means that alliance building techniques should be used throughout the assessment (Hilsenroth & Cromer, 2007), even if this means a somewhat longer assessment process.

The alliance is fostered when the clinician conducts the assessment in a way that conveys respect and demonstrates competence in assessing and treating personality disorder. The patient's perception of the relationship is also enhanced when the therapist is nurturing, collaborative, and understanding (Bachelor, 1995). Nurturance is conveyed by attentive, nonjudgmental

TABLE 3.4. Relationships between Domains, Goals, and Assessment

Domain	Treatment goals	Assessment
Symptoms	• Reduce symptoms	• Nature and severity of symptoms
Emotion/impulse control		
Undercontrol	• Control suicidal, parasuicidal, and other self-harming behavior	• Frequency and intensity of suicidal ideation • Frequency and nature of self-harm
	• Improve emotion/impulse regulation	• Emotional lability • Anxiousness • Aggression/hostility • Impulse control
	• Improve self-reflection	• Self-reflection abilities
	• Enhance ability to understand mental states	• Capacity to understand mental states of self and others
	• Increase effortful control	• Capacity for attention control
Overcontrol	• Reduce emotional constriction	• Restricted emotional expression
	• Improve self-reflection	• Self-reflection abilities
	• Enhance ability to understand mental states	• Capacity to understand mental states of self and others
	• Increase effortful control	• Capacity for attention control
Interpersonal	• Improve interpersonal relationships and behavior	• Interpersonal traits • Capacity for relationships • Interpersonal patterns • Interpersonal conflicts • Moral development • Capacity for cooperation • Capacity for empathy
Self and identity	• Increase self-esteem	• Level and stability of self-esteem
	• Modulate maladaptive self-schemas	• Core self-schemas
	• Promote more adaptive sense of self and identity	• Sense of self and identify
	• Develop a personal niche	• Assessment compatibility of personality and environment

listening and empathic attunement to the patient's feelings, problems, and situation.

Hilsenroth and Cromer (2007) identified three clinician behaviors that promote a positive alliance during assessment. First, the alliance is fostered by a longer and collaborative in-depth assessment that allows ample opportunity for the patient to voice concerns and discuss the cognitive and emotional aspects of these concerns. When discussing these issues, rapport is increased by using clear, concrete, and "experience-near" language and avoiding jargon. Second, detailed exploration of the patient's immediate concerns fosters the alliance and helps patients to commit to therapy. A key feature is to help the patient to discuss not only factual details about their concerns but also sources of distress while taking steps to ensure that patients are not overwhelmed by their distress. Third, it is important to seek constant feedback from patients about how they think the assessment is going and how they feel about discussing their problems. It also helps to incorporate a psychoeducational element by explaining features of the disorder as they are discussed during assessment and by helping patients to develop new insights into the problems they present.

CONCLUDING COMMENTS

The structured approach to assessment that we present as an alternative to the usual determination of categorical diagnoses is designed to be more clinically useful by focusing on functional impairments. It is not our intention to imply that the detailed methods we have discussed should be followed slavishly or that all aspects of the assessment should be completed prior to therapy. Instead, we seek to offer a scheme for thinking systematically about assessment in the context of therapy and about the relationship between assessment, treatment planning, and the interventions that are likely to be useful at different phases of treatment. Our goal was to outline the kinds of variables therapists should consider while recognizing that much of this information will be fleshed out during therapy. However, we think that it is helpful for the therapist to have a broad understanding of level of severity, salient personality traits and constellations, and critical impairments within each domain prior to starting therapy because this information is required to construct the formulation needed to negotiate the treatment contract.

Although our recommendations differ from traditional diagnostic assessment prior to therapy, the approach is consistent with emerging trends in the taxonomy of personality disorder and the emphasis being placed on understanding the functional impairments associated with these disorders. Like other recommendations, some of which we reviewed earlier, we advocate a broad but flexible assessment of all aspects of personality, including assets and liabilities and sources of resilience as well as vulnerability. We have also proposed a combination of functional and structural impairments. As indicated in the discussion of self-pathology, it is important to assess structural aspects of personality that have higher-order integrative functions. In some ways, our approach shows parallels to Kernberg's structural interview, which combines aspects of a traditional assessment, including chief complaint, current difficulties, and mental status information, with exploration of the individual's active and current representations of self in relationship to others. This focus enables the clinician to obtain a vivid picture of the patient's current functioning, the major focus of intervention, with less attention to personal history.

REFERENCES

Allport, G. W. (1961). *Pattern and growth in personality: A psychological interpretation.* New York: Holt, Rinehart & Winston.

American Psychiatric Association. (1980). *Diagnostic and statistical manual of mental disorders* (3rd ed.). Washington, DC: Author.

Bachelor, A. (1995). Clients' perception of the therapeutic alliance: A qualitative analysis. *Journal of Counseling Psychology, 42*, 323–337.

Bateman, A., & Fonagy, P. (2004). *Psychotherapy for borderline personality disorder: Mentalization-based treatment.* Oxford, UK: Oxford University Press.

Bateman, A., & Fonagy, P. (2006). *Mentalization-based treatment for borderline personality disorder.* Oxford, UK: Oxford University Press.

Berghuis, H., Kamphuis, J. H., Verheul, R., Larstone, R., & Livesley, W. J. (2012). The General Assessment of Personality Disorder (GAPD) as an instrument for assessing the core features of personality disorders. *Clinical Psychology and Psychotherapy, 20*(6), 544–557.

Beutler, L. E., Clarkin, J. F., & Bongar, B. (2000). *Guidelines for the systematic treatment of the depressed patient.* New York: Oxford University Press.

Beutler, L. E., & Groth-Marnat, G. (2003). *Integrative assessment of adult personality* (2nd ed.). New York: Guilford Press.

Bornstein, R. F. (1998). Reconceptualizing personality disorder diagnosis in DSM-V: The discriminant validity challenge. *Clinical Psychology: Science and Practice, 5*, 333–343.

Carver, C. S. (2011). Self-awareness. In M. R. Leary & J. P. Tangney (Eds.), *Handbook of self and identity* (2nd ed., pp. 50–68). New York: Guilford Press.

Carver, C. S., & Scheier, M. F. (1998). *On the self-regulation of behavior.* Cambridge, UK: Cambridge University Press.

Cervone, D., & Shoda, Y. (1999). Social-cognitive theories and the coherence of personality. In D. Cervone & Y. Shoda (Eds.), *The coherence of personality: Social-cognitive bases of consistency, variability, and organization* (pp. 3–33). New York: Guilford Press.

Clark, L. A. (1990). Toward a consensual set of symptom clusters for assessment of personality disorder. In J. Butcher & C. Spielberger (Eds.), *Advances in personality assessment* (Vol. 8, pp. 243–266). Hillsdale, NJ: Erlbaum.

Clark, L. A. (1993). *Manual for the Schedule for Non-adaptive and Adaptive Personality (SNAP).* Minneapolis: University of Minnesota Press.

Clark, L. A., & Livesley, W. J. (1994). Two approaches to identifying the dimensions of personality disorder. In P. T. Costa & T. A. Widiger (Eds.), *Personality disorders and the five-factor model of personality* (pp. 261–277). Washington, DC: American Psychological Association Press.

Clarkin, J. F., Howieson, D. B., & McClough, J. (2008). The role of psychiatric measures in assessment and treatment. In R. E. Hales, S. C. Yudofsky, & G. O. Gabbard (Eds.), *The American Psychiatric Publishing textbook of psychiatry* (5th ed., pp. 73–110). Washington, DC: American Psychiatric Publishing.

Clarkin, J. F., Yeomans, F. E., & Kernberg, O. F. (2006). *Psychotherapy for borderline personality: Focusing on object relations.* Washington, DC: American Psychiatric Publishing.

Cloninger, C. R. (1987). A systematic method for the clinical description and classification of personality variants. *Archives of General Psychiatry, 44,* 573–588.

Cloninger, C. R. (2000). A practical way to diagnose personality disorder: A proposal. *Journal of Personality Disorders, 14,* 99–106.

Costa, P. T., & Widiger, T. A. (Eds.). (1994). *Personality disorders and the five factor model of personality.* Washington DC: American Psychological Association.

Crawford, M. J., Koldobsky, N., Mulder, R., & Tyrer, P. (2011). Classifying personality disorder according to severity. *Journal of Personality Disorders, 25,* 321–330.

Davidson, K. M. (2008). *Cognitive therapy for personality disorders: a guide for clinicians* (2nd ed.). Hove, UK: Routledge.

Dimaggio, G., Carcione, A., Nicolò, G., Lysaker, P. H., d'Angerio, S., Conti, M. L., et al. (2013). Differences between axes depend on where you set the bar: Associations among symptoms, interpersonal relationship and alexithymia with number of personality disorder criteria. *Journal of Personality Disorders, 27,* 371–382.

Eysenck, H. J. (1987). The definition of personality disorders and the criteria appropriate to their definition. *Journal of Personality Disorders, 1,* 211–219.

Eysenck, H. J., & Eysenck, M. W. (1985). *Personality and individual differences: A natural science approach.* New York: Plenum Press.

Giesen-Bloo, J., van Dyck, R., Spinhoven, P., van Tilberg, W., Dirksen, C., van Asselt, T., et al. (2006). Outpatient psychotherapy for borderline personality disorder: Randomized trial of schema-focused therapy vs. transference-focused therapy. *Archives of General Psychiatry, 63,* 649–658.

Harkness, A. R. (1992). Fundamental topics in the personality disorders: Candidate trait dimensions from the lower regions of the hierarchy. *Psychological Assessment, 4,* 251–259.

Harter, S. (2012). *The construction of the self.* New York: Guilford Press.

Hentschel, A. G., & Livesley, W. J. (2013a). The General Assessment of Personality Disorder (GAPD): Factor structure, incremental validity of self pathology, and relations to DSM-IV personality disorders. *Journal of Personality Assessment, 95,* 479–485.

Hentschel, A. G., & Livesley, W. J. (2013b). Differentiating normal and disordered personality using the General Assessment of Personality Disorder (GAPD). *Personality and Mental Health, 7,* 133–142.

Hilsenroth, M. J., & Cromer, T. D. (2007). Clinical interventions related to alliance during the initial interview and psychological assessment. *Psychotherapy: Research, Theory, and Practice, 44,* 205–208.

Hopwood, C. J., Malone, J. C., Ansell, E. B., Sanislow, C. A., Grilo, C. M., McGlashan, T. H., et al. (2011). Personality assessment in DSM-5: Empirical support for rating severity, style, and traits. *Journal of Personality Disorders, 25,* 305–320.

Hopwood, C. J., Wright, G. C., Ansell, E. B., & Pincus, A. L. (2013). The interpersonal core of personality pathology. *Journal of Personality Disorders, 27*(3), 270–295.
Kernberg, O. F. (1984). *Severe personality disorders: Psychotherapeutic strategies.* New Haven, CT: Yale University Press.
Kiesler, D. J. (1986). The 1982 interpersonal circle: An analysis of DSM-III personality disorders. In T. Millon & G. L. Klerman (Eds.), *Contemporary directions in psychopathology: Toward the DSM-IV* (pp. 571–597). New York: Guilford Press.
Kohut, H. (1971). *The analysis of the self.* New York: International Universities Press.
Leary, T. (1957). *Interpersonal diagnosis of personality: A functional theory and methodology for personality evaluation.* New York: Ronald Press.
Leising, D., & Zimmerman, J., (2011). An integrative conceptual framework for assessing personality and personality pathology. *Review of General Psychology, 15,* 317–330.
Linehan, M. M. (1993). *Cognitive-behavioural treatment of borderline personality disorder.* New York: Guilford Press.
Livesley, W. J. (1998). Suggestions for a framework for an empirically based classification of personality disorder. *Canadian Journal of Psychiatry, 43*, 137–147.
Livesley, W. J. (2003). Diagnostic dilemmas in the classification of personality disorder. In K. Phillips, M. First, & H. A. Pincus (Eds.), *Advancing DSM: Dilemmas in psychiatric diagnosis* (pp. 153–189). Arlington, VA: American Psychiatric Association Press.
Livesley, W. J., & Jackson, D. N. (2009). *Dimensional Assessment of Personality Pathology—Basic Questionnaire technical manual.* Port Huron, MI: Sigma Press.
Livesley, W. J., Jackson, D. N., & Schroeder, M. L. (1992). Factorial structure of personality disorders in clinical and general population samples. *Journal of Abnormal Psychology, 101*, 432–440.
Livesley, W. J., & Jang, K. L. (2000). Toward an empirically based classification of personality disorder. *Journal of Personality Disorders, 14*, 137–151.
Livesley, W. J., Jang, K. L., & Vernon, P. A. (1998). The phenotypic and genetic architecture of traits delineating personality disorder. *Archives of General Psychiatry, 55*, 941–948.
MacKinnon, R. A., Michels, R., & Buckley, P. J. (2009). *The psychiatric interview in clinical practice* (2nd ed.). Washington, DC: American Psychiatric Publishing.
McAdams, D. P. (1994). Can personality change?: Levels of stability and growth in personality across the life span. In T. F. Heatherton & J. L. Weinberger (Eds.), *Can personality change?* (pp. 299–313). Washington, DC: American Psychological Association Press.
McAdams, D. P., & Pals, J. L. (2006). A new big five: Fundamental principles for an integrative science of personality. *American Psychologist, 61*, 204–217.
Millon, T. (1996). *Personality and psychopathology: Building a clinical science.* New York: Wiley
Mischel, W., & Morf, C. C. (2003). The self as a psycho-social dynamic processing system: A meta-perspective on a century of the self in psychology. In M. R. Leary & J. P. Tangney (Eds.), *Handbook of self and identity* (pp. 15–43). New York: Guilford Press.
Mischel, W., & Shoda, Y. (1995). A cognitive-affective system theory of personality:

Reconceptualizing situations, dispositions, dynamics, and invariance in personality structure. *Psychological Review, 102*, 246–268

Mulder, R. T. (2012). Cultural aspects of personality disorder. In T. A. Widiger (Ed.), *Oxford handbook of personality disorders* (pp. 260–274). Oxford, UK: Oxford University Press.

Mulder, R. T., Newton-Howes, G., Crawford, M. J., & Tyrer, P. J. (2011). The central domains of personality pathology in psychiatric patients. *Journal of Personality Disorders, 25*, 364–377.

Parker, G., & Barrett, E. (2000). Personality and personality disorder: Current issues and directions. *Psychological Medicine, 30,* 1–9.

Parker, G., Hadzi-Pavlovic, D., Both, L., Kumar, S., Wilhelm, K., & Olley, A. (2004). Measuring disordered personality functioning: To love and to work reprised. *Acta Psychiatrica Scandinavica, 110,* 230–239.

Pincus, A. L., & Hopwood, C. J. (2012). A contemporary interpersonal model of personality pathology and personality disorder. In T. A. Widiger (Ed.), *Oxford handbook of personality disorders* (pp. 372–398). New York: Oxford University Press.

Piper, W. E., & Joyce, A. S. (2001). Psychosocial treatment outcome. In W. J. Livesley (Ed.), *Handbook of personality disorders* (pp. 323–343). New York: Guilford Press.

Read, S. J., Jones, D. K., & Miller, L. C. (1990). Traits as goal-based categories: The importance of goals in the coherence of dispositional categories. *Journal of Personality and Social Psychology, 58,* 1048–1061.

Rutter, M. (1987). Temperament, personality and personality disorder. *British Journal of Psychiatry, 150*, 443–458.

Sanderson, C., & Clarkin, J. F. (2013). Further use of the NEO-PI-R personality dimensions in differential treatment planning. In T. A. Widiger & P. T. Costa (Eds.), *Personality disorders and the five factor model of personality* (3rd ed., pp. 325–348). Washington, DC: American Psychological Association.

Shapiro, D. (1981). *Autonomy and rigid character.* New York: Basic Books.

Sheldon, K. M., & Elliot, A. J. (1999). Goal striving, need satisfaction, and longitudinal well-being: The self-concordance model. *Journal of Personality and Social Psychology, 76,* 482–497.

Soloff, P. H. (2000). Psychopharmacology of borderline personality disorder. *Psychiatric Clinics of North America, 23,* 169–190.

Svrakic, D. M., Whitehead, C., Przybeck, T. R., & Cloninger, C. R. (1993), Differential diagnosis of personality disorders by the seven-factor model of temperament and character. *Archives of General Psychiatry. 50,* 991–999.

Toulmin. S. (1978). Self-knowledge and knowledge of the "self. " In T. Mischel (Ed.), *The self: Psychological and philosophical issues* (pp. 291–317). Oxford, UK: Oxford University Press.

Trull, T., & Durrett, C. (2005). Categorical and dimensional models of personality disorder. *Annual Review of Clinical Psychology, 1,* 355–380.

Tyrer, P., Crawford, M., Mulder, R., Blashfield, R., Farnam, A., Fossati, A., et al. (2011). The rationale for the reclassification of personality disorder in the 11th revision of the International Classification of Diseases (ICD-11). *Journal of Personality and Mental Health, 5,* 246–259.

Tyrer, P., & Johnson, T. (1996). Establishing the severity of personality disorder. *American Journal of Psychiatry, 153,* 1593–1597.

Vaillant, G. E., & Perry, J. C. (1980). Personality disorders. In H. Kaplan, A. M.

Freedman, & B. Sadock (Eds.), *Comprehensive textbook of psychiatry* (3rd ed., pp. 1562–1590). Baltimore: Williams & Wilkins.

Verheul, R., Andrea, H., Berghout, C. C., Dolan, C., Busschback, J., van der Kroft, P., et al. (2008). Severity indices of personality problems (SIPP-118): Development, factor structure, reliability, and validity. *Psychological Assessment, 20,* 23–34.

Verheul, R., & Widiger, T. A. (2004). A meta-analysis of the prevalence and usage of the personality disorder not otherwise specified (PDNOS) diagnosis. *Journal of Personality Disorders, 18,* 309–319.

Wakefield, J. C. (2008). The perils of dimensionalization: Challenges in distinguishing negative traits from personality disorders. *Psychiatric Clinics of North America, 31,* 379–393.

Westen, D., & Arkowitz-Westen, L. (1998). Limitations of Axis II in diagnosing personality pathology in clinical practice. *American Journal of Psychiatry, 155,* 1767–1771.

Widiger, T. A., Costa, P. T., Jr., & McCrea, R. R. (2002). A proposal for Axis II: Diagnosing personality disorders using the five-factor model. In P. T. Costa, Jr. & T. A. Widiger (Eds.), *Personality disorders and the five-factor model of personality* (2nd ed., pp. 431–456). Washington, DC: American Psychological Association.

Widiger, T. A., & Lowe, J. R. (2012). Personality disorders. In M. M. Anthony & D. H. Barlow (Eds.), *Handbook of assessment and treatment planning for psychological disorders* (2nd ed., pp. 571–605). New York: Guilford Press.

Widiger, T. A., & Simonsen, E. (2005). Alternative dimensional models of personality disorder. *Journal of Personality Disorders, 19,* 110–130.

Widiger, T. A., Trull, T. J., Clarkin, J. F., Sanderson, C., & Costa, P. T., Jr. (1994). A description of the DSM-III-R and DSM-IV personality disorders with the five-factor model. In P. T. Costa & T. A. Widiger (Eds.), *Personality disorders and the five-factor model of personality* (pp. 41–56). Washington DC: American Psychological Association.

Wiggins, J. S. (1982). Circumplex models of interpersonal behavior. In J. P. Kendall & J. N. Butcher (Eds.), *Handbook of research methods in clinical psychology* (pp. 183–221). New York: Wiley.

Wiggins, J. S., & Pincus, A. L. (1989). Conceptions of personality disorder and dimensions of personality. *Psychological Assessment, 1,* 305–316.

Young, J. E., Klosko, J. S., & Weishaar, M. E. (2003). *Schema therapy: A practitioner's guide.* New York: Guilford Press.

chapter 4

Formulation and Treatment Planning

John F. Clarkin and W. John Livesley

An important function of diagnostic assessment is to construct a formulation that explains the origins and development of a patient's problems to use in planning treatment, establishing collaborative treatment goals, and negotiating the treatment contract. Although most psychotherapists probably consider case formulation an essential clinical task, the specialized therapies for personality disorder differ in the use of case formulation. As noted by Livesley and Clarkin (Chapter 3, this volume), some manualized therapies make little use of assessment and formulation, whereas others, especially the cognitive therapies and transference-focused psychotherapy (TFP), build treatment around case formulation. With integrated modular treatment (IMT), formulation is the blueprint for therapy and for promoting more integrated personality functioning. Discussion of the formulation with the patient bridges assessment and treatment and offers an important opportunity to engage the patient in collaborative therapeutic work.

FORMULATION

A comprehensive case formulation weaves together the diverse biological, psychological, and social factors that contributed to the patient's clinical presentation into a narrative account of her or his life and personality. This narrative explains her or his current problems and defines the major issues for treatment. Essentially, a formulation is a hypothesis about the origins, precipitants, and perpetuating influences on the patient's problems (Eells, 1997). Before considering the contents and structure of a useful formulation, we need to consider the functions of a formulation because these functions influence its focus and structure.

Therapeutic Functions of Formulation

The value of a case formulation for the therapist is that it organizes clinical information so as to make it readily accessible during treatment. The formulation also helps patients to understand their problems and distress. This is important because many patients with personality disorders have limited understanding of why they are so distressed and their lives so chaotic, and this compounds their distress and demoralization. The formulation offers meaning that often helps to settle and contain reactivity and defines the salient issues that need to be addressed in the early phase of treatment.

The formulation also provides a road map for treatment. Effective formulations have descriptive and prescriptive components. The description of the origins and nature of the patient's problems helps to establish the main treatment pathway. The prescriptive element establishes the overall intensity of therapy (frequency of sessions and duration of treatment), the broad sequence in which problems will be addressed, and the treatment modules that will be used at different phases of treatment. Thus the formulation provides the therapist with a broad perspective on the likely course of therapy. This perspective provides a context for working with the patient to negotiate the treatment contract. Because the formulation provides patients with an organized account of their problems, it forms the basis for psychoeducation about the nature and origin of their difficulties. Psychoeducation begins when the formulation is discussed with the patient with an explanation of the nature of his or her difficulties and how treatment may be helpful.

With IMT, integration is both an operational task—the coordinated use of a combination of interventions selected from different treatment models—and a therapeutic goal—the development of more integrated personality functioning. With longer-term therapy, the achievement of greater personal coherence is linked to the construction of a more adaptive sense of self and identity. Livesley and Clarkin (Chapter 3, this volume) noted that self/identity impairment helps to define personality disorder. For many patients, it is not sufficient to decrease symptoms, increase emotion regulation, or resolve impaired interpersonal functioning. They also need to develop a more satisfying and meaningful lifestyle and a more adaptive sense of self. This is where a good formulation is helpful: It provides the blueprint for constructing a more adaptive self-narrative. Collaborative discussion and modification of the formulation immediately following assessment forms the basis for a therapy-long process of revising the formulation with the patient as new material and new understanding emerge with treatment.

Ongoing reformulation is an important process. Contemporary personality research documents the role of personal narratives in integrative personality functioning (McAdams & Pals, 2006). People construe their lives as ongoing stories that establish their identities, shape their behavior, and help them to integrate with their culture and community. Self-narratives are seriously impoverished in individuals with personality disorder. The *descriptive* component of the formulation lays out the essential details of the patient's life and personality and draws together a wide variety of facts to create a coherent narrative that resembles the autobiographical sense of self. Thus the formulation is the first step in a therapy-long endeavor to help patients construct a coherent personal narrative that promotes more integrated functioning. For this reason, it is important that the formulation is discussed collaboratively with the patient and revised throughout treatment. When first discussed with the patient, the narrative is essentially a set of hypotheses that are subsequently modified as new information emerges during treatment. In the process, the formulation is "metabolized" until it becomes part of the patients' understanding of themselves and their lives.

Structure and Contents of the Formulation

Although the formulation describes the main facts of a person's life, these facts are inevitably influenced by the clinician's conceptual models of personality disorder and therapy. Hence the formulations of specialized therapies differ substantially in content and focus. With IMT, the formulation is guided by the traditional contents of a psychiatric history and a description of personality pathology in terms of severity, salient traits, and domains of dysfunction. The goal is to understand these impairments in the context of the individual's life history. This descriptive component of the formulation usually involves (1) an account of presenting problems, current concerns, and contemporary situational factors, along with a brief history of these problems; (2) discussion of possible vulnerability factors, including genetic predisposition, other co-occurring mental disorders, psychosocial influences, and any medical conditions; (3) a developmental history organized around events and relationships that are believed to have contributed to problems; (4) a description of personality, including strengths and liabilities based on level of severity of personality, major traits, and domains; and (5) a consideration of how personality factors and life events interacted to create and perpetuate current problems. This narrative is accompanied with diagnostic information covering both personality disorder and other mental disorders.

An effective formulation is more than a simple list of possible causal factors, developmental experiences, and psychopathology. Rather, this information is given shape and structure through a narrative that welds together key factors and highlights salient issues. The formulation should also discuss potential targets for change. The four domains of impairment (symptoms, regulation and modulation, interpersonal, and self/identity) provide a convenient way to organize a discussion of these targets. A summary of major symptoms can be followed by a description of emotion and impulse dysregulation and the factors contributing to these difficulties. Description of interpersonal problems should include repetitive maladaptive interpersonal patterns, associated schemas, and key conflicts that contribute to presenting symptoms and problems. As with the control and modulation domain, it is useful to identify important psychosocial events that contributed to these problems and current relationships that may either perpetuate or modulate these problems. Finally, the formulation should include a brief description of self- and identity pathology, including core self-schemas. Description of domains of impairment leads naturally to the prescriptive aspects of the formulation. As we discuss later, domains are closely tied to the selection of specific treatment modules (see later discussion, as well as Livesley & Clarkin, Chapters 2 and 3, this volume) and to the sequence in which problems are addressed.

When constructing a case formulation, the clinician needs to balance the comprehensiveness and specificity of the formulation against pragmatic considerations regarding the length of the assessment process and the need to start treatment. This is a challenge because most patients with personality disorder have complex histories with multiple problems linked to diverse etiological factors. Pragmatic considerations suggest that comprehensiveness may need to be sacrificed, at least temporarily, to avoid an excessively lengthy assessment process. What is needed is a formulation with sufficient detail to map the broad structure of therapy that can be elaborated as therapy unfolds. It is also important to focus on key themes and avoid excessive detail that may be confusing and lead to a formulation that lacks clarity and focus (Eells, 1997).

Form of the Formulation

A practical issue is whether the formulation should be written out and whether the patient should have a written copy. Several authors concur that a written formulation is helpful (Davidson, 2008; Perry, Cooper, & Michels, 1987; Ryle, 1997, 2001). Constructing a written account forces clarity and conciseness and a more critical evaluation of the information. It can also be used by therapists to refresh their memory about salient issues. It is helpful to share the written formulation with the patient and to invite the patient's comments and input. This means that the formulation needs to be expressed in clear, nontechnical language that reflects observable behavior and uses the patient's own language whenever possible (Hilsenroth & Cromer, 2007). Ryle (1997) suggests writing a "reformulation" letter that links the patient's problems to her or his history. The contents of the letter are usually discussed with the patient, written out, and then given to the patient. Subsequently, the letter is discussed further and revised if necessary during the last assessment session. This is a useful process that focuses the patient's attention on key issues, fosters collaboration, and models openness and flexibility.

The danger is that the patient may be overwhelmed by the information. This may mean that the patient should be initially presented with a summary that contains sufficient information to negotiate a meaningful contract and that further information is gradually presented as therapy progresses. Decisions about the amount and type of information to share with the patient are influenced by the patient's cognitive capacity to manage information, his or her current level of initial distress and impairment, and the nature of the clinician's formulation and the degree to which the patient is aware of the nature of the contents.

A further refinement to the use of a written formulation is the use of diagrams to explain key themes (Livesley, 2003; see Salvatore, Popolo, & Dimaggio, Chapter 19, this volume). Construction of a diagram also forces the clinician to be clear and concise. Diagrams are also easier for patients to understand and enable them to see at a glance how different thoughts, emotions, and events are connected. Patients can also take a diagram away with them and modify it between sessions. This helps them to take "ownership" of the formulation and promotes a sense of agency.

Role of Formulation in Engagement

Sitting with patients to review the results of the assessment and formulation and asking for their input about how the formulation could be modified to provide a better description and understanding of their problems is a crucial part of the treatment process that incorporates many of the common mechanisms of therapeutic change. The process engages the patient in a collaborative exchange that helps the patient to begin to see treatment as a collaborative venture. This is especially helpful with patients who approach treatment somewhat passively, seeing the therapist as the expert who provides treatment and themselves as the passive recipients of care. An active exchange so early in the process restructures these expectations and builds the alliance. The alliance is also fostered by the clinician's explaining the nature of the patient's problems and the way therapy may help the patient to make changes (Hilsenroth & Cromer, 2007). This paves the way for a collaborative discussion of treatment goals and what the patient would like to achieve in treatment.

TREATMENT PLANNING

Integrated modular treatment may be delivered along multiple pathways in various settings, including hospital inpatient units, day hospitals, outpatient services, community care teams, forensic services, and office practice. Whatever the setting, pathways vary according to decisions about treatment intensity, duration, and intervention strategies. We should note, however, that given the complexity of personality pathology and the limited information obtained through routine assessment, it is not possible to map out a fixed treatment plan of the type used by protocol-driven therapies. All that is necessary at this stage is to make initial decisions about treatment intensity based on severity and about broad treatment pathways based on trait constellations. It is also possible to develop general ideas about what specific treatment modules will be needed based on an evaluation of domains of impairment. A general plan covering these issues provides a broad perspective that is useful when discussing treatment options with the patient.

Severity and Treatment Intensity

An evaluation of severity is the first step in assessing personality disorder because of its implications for treatment goals and intensity. With increasing severity, emphasis is placed on containment and stabilization rather than more definitive change, achieved through the use of more supportive and behavioral interventions. Severity also influences treatment intensity. In the current context, intensity refers to the degree to which general treatment modules (see Livesley & Clarkin, Chapter 2, this volume) that focus on relationship dimensions and generic interventions for promoting motivation, self-agency, and self-reflection are supplemented with more specific change-focused intervention modules. The distinction is similar to the traditional psychodynamic distinction between supportive versus expressive interventions.

Interventions based on general treatment modules are inherently supportive and place minimal stress on the treatment alliance. In contrast, specific treatment modules invariably impose some strain on the patient and the treatment relationship due to the implied expectation of change. This strain increases with the use of modules that are more exploratory and emotionally arousing. Consequently, a critical decision for all treatments, regardless of duration, concerns the use of specific interventions that have the potential to strain the alliance and to be destabilizing. This decision hinges on the severity of personality disorder and the presence of specific markers of severity, such as high levels of cognitive dysregulation, severely impaired effortful control, and a tendency to dissociate when stressed. Increasing severity suggests greater reliance on general modules and more cautious use of specific modules. When specific interventions are used in treating severe disorder, greater emphasis is placed on behavioral interventions to deal with specific problems, such as deliberate self-harm.

Treatment Pathways and Trait Constellations

A central problem in establishing treatment plans and discussing these plans with the patient is the dearth of empirical evidence about typical treatment trajectories and the factors that are important in tailoring treatment to the personality characteristics of individual patients. Thus, in discussing treatment pathways, we are forced to extrapolate from modest findings emerging from longitudinal studies about the typical course of personality disorder and to rely heavily on clinical observation and experience. Our ideas about treatment pathways and trait constellations should therefore be considered, at best, hypotheses about how personality traits may influence course and outcome.

We propose that outcome differs across the emotional dysregulation, dissocial behavior, and social avoidance constellations discussed by Livesley and Clarkin (Chapter 3, this volume) and that each constellation requires a somewhat different treatment pathway. Earlier chapters described a stage model of therapy—the idea that treatment typically passes through five phases involving safety, containment, regulation and control, exploration and change, and synthesis and integration, with each phase focusing on specific problems related to a given domain of impairment. The hypothesis advanced is that progress through these phases differs across trait constellations.

Although data are limited, the evidence available suggests that outcome is better for patients with emotionally unstable and impulsive traits (in DSM-IV/DSM-5 terms, borderline and antisocial personality disorders) than for patients with socially withdrawn traits (DSM-IV/DSM-5 schizoid personality disorder; Paris, 2003). This idea is consistent with the traditional clinical view that borderline and antisocial disorders tend to "burn out" over time, a view supported by empirical research on change in normal personality traits that shows that people become less reactive, emotional, and impulsive with age and more responsible (Tickle, Heatherton, & Wittenberg, 2001). These observations point to a poorer outcome for patients with high levels of social withdrawal. Based on these ideas, we suggest two broad treatment pathways based on trait constellations: (1) a pathway for patients with the emotional dysregulation and dissocial constellations of traits who can probably be treated with a common pathway, at least in the early phases of treatment, and (2) a somewhat different pathway for patients with the socially avoidant and emotionally constricted constellation.

Pathways for Emotionally Dysregulated and Dissocial Trait Constellations

The initial treatment pathway for patients with these traits involves a relatively prolonged engagement phase (containment and earlier control and regulation phases), with high therapist activity to contain and settle the unstable emotions and impulses associated with suicidality, deliberate self-harm, violence, acting-out tendencies, and aggressiveness. Once containment is achieved and crisis behaviors settle, attention can be given to building emotion and impulse control. This is usually a lengthy process, although considerable variation occurs across patients. Although the self-regulation impairments associated with the emotionally dysregulated and dissocial constellations differ, there are important commonalities that can be treated using the same specific treatment modules (see Livesley, Chapter 11, this volume). Both constellations are associated with problems in identifying and labeling emotions, accepting and tolerating emotions, anger management, effortful control, emotion regulation, and so on.

Following improved emotion and impulse control and greater stability, the subsequent treatment pathway differs according to level of severity (defined in terms of self- and interpersonal pathology; see Livesley & Clarkin, Chapter 3, this volume). For patients with severe disorder, subsequent treatment is based on an evaluation of the extent to which the patient is likely to benefit from further treatment. There are three main options. First, for some patients, treatment may terminate at this point, either because they are satisfied with the progress made or because the therapist thinks that further progress is unlikely. Second, with patients with severe disorder, intensive treatment gives way to a more supportive and rehabilitative approach designed to maintain changes and help the individual to manage personality vulnerabilities. For many of these patients, occasional supportive sessions are sufficient to ensure that improvement is maintained. With other patients, a more active rehabilitative approach may be warranted that acknowledges the severity of the underlying impairments and focuses on helping the patient to manage them more effectively. This approach often involves a frank but supportive discussion of treatment options with a focus on helping the patient to accept his or her vulnerabilities and manage his or her life and relationships accordingly. With one patient this occurred after 3 years of biweekly and, later, weekly sessions. The patient had long history of emotional instability and seriously impaired and highly conflicted relationships with men. During therapy, the patient acquired greater mastery over her emotions but nevertheless recognized that she was highly vulnerable in close relationships due to severe boundary difficulties and a highly fragile self. She decided that these difficulties were unlikely to change and that she lacked the energy to work on them in therapy. She thought that she could manage better if she did not live with anyone again. After exploring these problems at length over several sessions, a new contract was established that involved less intense treatment. This focused on helping her establish a lifestyle and construct a personal niche that she found satisfying and supportive without the need for an enduring intimate relationship.

With the less severe forms of disorder, however, improved emotion regulation makes it possible for treatment to focus increasingly on interpersonal problems and impairments. At this point, the pathways of care for these two constellations diverge. With emotion dysregulation, the focus will largely be on interpersonal behaviors mediated by fearfulness and threat, such as abandonment anxiety, rejection sensitivity, and submissive dependency. With the dissocial pattern, the focus is on promoting more prosocial behaviors, developing empathy, reducing interpersonal hostility and sadistic tendencies, and modulating narcissistic grandiosity.

Pathway for the Socially Avoidant Trait Constellations

The pathway proposed for patients with constricted emotions and social withdrawal involves shorter safety and containment phases, with a prolonged emphasis on engagement and a somewhat different level of therapist activity. The emphasis is almost entirely on establishing contact with the patient and building a reasonable working treatment alliance with less concern with containment. Progress is often slow. A low-key nonintrusive approach is needed to avoid activating further avoidance and withdrawal. With lower levels of severity, the formation of a modest alliance may make it possible to move to the control and regulation phase with a focus on psychoeducation about the nature and adaptive value of emotions, followed by attempts to focus on any emotions that may be activated in session. The goal is to promote emotion recognition and tolerance in the context of a supportive relationship and to reduce emotional constriction. Subsequently, treatment may follow the phases of change described earlier, but emotional and interpersonal changes are likely to be modest.

With high-severity cases, the establishment of modest engagement and rapport provides an opportunity to adopt a more social-engineering and rehabilitative-management strategy to help the patient to accept that he or she does not have a great need for people, to be comfortable with this fact, and to establish a lifestyle that is compatible with these traits. Many socially avoidant individuals do not want to be sociable; they largely seek help because others think they should change their ways. With such individuals it is probably more productive to help them to accept their personality traits and to find a niche that allows them to feel comfortable and accepted.

Domains and the Use of Specific Treatment Modules

A key feature of IMT, noted by Livesley and Clarkin (Chapter 3, this volume), is the emphasis on decomposing personality disorder into specific domains of impairment (symptoms, regulation and modulation, interpersonal, and self/identity) and on linking these domains to specific intervention modules. This process greatly facilitates the selection of interventions and provides the foundation for coordinating the use of specific interventions. The assumption is that domains differ in amenability to change and that these differences provide a rationale for addressing domains in a sequential manner, beginning with the most changeable of symptoms and progressing first to control and modulation of emotions and impulses and then to interpersonal impairments before terminating with the treatment of the most stable aspects of personality pathology, namely self and identity problems.

The treatment of each domain is based on the idea of technical eclecticism (see Livesley, Dimaggio, & Clarkin, Chapter 1, this volume). That is, interventions are selected from all therapeutic models as needed to treat the problems of specific patients. Ideally, selection would be based on evidence of efficacy. Unfortunately, outcome research has not progressed to the point of establishing the best ways to treat the different components of personality disorder, forcing us to rely largely on a rational analysis of the methods that appear relevant to each domain. The use of specific interventions is guided by the principle that specific interventions are used only when the therapeutic alliance is satisfactory and the patient is motivated to work on changing the problem at hand. The following sections discuss the range of interventions that may be considered for treating each domain. This discussion is intended to illustrate the kinds of interventions the therapist may wish to consider rather than offering a proscribed list of strategies. The selection of specific interventions is the least proscribed component of IMT, providing an opportunity for the therapist to be creative in selecting interventions that best fit the patient's problems and personality and the preferred intervention strategy.

Figures 4.1–4.4 suggest some therapeutic models that therapists may find useful sources of specific interventions for treating each domain, along with suggestions about actual interventions. In the symptom domain, relatively few specific interventions are suggested for the initial stages of therapy (see Figure 4.1). Reliance is placed instead on generic interventions to provide the support needed to contain distress and reactivity, plus medication where indicated. In this context, it should be noted that medication is conceptualized as a specific intervention and hence used in the context of general intervention strategies, particularly those concerned with establishing engagement and an effective alliance (see Silk & Friedel, Chapter 10, this volume).

For containment and improvements to the alliance, more specific interventions are added as therapy progresses to treat dysregulation of emotions and impulses (see Figure 4.2). In other chapters, we have referred to this phase of treatment as *control and regulation*, a term that requires a little explanation. The goal is not to limit and constrain emotion expression but rather to achieve more modulated and nuanced expression of the full range of emotions both in individuals with emotional dysregulation and those with emotional constriction. This achievement requires the acquisition of emotion-regulating skills needed to self-regulate emotional expression and an increased capacity to process emotions as they occur in an interpersonal context. Thus, although a skill-building approach is considered a necessary component of therapy, it is

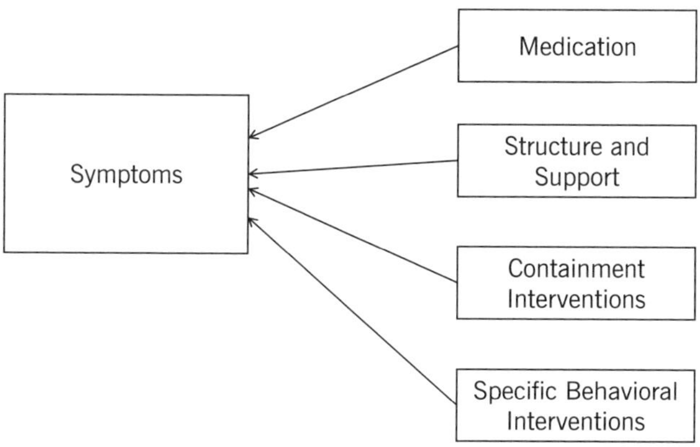

FIGURE 4.1. Symptom domain and intervention modules.

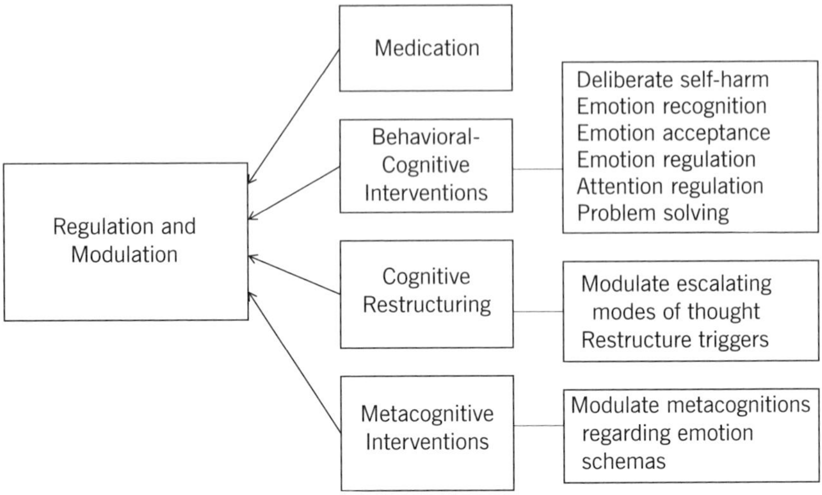

FIGURE 4.2. Regulation and modulation domain and intervention modules.

not considered sufficient: Patients also need to develop the ability to reflect on their emotional experiences and to understand the interpersonal contexts that evoke emotions and the way these emotions influence thoughts and action. To achieve these goals, therapists may need to draw upon several therapies to assemble the range of interventions needed. Figure 4.2 points to the central role of cognitive-behavioral therapies as a source of skill-building methods (see Livesley, Chapter 11; Ottavi et al., Chapter 13, this volume), cognitive restructuring methods to modulate schemas associated with emotional arousal and expression (see Leahy, Chapter 12, this volume) and metacognitive therapies (see Bateman & Fonagy, Chapter 7; Dimaggio et al., Chapter 8, this volume). However, the therapist may also want to draw upon other treatment models, such as the acceptance-based behavioral therapies (Hayes, Strosahl, & Wilson, 1999: Roemer & Orsillo, 2009), for strategies to promote emotional tolerance and acceptance and greater self-compassion. Treatment of the interpersonal domain usually requires an even greater repertoire of methods drawn from a wider range of therapies (see Figure 4.3). Mentalizing and other metacognitive interventions continue to play a major role along with those from cognitive therapy, including schema-focused therapy. However, these methods usually need to be supplemented with methods from interpersonal reconstructive (Benjamin, 2003) and psychodynamic therapy to address repetitive maladaptive interpersonal patterns and avoidance behaviors as they emerge in treatment. Specific interventions to deal with the interpersonal aspects of trauma and adversity are also important in this phase of treatment. Finally, changes to self-pathology usually require an array of methods to construct a new self-narrative and develop a personal niche that supports adaptive personality

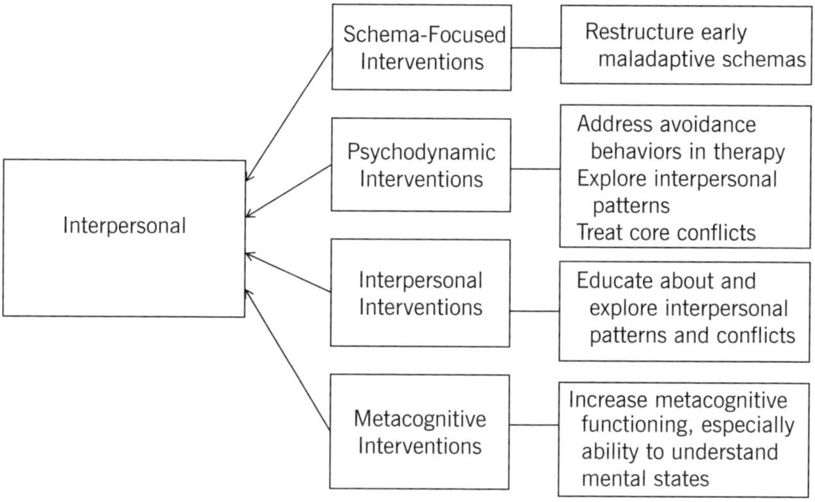

FIGURE 4.3. Interpersonal domain and intervention modules.

functioning. Unfortunately, we know little about how to help patients to construct a new sense of self and identity. Relatively little empirical attention has been given to this important treatment task, and the only therapy that discusses the problem in depth is TFP (see Clarkin, Yeomans, De Panfilis, & Levy, Chapter 18, this volume). The therapeutic task is somewhat different from that of other treatment phases, which are largely concerned with identifying and changing maladaptive personality processes and structures. Here the task is less analytic and more synthetic—the synthesis of a new and more adaptive self-system (Livesley, 2003). Figure 4.4 contains some suggestions that we have found useful in helping the relatively small number of patients who reach this stage of therapy.

CASE EXAMPLES

The following three case vignettes illustrate the presentations that characterize patients with different levels of severity of personality disorder.

Case Example 1

Darlene is a 24-year-old single unemployed white female. She sought treatment at a university hospital outpatient clinic dressed in sweat pants and torn T-shirt after having been administratively discharged from a local day hospital for having a sexual relationship with a male patient in the program. The current episode of emotional upset began following the death of her father

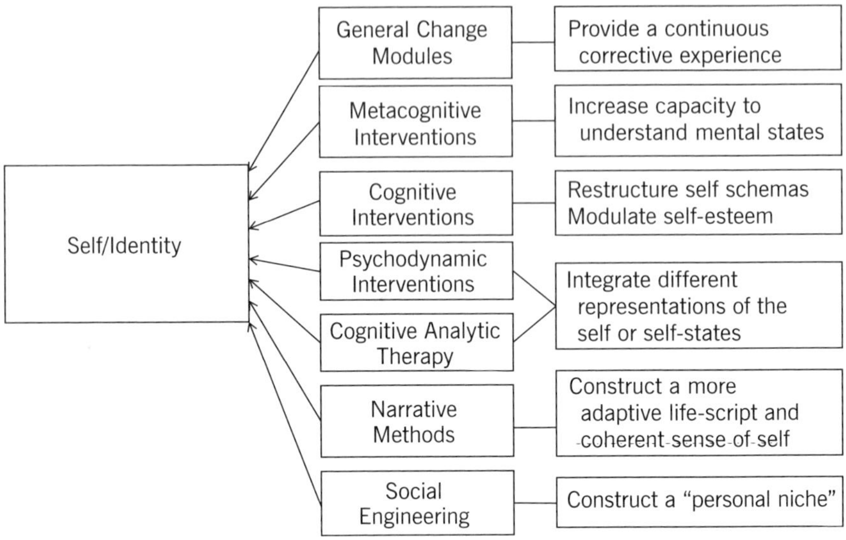

FIGURE 4.4. Self domain and intervention modules.

from terminal cancer 3 weeks previously with a suicide attempt (overdose with medication) that resulted in a brief inpatient hospitalization followed by discharge to the day hospital.

Darlene was financially supported by her mother and stepfather. She had had brief and chaotic relationships with men whom she usually met in bars and had one-night stands with. Some relationships lasted several weeks, but these typically ended with a fight, after which she would go to a bar to meet and have sex with another man.

Darlene was raised by affluent parents on the West Coast. She describes her mother as distant and emotionally cold and holds her responsible for taking Darlene away from her father when they divorced; she was 11 years old at the time. Darlene completed high school and attended a prestigious university on the West Coast. During this time, she abused alcohol and drugs, and at one point she was dependent on heroin. She was arrested for driving under the influence twice and expressed no concern that she could have seriously injured someone. Darlene attended the university for 4 years but did not complete a degree program. At age 21, she was involved in a serious car accident and sustained back injuries. She was provided with a prescription for pain killers, which she still uses for infrequent back pain. In her past treatments, she has received diagnoses of major depression, substance abuse disorder, and BPD.

Case Formulation

Darlene clearly suffers from a personality disorder manifested in a confused and fragmented sense of self with no clear goals or inner direction. Her relationships with others are brief and filled with angry conflicts. These deficits in self- and relationship functioning are long-standing. The level of personality disturbance is severe. She meets a number of criteria for borderline, narcissistic, and antisocial personality disorders. She exhibits a number of domains of dysfunction, including past symptoms of depression and substance abuse, current poor regulation of anger, serious difficulties in relating to others, and lack of investment in work and enduring relationships.

The immediate treatment concern will be to establish a structured treatment framework with Darlene, to assess her ability to form more than a superficial relationship with the therapist, and to assist her in making a motivated attempt to change. If a treatment structure can be established in which she can achieve some motivation for change, the modules of treatment that focus on the containment of destructive behaviors will be most important. Only if these modules of treatment are successful in helping Darlene to control destructive behavior can the therapist move on to modules to help her coalesce a coherent conception of herself with meaningful life goals.

Case Example 2

Elvera is a 34-year-old single Hispanic woman with a chief complaint of inability to control her moods and anger, so out of control at times as to interfere with satisfying friendships and close relationships. She is employed as a legal assistant. Elvera's anger drives her to rages at her mother, to destroying objects in her apartment, and to anger at her boss that she is able to stifle and not act upon. She has a history of cutting her wrists superficially during episodes of intense anger and upset. She has had several brief individual psychotherapy treatments in the past.

Elvera had a chaotic childhood. It would appear from her account that her mother had periods of psychosis, at times unreachable, at other times quite paranoid, thinking that someone would invade the house and steal the children. The father was physically abusive, with severe physical and psychological punishments toward the children.

Elvera successfully completed high school and entered the work world. She has no history of drug or alcohol abuse. She has a history of brief relationships with men, with no relationships lasting longer than 6 months. She tends to be suspicious about her friends, constantly assuming that they do not have her interests or welfare in mind. Elvera is constantly fearful of being rejected by others and, at the same time, does not trust her own judgment and accurate perception of others. She is very confused about her own desires and goals, with shifting ideas of career goals fluctuating among being a photographer, an artist, and an actress.

Case Formulation

Elvera demonstrates difficulties in achieving a coherent, positive sense of self, with related difficulties in understanding the experience and motives of others, leading to major problems in relating to others. She has a personality disorder of a moderate degree of severity, meeting a mixed group of criteria for paranoid, borderline, avoidant, and narcissistic personality disorders. In terms of domains of difficulty, Elvera's symptoms include rage outbursts with a past history of wrist cutting. There are major problems in regulation of affect, especially anger. Her friendships and heterosexual relations are distant, impaired by a sense that others are not really concerned about her. Treatment modules to improve affect regulation, followed by modules to improve self-perception, appropriate personal goals, perception of others, and interpersonal relations will be essential.

Case Example 3

Sandra presented for assessment prior to treatment at the age of 36 years with self-harming behavior, unstable emotions and moods, and intense distress that began shortly after she learned that her daughter had been abused by a friend and neighbor. At the first interview, she was very distressed and had difficulty organizing her thoughts. Sandra also reported feeling confused and that she had what seemed to be pseudohallucinations. She also said that, several days before, she had heard a voice saying that she was bad, although the voice was not experienced as external to herself.

Personal History

Subsequent assessment interviews revealed a history of problems dating to mid-teenage years involving deliberate self-injury, unstable moods, rapid emotional changes, and difficult interpersonal relationships that led to frequent crises and a series of brief inpatient admissions. Over the years, Sandra had seen many clinicians but had never stayed in treatment for more than a few months. She was very negative about previous therapy and pessimistic about the prospects of receiving help. The unstable moods and self-harming behavior had escalated following the incident involving her daughter. Sandra felt very guilty about what had happened and felt that she had let her daughter down.

Sandra described growing up in a large dysfunctional and unstable family, with extensive emotional and physical abuse from her mother and her older siblings and extensive sexual abuse perpetrated by her mother's partner; her parents had separated when she was young. Following the abuse of her daughter, Sandra began recalling her own experiences, and for nearly a year she experienced intrusive memories of the abuse and frequent flashbacks that were extremely distressing and led to dissociative reactions.

Sandra lived with her partner and three children, two boys from the relationship with her partner and a teenage daughter from an earlier relationship. At the time of the assessment, she had not worked for nearly a year. Before her current difficulties began, she had worked part time at a local supermarket. She had had numerous similar jobs in the past, none lasting very long. Although Sandra was in a steady relationship, the relationship was dysfunctional. She found her partner hypercritical, emotionally abusive, and unsupportive. She also felt that neither he nor her large extended family appreciated what she did for them. Sandra remained in the relationship because she could not tolerate the idea of being alone, and she was very afraid that her partner would leave her. Nevertheless, she was extremely frustrated that he did not seem to appreciate her because she thought that she worked hard to build a good home for him and the children. Sandra was house-proud and went to considerable effort to cater to her partner's needs, even at some cost to herself. Her feeling of being unappreciated and neglected were not unusual: Her life was a series of abusive and failed relationships.

Sandra's relationship with her extended family was intense, almost to the point of being enmeshed, and highly conflicted. She was the youngest of a large family, all of whom interfered regularly in her life and disapproved of her behavior, sometimes violently. They also made extensive demands of her, expecting her to babysit and assist with all manner of chores. Sandra was unable to resist these demands even when they were unreasonable and often felt exhausted trying to meet the often conflicting needs of her partner, children, and extended family.

Sandra's social life was similarly unstable: Friendships were formed rapidly and equally rapidly broken. As with her family, she frequently felt disappointed in her friends and acquaintances, who invariably failed to meet her expectations. When assessed, she had no close friends and no social support outside the family. Sandra was concerned about her lack of friends. However, she also noted that, although she often felt overwhelmed and exhausted by her chaotic life, it was as if she needed the turmoil because she was easily bored and often looked for excitement. Looking to the future, Sandra said that she would like a different job that was more satisfying, but she was unsure of what she really wanted to do or, indeed, what she wanted from life.

Diagnosis and Assessment

Mental state examination and evaluation of personality indicated that Sandra met most criteria for BPD and criteria for DSM-IV dependent personality disorder. She was not considered to have an Axis I disorder, although depressive symptoms were noted. Assessment was structured by the three-level system described by Livesley and Clarkin (Chapter 3, this volume). Sandra was considered to have severe personality disorder, showing both severe self-pathology and chronic interpersonal difficulties. She had a poorly developed and unstable sense of self. She was unsure about who she was, and the interview revealed substantial evidence of boundary problems: Sandra described several episodes in which she inappropriately revealed detailed personal information to strangers and then felt alarmed about what she had done; she defined herself by the way others treated her; and she seemed to adopt the opinions of her family without question, as if she was uncertain about her own thoughts and feelings. The interview also produced extensive evidence of her difficulty with close relationships.

Evaluation of trait domains and primary traits was guided by the four-factor structure (emotional dysregulation, dissocial, social avoidance, and compulsivity) described by Livesley and Clarkin (Chapter 3, this volume; see Table 3.2). Assessment was initially based on the assessment interviews and later confirmed with a self-report questionnaire. Sandra had most of the emotional dysregulation cluster of traits, with anxiousness, emotional intensity and reactivity, submissiveness, insecure attachment, and cognitive dysregulation being most notable. She had a relatively high level of a single trait, sensation seeking, from the dissocial factor. She was also moderately compulsive and conscientious.

Assessment of the four domains—symptoms, control and modulation, interpersonal, and self/identity—was also based on the clinical interview. Symptoms included anxiety, sadness and dysphoria, low mood, and self-harming acts. Sandra also complained of a voice saying that she was bad. Careful assessment determined that this was not a true hallucination but rather a pseudohallucination; Sandra noted that the voice was not coming from outside herself. She also showed other features of cognitive dysregulation, such as the tendency for thoughts to become disorganized when she was distressed and difficulty thinking clearly, that caused her to feel confused. Sandra also dissociated fairly frequently when extremely distressed.

Within the regulation and modulation domain, Sandra showed most features of emotional dysregulation (see Livesley, Chapter 11, this volume), with unstable emotions and unpredictable mood changes. When highly distressed she found it difficult to decenter from the feelings and unable to reflect on her experiences. Instead, Sandra was trapped in what felt like endless distress. Emotional arousal readily caused impaired cognitive functions, which further decreased her control over emotions, leading to the emotional state. She seemed to self-regulate distress with deliberate self-harming actions but showed no understanding of the links between the two. Sandra also had impaired metacognitive functioning. Self-reflection was limited and severely affected by emotional arousal. She also found it difficult to understand the mental states and actions of others.

Interpersonal pathology was closely linked to traits of anxious attachment and submissiveness. Sandra longed for closeness, especially to be loved by her mother, but lived in a state of fear that those close to her would abandon or reject her. Despite yearning for closeness, she found no support or comfort from contact with either her partner or her family of origin. Instead, she was frequently locked in a position of hostile dependency. Schemas of abandonment and rejection were in an almost chronic state of activation and linked to schemas of incompetence and inability to manage without the support of others. The interview also suggested that interpersonal crises were also fueled by the need for excitement and stimulation; Sandra noted that she seemed to feel more alive when fighting with her partner.

Substantial interpersonal problems were also linked to Sandra's submissive tendencies. Despite an angry demeanor, she was very subservient. She was a "people pleaser" who found it difficult to resist the demands of others. She was afraid of saying "no," fearing it would lead others to be angry with her and cause them to reject her. Sandra was also a "compulsive caregiver" who spent considerable amounts of time looking after others and seeking to meet their needs.

As noted before, Sandra showed substantial problems in the self/identity domain. In addition to core impairments consistent with a diagnosis of severe personality disorder, she held core self-schemas that she was bad and fundamentally flawed. Sandra also felt intense guilt linked to childhood sexual abuse and believed that she deserved the bad things that happened to her. Her self-esteem was almost constantly poor.

Formulation

Despite the complexity of Sandra's problems, the assessment process was telescoped into a short time frame because she needed immediate help given her decompensated state. Consequently, the initial formulation was also relatively brief. Diagnostically, it was clear that Sandra had severe personality disorder and that the primary form of disorder was emotion dysregulation (BPD). The disorder seemed to arise from the interaction of genetic and environmental risk factors. The family history included an older sibling with very similar problems and several brothers with anger problems and unstable moods. Several other family members also had problems with trait anxiety. Multiple psychosocial risk factors seemed to have contributed to the development of disorder, with three factors standing out. First, Sandra had severe attachment problems with high levels of attachment insecurity. She described her mother as unloving and inattentive throughout most of her childhood. Indeed, she seemed to have been cared for largely by an older sister. These problems probably added to both emotional control difficulties and self-pathology because there seemed little opportunity in the family of origin to acquire emotion regulation skills or a coherent self-structure. Second, the sexual abuse probably contributed to problems both at a biological level, by increasing stress responsivity (Sandra recalled the intense fear she felt at the time), and at psychological levels, by laying down schemas related to insecurity, powerlessness, mistrust, and self-derogation. Third, family dynamics simply added to these problems by reinforcing maladaptive coping mechanisms, contributing to schemas of self-blame and low self-worth, and systematically invalidating Sandra for most of her life.

The current presentation was precipitated by the abuse of her daughter that awoke memories of Sandra's own experiences of abuse, which were never far below the surface, and her feelings of guilt and worthlessness. These feelings overwhelmed her poor coping capacity, which was heavily dependent on feeling that she was a good mother. Problems were perpetuated by Sandra's own personality characteristics that made her vulnerable to stress and by several factors in her current situation, most notably the difficulties she had described with her family of origin and her partner.

The formulation also noted several complicating factors, especially Sandra's tendency to decompensate cognitively under stress and dissociative tendencies that were likely to have an impact on treatment. These features suggested that it would be important to regulate emotional arousal to ensure that Sandra was not overwhelmed and to improve her emotion regulation before the traumatic events of her life were addressed in depth. Offsetting these liabilities was the presence of moderate levels of compulsivity, which seems to improve prognosis of patients with BPD, probably because it leads to a more conscientious attitude to treatment.

At the end of the assessment, Sandra was given only a brief formulation to avoid overwhelming her. She had previously told the clinician that she had been told she had BPD, and she asked about this. The clinician said that he did not find this diagnosis very helpful, but, given the things Sandra had told him, he could understand why she had been given the diagnosis. He went on to explain that he thought that her personality problems primarily involved difficulty controlling emotions and that the emotional dysregulation affected her relationships with others. It was noted that the incident involving her daughter seemed to have triggered memories of her own abuse, causing distress that often seemed to Sandra to be uncontrollable. When the feelings became intolerable, she hurt herself, and this seemed to be the only way she could find to stop the mental pain. Sandra was asked what she thought about this. She agreed that this is what seemed to happen. Following a short discussion of the formulation, she was offered immediate treatment with twice-weekly appointments.

Treatment Planning

The initial plan was to focus on containing reactivity and distress and on reducing self-harming behavior. This plan was formulated in the context of an understanding that the initial phase of therapy was likely to be prolonged and difficult. Because of previous experiences and developmental events, Sandra was extremely mistrustful, which was likely to lead to difficulty building an alliance. It was also anticipated that distrust would continue to be a problem throughout therapy. Given Sandra's propensity to dissociation and cognitive dysfunction when distressed, it was decided that treatment should proceed slowly, with the main emphasis on support and validation with a primary focus on current functioning. It was also decided that, if distressing material related to abuse and trauma emerged early in treatment, the therapist would listen to the material and validate it but refrain from working with it until considerable improvement in emotion regulation had occurred and a reasonable level of stability had been achieved. Sandra had major interpersonal problems that would have to be addressed at some point, but at this time it was decided that these would not become a major focus for a while. Clarkin, Livesley, and Dimaggio (Chapter 20, this volume) provide a more detailed description of Sandra's subsequent treatment.

CONCLUDING COMMENTS

The diagnostic assessment comes to fruition in the construction of a formulation that begins to relate the origins and development of a patient's problems to a plan for treatment, establishing collaborative treatment goals, and negotiating the treatment contract. With IMT, the case formulation is the essential blueprint for the sequencing of therapy toward promoting more integrated personality functioning. The case examples utilized in this chapter illustrate the levels of severity as they affect the integrated treatment plan. The treatment of the third case, that of Sandra, is discussed by Clarkin and colleagues (Chapter 20, this volume) to illustrate the practical application of an integrated approach.

REFERENCES

Benjamin, L. S. (2003). *Interpersonal reconstructive therapy: An integrative, personality-based treatment for complex cases*. New York: Guilford Press.

Davidson, K. (2008). *Cognitive therapy for personality disorders* (2nd ed.). London: Routledge.

Eells, T. D. (1997). Psychotherapy case formulation: History and current status. In T. D. Eells (Ed.), *Handbook of psychotherapy case formulation* (pp. 1–25). New York: Guilford Press.

Hayes, S. C., Strosahl, K. D., & Wilson, K. G. (1999). *Acceptance and commitment therapy: An experiential approach to behavioral change*. New York: Guilford Press.

Hilsenroth, M. J., & Cromer, T. D. (2007). Clinical interventions related to alliance during the initial interview and psychological assessment. *Psychotherapy: Research, Theory, and Practice. 44*, 205–218.

Livesley, W. J. (2003). *Practical management of personality disorder*. New York: Guilford Press.

McAdams, D. P., & Pals, J. L. (2006). A new Big Five: Fundamental principles for an integrative science of personality. *American Psychologist, 61*, 204–217.

Paris, J. (2003). *Personality disorders over time*. Washington, DC: American Psychiatric Publishing.

Perry, S., Cooper, A. R., & Michels, R. (1987). The psychodynamic formulation: Its purpose, structure, and clinical application. *American Journal of Psychiatry, 144*, 543–550.

Roemer, L., & Orsillo, S.M. (2009). *Mindfulness and acceptance-based behavioral therapies in practice.* New York; Guilford Press.

Ryle, A. (1997). *Cognitive analytic therapy and borderline personality disorder.* Chichester, UK: Wiley.

Ryle, A. (2001). Cognitive analytical therapy. In W. J. Livesley (Ed.), *Handbook of personality disorders* (pp. 400–413). New York: Guilford Press.

Tickle, J. J., Heatherton, T. F., & Wittenberg, L. G. (2001). Can personality change? In W. J. Livesley (Ed.), *Handbook of personality disorders* (pp. 242–258). New York: Guilford Press.

chapter 5

Establishing a Treatment Framework and Therapeutic Alliance

Paul S. Links, Deanna Mercer, and Jon Novick

Psychotherapy is understood to be a necessary element of treating patients with personality disorders (Goin, 2001). Two related processes are essential features of any psychotherapy: the establishment of the treatment framework or contract and creating an effective therapeutic alliance. This chapter begins by defining these concepts and introducing two evidence-based psychotherapies for patients with borderline personality disorder (BPD). The two therapies chosen as exemplars of current evidence-based therapies are dialectical behavior therapy (DBT; Linehan, 1993a) and general psychiatric management (GPM; McMain et al., 2009). From these two efficacious therapies, we have tried to capture those strategies needed to create an effective treatment framework and therapeutic alliance when treating patients with personality disorders. The chapter concludes with a synthesis of those elements that seem essential for psychotherapists to use in creating an effective treatment framework (or contract) and therapeutic alliance.

DEFINITIONS

Establishing the treatment framework in psychotherapy involves articulating (1) the goals of the therapy, (2) the roles of the patient and therapist in achieving these goals, and (3) housekeeping tasks such as setting out the time and place for the sessions, the beginning and end of sessions, the handling of emergencies and contacts between sessions, missed sessions, and billing and payment for therapy (Goin, 2001). For our purposes, the development of a treatment framework is equivalent to setting out a treatment contract (Kernberg, Selzer, Koenigsberg, Carr, & Appelbaum, 1989). It is important to remember that the establishment of a treatment contract or framework marks the end of the assessment and the beginning of the treatment phase of the therapy.

The therapeutic alliance was initially characterized by Freud as the "unobjectionable positive transference" that serves as an important motivator for the patient's collaboration with therapy (Bender, 2005). Of the contemporary definitions, Gutheil and Havens (1979) characterized the alliance as arising from the split in the ego that allows the analyst to work with the healthier elements in the patient against resistance and, in particular, personality pathology. Bordin (1979) provided a more pantheoretical definition of the therapeutic alliance involving the bond and agreement between the therapist and patient on the tasks each is to perform in the therapy and the goals of the therapy. The bond in therapy is the quality of the relationship formed between the patient and therapist that mediates whether the patient will take up the tasks inherent in working toward the goals of the therapy. As others (Bender, 2005) have acknowledged, the tasks of therapy (developing an effective patient–therapist bond and agreement on tasks and goals of therapy) are often more difficult to establish in patients with personality disorders. In our experience, successful therapy with these patients requires specific strategies and interventions to aid in the successful implementation of therapy.

Personality disorders may affect the development of the treatment framework and therapeutic alliance in several ways. First, the patient's personality functioning may undermine the helpfulness of the therapist by challenging the parameters of the treatment contract. For example, the patient may arrive late, insist on extending session times, or miss making payments. Second, more time is often required to establish an effective working alliance. In this regard, Gunderson (2001; Gunderson & Links, 2008) suggested that one of the goals of therapy was to establish the working alliance and described how the alliance develops through a series of stages in long-term psychotherapy. The first stage, the contractual alliance, involves establishing treatment goals and defining the therapist and patient roles in achieving these goals. Next, the relational alliance develops as the patient experiences the therapist as caring, understanding, genuine, and likeable. In the third stage, the working alliance is formed, and the patient joins with the therapist as a reliable participant in the therapy and in understanding him- or herself.

The third way personality disorder may affect the alliance is by creating alliance strains and ruptures (Bender, 2005). Alliance strains and ruptures are an expected part of any therapy; however, they are more frequent and more difficult to repair when working with patients with personality disorders. They also contribute to the high dropout rates of somewhere between 40 and 60% observed in patients with BPD (Gunderson et al., 1989; Skodol, Buckley,

& Charles, 1983). Paradoxically, authors such as Lewis (2000) have proposed that in successful therapy, the rupture and repair of affective bonds within attachment relationships such as the therapy relationship is the most powerful healing aspect of therapy. Bennett, Parry, and Ryle (2006) found when using task analysis of cognitive analytic therapy that therapists with good outcome cases were able to identify the same dysfunctional interpersonal behaviors that led to relationship strains or disruptions in therapy as those that occurred in patients' relationships outside of therapy. Furthermore, effective therapists were able to identify a very high proportion of these behaviors. Bennett and colleagues suggested that these ruptures (regardless of the type of therapy that was being performed) could be successfully resolved by (1) recognizing these metacommunications (the therapist recognizing the patient's true meaning in other forms of communication beyond what is verbally expressed), (2) focusing the patient's attention on the immediate therapy experience, and (3) collaborating with the patient in exploring this behavior. Also important in this process was the therapists' willingness to acknowledge their own contributions to the rupture. Projective identification is an example of a personality disorder behavior that can strain and ultimately rupture the therapeutic alliance. In projective identification, the therapist is gently (or not so gently) drawn into identifying with and playing the role of a person from previous dysfunctional interpersonal dyads. This process, in which the therapist is drawn into playing reciprocal roles, acts to reinforce the patient's dysfunctional interpersonal behaviors. Therefore, therapy with patients with personality disorders must include strategies to resolve and repair alliance ruptures to prevent dropouts, to strengthen the therapeutic alliance, and to facilitate therapeutic change.

We now examine two forms of evidence-based psychotherapies for patients with BPD to explore the treatment contracts that would typically be developed with a patient with a personality disorder.

DIALECTICAL BEHAVIOR THERAPY

DBT is the manualized cognitive-behavioral outpatient treatment for patients with BPD and recurrent suicidal behavior (Linehan, 1993a, 1993b; Linehan, Armstrong, Suarez, Allmon, & Heard 1991). Although DBT is a behavioral treatment that aims to help patients to develop more effective coping strategies, the overarching goal is to "offer the promise of a life worth living for highly suicidal people with borderline personality disorders" (Linehan, 2007, p. xi).

When Linehan began her work with highly suicidal women with BPD, she was convinced that behavioral approaches should work for the problems in living experienced by patients with BPD. However, she found that the highly change-oriented approach of behavior therapy led patients to either attack or withdraw from the therapist. Linehan recognized the necessity of building a strong therapeutic alliance with patients to improve their motivation to engage in therapy. She also found that acceptance strategies—strategies that allow the therapist to accept patients just as they are within a context of trying to teach them to change—facilitated the therapeutic alliance and improved motivation to participate in problem-solving strategies. Linehan's personal experience in Zen provided a method for acceptance in the form of mindfulness. The mindfulness techniques included focusing on the moment and nonjudgmental awareness of one's experiences, including thoughts, emotions, and behaviors.

The last step in the development of DBT was to pull together behavioral problem-solving strategies and acceptance strategies. Linehan found that moving quickly and flexibly between these two strategies and finding ways to see them both as "true" was critical to successful treatment. This pulling together of seeming opposites and searching for a synthesis between acceptance on the one hand and change on the other is the heart of dialectical philosophy and permeates DBT.

Treatment Contract

To address the problem of challenging the parameters of the treatment, DBT clearly spells out the contract. The pretreatment period involves establishing the patient's goals for a life worth living, getting agreement on working toward these goals, and stopping suicide and life-threatening behaviors in order to build a life worth living. It also requires that the patient make an explicit agreement to work on any factors that get in the way of successful therapy (therapy-interfering behaviors). A unique feature of DBT is that the therapist is also required to make a commitment to reducing and stopping any therapy-interfering behaviors. For example, a therapist may be chronically late for sessions, and as a result his or her patient may be irritated and upset by the time the session starts. As a result, the first 15 minutes of each session are spent soothing the patient. A DBT therapist would identify that this is his or her therapy-interfering behavior and would clearly state a plan to deal with this behavior—for example, "I recognize that my being late gets in the way of your being able to participate in our sessions. I will move our appointment to the first appointment of the day, as that is when I am less likely to be running behind." In our experience, this two-way agreement about dealing with therapy-interfering behaviors makes it easier to get commitment from the patient. DBT also requires that patients agree to work on reducing any behaviors that significantly interfere with quality of life—that is, those behaviors that would make it impossible for the average person to have a decent quality of life, such as untreated depression, living in a physically abusive relationship, or unstable housing. Lastly, patients commit to increasing skillful behaviors in order to achieve these goals.

Besides making the goals of therapy and the roles of the patient clear, DBT also spells out the principles and main strategies and structure of the individual, group, telephone coaching, and therapist consultation modes of DBT. For example, a therapist knows that he or she is doing DBT when he or she is fulfilling the five functions of DBT: (1) teaching skills, (2) helping the patient generalize those skills to the natural environment, (3) improving patient motivation, (4) teaching the patient to structure the environment, and (5) improving therapist skill and motivation. With clear goals and tasks, the therapist is able to spot quickly (although not always as quickly as the therapist would like!) when therapy is going off track and take remedial action. Although working within this structure does not prevent all instances of patients pushing the limits of therapy—or ultimately burning out the therapist—it does provide a "container" for therapy. When the therapy moves outside of this "container," it signals to the therapist to pull back in order to avoid burning out. Lastly, the treatment contract spells out the duration of therapy (e.g., 1 year), the frequency of appointments (e.g., once per week), the reasons to call a therapist (e.g., crisis, skills coaching, situations in which there has been a conflict or misunderstanding between the therapist and the patient and the patient wishes to restore a sense of security in the relationship before the next session), the rules of dropout (e.g., four missed sessions in a row), and guidelines for group skills training.

GENERAL PSYCHIATRIC MANAGEMENT

To determine the effectiveness of DBT, we completed a large randomized controlled trial involving real-world settings and evaluating the clinical and cost effectiveness of DBT compared with consensus-based best-practice therapy (McMain et al., 2009). Our study attempted to improve upon earlier research by using a rigorous, active, and recommended comparison treatment. In 2001, the American Psychiatric Association developed a practice guideline for the treatment of patients with BPD. The guideline represented a comprehensive set of evidence-based "best-practice" recommendations for the psychiatric community (American Psychiatric Association, 2001; Oldham, 2005). For our study, we implemented the guidelines in a general hospital psychiatric outpatient setting and called the therapy general psychiatric management (GPM). The guidelines indicate that the primary treatment for BPD is psychotherapy, complemented by symptom-targeted pharmacotherapy. Therefore, GPM included both psychotherapy and symptom-targeted pharmacotherapy. This chapter describes the essential elements of GPM used to establish the treatment framework and create the therapy alliance.

Overall, GPM consisted of psychotherapy management using dynamically informed psychotherapy and case management based on the care promoted in the American Psychiatric Association's (2001) practice guidelines for the treatment of BPD and symptom-targeted medication management. For the initial study, the GPM psychotherapy component was based on a psychotherapeutic/psychodynamic approach drawn from the writings of Gunderson (2001; Gunderson & Links, 2008), and DBT strategies were prohibited from use. The psychotherapy component emphasized the relational aspects of the disorder and attributed difficulties to a deficit model focusing on the consequences of precarious early attachment relationships (Gunderson, 2001). Although Gunderson formulated intolerance of aloneness as the core dynamic of BPD, we focused therapy on exploring the consequences of disturbed attachment relationships on the patients' emotional processing. GPM also included medication management based on the symptom-targeted approach presented in the guideline. Because patients were selected for parasuicidal behavior and the primary outcome for the randomized controlled study was prevention of these behaviors, two algorithms—one related to mood lability and the other to impulsivity/aggressiveness—were prioritized as symptom targets for pharmacotherapy.

The typical treatment contract in GPM included weekly individual sessions during which medication management was reviewed. Most often the sessions ran for 50 minutes, and the therapist was available for intersession crises. After hours, the patient was encouraged to use the emergency department affiliated with the therapist's general hospital.

In the next section we discuss common strategies drawn from both DBT and GPM to establish and maintain the treatment contract and framework, as well as the shared strategies needed to ensure an effective therapeutic alliance.

COMMON STRATEGIES

Facilitating Adherence to the Treatment by Increasing Therapist Activity

Keeping the patient in therapy was seen as a priority for both therapies. Indeed, one reason that DBT is effective may be its success in maintaining the patient in therapy. Special attention is given to increasing adherence to treatment, with an active focus on therapy-interfering behavior, and to ensuring that the therapist holds this as a primary treatment responsibility. The emphasis on establishing a treatment contract by clearly defining what is required of the patient (i.e., commitment to building a life worth living and stopping suicidal and parasuicidal behavior, therapy-interfering behavior, and quality-of-life-destroying behaviors) is consistent with the research by Yeomans and colleagues (1994) on transference-focused psychotherapy (TFP), which showed that the use of a treatment contract as part of a structured treatment model resulted in a substantial reduction in dropout rates.

The two main strategies in DBT, acceptance and change strategies, both improve adherence to treatment. Acceptance strategies help patients feel understood (and ultimately help patients to understand themselves) and improve patients' motivation to participate in the treatment. DBT change strategies (skills training, exposure therapy, cognitive modification, and structuring the environment) clearly describe the activity required for change. Providing specific ways to accomplish change improves patient ability to participate in treatment.

Similarly, in GPM, the therapist is instructed to be active and engaging to facilitate adherence to treatment and to encourage a strong attachment relationship between patient and therapist (Bateman & Fonagy, 2000). Therapy has to be seen as a collaborative exercise, and the clinician must remove the pejorative inferences that others have often attributed to the patient's suicidal behavior. The patient is approached as a competent adult who should be an active participant in all aspects and phases of treatment. Assisting the patient's active involvement in therapy will also foster the patient's sense of empowerment and validation and speaks to the healthier aspects of the patient that are thereby indirectly or implicitly highlighted and referenced.

Case Example

A 26-year-old woman demonstrated frequent impulsive behavior throughout her first 9 months in therapy. However, her therapy attendance became even more sporadic when she was charged with stealing money from her parents. The therapist actively maintained phone contact with the patient during this period, often calling the patient when she failed to make scheduled appointments. This active outreach to the patient was seen as encouraging her recognition of the need for therapy. In addition, the contacts were made to counter the patient's projection that the entire world was unreliable and untrustworthy.

Educating the Patient about the Disorder

Providing education about the disorder and its treatment is an important part of the clinician's therapy with the patient and an essential element in building the alliance. The biosocial model is useful for this purpose. In the case of BPD, the biosocial model suggests that problems are a consequence of pervasive emotion dysregulation, which leads to extreme responses to day-to-day stresses. This is particularly the case when the stress is interpersonal. Emotion dysregulation develops as a result of biological factors—the emotionally vulnerable temperament—and social factors—the interaction with an environment that lacks the capability to teach the emotionally vulnerable child the skills to manage her or his emotions. In addition, the environment may act in ways that either enhance or worsen the individual's emotional vulnerability. The message to the child who struggles with intense and long-lasting emotional reactions that her or his emotional reaction is wrong and that she or he ought to change creates additional problems. The types of environments that are implicated in the biosocial theory vary from the more benign, such as families that are overwhelmed and are unable to respond to the special needs of an emotionally intense child, to abusive environments that put extreme emotional demands on a child.

In our experience, the biosocial theory is a turning point for therapists, patients, and family members. Recognizing that the person with BPD is emotionally intense for reasons other than his or her own desire allows others to show effective compassion—the ability to be both compassionate and understanding—and helps the therapist to develop an effective treatment plan. Insights that flow naturally from the biosocial theory include the individual's and therapist's recognition that the patient needs to learn skills to manage intense emotions; they also enable families to recognize that their family member has special emotional needs that make it difficult for him or her to respond to stressful situations in the calm, cool, and collected manner that they and the person with BPD would like. These special skills take time to master and effort to learn; and because what is needed to be learned is known (i.e., there is a treatment that teaches these skills), there is hope that the person can build a different way of living.

Educating the patient fits with the more recent approach of discussing the personality disorder diagnoses with patients. Generally, patients feel validated to know that their condition really exists and is taken seriously; they feel comforted to know that they are not alone in their struggles. This education also speaks to the healthier, observing part of the patient's ego, making room for a more objective stance toward his or her experiences and reducing inner judgments. Information is provided about the cause and course of the disorder and the various options for treatment. For example, it is useful to inform patients that follow-up studies show that priority should be given to treating any comorbid substance abuse disorder and that resolution of a substance abuse disorder may greatly improve the course of the BPD, whereas the persistence of substance abuse will undermine therapy (Links, Heslegrave, Mitton, van Reekum & Patrick, 1995; Zanarini, Frankenburg, Hennen, Reich, & Silk, 2005).

Case Example

A 30-year-old man with BPD seemed to misrepresent his alcohol dependence problems to his therapist when he first presented for treatment. However, it was rapidly apparent that the patient met criteria for comorbid alcohol dependence. The patient more readily accepted his diagnosis of BPD than his alcoholism. A major focus of the early sessions was to educate the patient about the impact of comorbid alcohol dependence on the BPD symptoms. To motivate the patient toward attending a program for his alcohol problems, the therapist repeatedly related his active BPD symptoms to abuse of alcohol.

Crisis and Safety Monitoring

These strategies are discussed by Links and Bergmans (Chapter 9, this volume). The therapist should anticipate that strategies to manage crises will be utilized in the early months of therapy to maintain the patient's engagement in treatment and reduce suicidal and other unsafe behaviors. If these behaviors do not reduce in frequency, the therapist should seek supervision or the advice of a consultant.

Involving More Than One Therapist

As the treatment of patients with personality disorders calls for an eclectic array of treatment methods, there is often value in the patient's use of different providers for different aspects of care. For example, one therapist may address a particular intervention while another may address a different intervention or need. Not all therapists or providers can do all the types of interventions that are helpful for a particular patient. For example, a patient may be in a group and also may have an addiction worker, a benefits worker, and a more "expressive" therapy with another individual therapist. Unlike some more "proprietary" treatment approaches that do not like to blend modalities, the use of different resources to meet the patient's overall needs seems of particular value with the most challenging patients with personality disorders. The advantages of encouraging the patient to use more than one therapist include (1) that the patient becomes reliant on more than one source of support, thus diluting the transference response to any one therapist; (2) that having multiple therapists lessens the risk of therapist "burnout"; and (3) that this approach can enhance the patients' connections to their communities or to the healthier aspects of themselves. Although splitting (one therapist seen as good while the other is seen as bad) can occur between therapists, this usually can be avoided when open communication between the therapists is established as part of the original treatment contract with the patient.

Establishing and Maintaining a Therapeutic Framework to Enhance the Alliance

The idea that therapy requires collaboration between therapist and patient is a given in all therapies. Research on common factors in psychotherapy demonstrates that the bond between a therapist and a patient has a substantial impact on outcome. However, the intense emotional responses of patients with BPD can make it difficult for therapists to intuitively use the skills that they would normally use to develop a strong bond with their patients.

Case Example

M was a 35-year-old woman who had been in DBT for the past 6 months. In previous therapy, M had deteriorated rapidly, with 20 hospital days in a period of 3 months, despite the fact that the previous therapist saw her more frequently and responded to frequent crisis calls. The reason for this deterioration was explored when M started DBT. It was thought to be due to premature exploration of traumatic experiences (premature because M was not felt to have the skills to cope with the intense emotions that arise during exploration of traumatic experiences). As DBT progressed, the therapist noticed several behaviors that caused her (the therapist) increasing worry. These included M's drawings, which depicted the therapist as rescuing M. In addition, M spoke openly about wanting the therapist to hug her, "like a mother would." At the same time, M appeared to be making progress, with fewer admissions to the hospital and no episodes of self-harm. The therapist came increasingly to suspect that M was hoping for "adoption" (for the therapist to be a primary maternal figure in the patient's life) and felt very uncomfortable in responding to any of M's behaviors with her (the therapist's) usual warmth. This was problematic for the therapy because the therapist's warmth was clearly a positive reinforcement for effective behaviors by M (completing homework, engaging more actively in session), but it also seemed to reinforce ineffective behaviors (investing in the hope that the therapist would play a more active role in M's life). Not responding with warmth was a major change in style for the therapist and reduced her own motivation to continue the therapy. In addition, as the therapist withdrew her warmth, M became increasingly anxious and increased the frequency of requests for telephone coaching.

It is clear in the preceding example that the therapy with M quickly became less effective as the therapist withdrew her warmth. In this situation, DBT requires the therapist to address her own limits (the therapist clearly did not want to adopt M). The therapist did address this with M (with a lot of support and coaching from her DBT team), validating the desire for adoption as understandable given the abusive upbringing that M had experienced and highlighting that this was not possible and that M and her therapist needed to help M find ways to accept the therapist's limits.

As an overall principle, to maintain the alliance, the therapist attends to the patient's preferences, which may include establishing the frequency of sessions, as well as the selection of issues or content discussed in the sessions. Therapists should be open and available to deal with the patient's agenda, although the therapist has to ensure that the therapy remains effective and fosters the patient's feelings of self-efficacy. The therapist should understand that some patients entering therapy will be capable of more expressive or extended therapy, whereas others require a preparatory phase, paving the way for more extensive work in the future, such as working on the history of previous trauma.

The importance of respecting boundaries during the initial stages of therapy has been increasingly described in the literature. Some authors have described this as "optimal" distance (Gabbard & Wilkinson, 1994). In addition to creating a safe place for therapy to unfold and survive, a stable frame can also play an important role in helping patients create more stable inner experiences. A clinical example may help to describe what is meant by maintaining boundaries but also how the tactful use of rigidity or flexibility can be therapeutically advantageous.

Case Example

A depressed patient with BPD agreed to be financially responsible for missed sessions, regardless of cause, if sufficient notice was not given to the therapist. Six months into the 12-month treatment contract of weekly sessions, the patient missed an appointment and was billed. After paying for the initial appointment, she then missed two more appointments for different reasons. Because her mood was also improving, the therapist wondered whether the patient was engaging in a flight into health, experiencing a hypomanic response, paying for sessions rather than attending them, or acting out some other unidentified object relationship. From the vantage point of the frame, it was hypothesized that the patient's improved mood might be related to the firm stance taken by the therapist in respecting the initial contract arrangement. The next session offered an occasion to confirm this last hypothesis, as the patient arrived with a small gift. When therapist and patient explored the various aspects of the attempt at gifting, the patient explained that even as she was purchasing the gift, she knew her therapist "probably has a policy about this." It appeared as though the patient was testing the strength and the stability of the frame over the course of treatment, and this seemed to allow certain gains in the patient. She became more self-assertive, independent, and autonomous. As she became less dependent, significant others in her life appeared to increasingly seek her company, as well as respect her wishes. As her treatment boundaries and responsibilities were respected, her self-respect increased, and her boundaries with significant others improved.

This vignette demonstrates how maintenance of the frame can play a mutative role in addition to protecting the work and preventing boundary violations. Conversely, Gabbard and Lester (1996) have written about the value in certain boundary "transgressions." Although no one is promoting the purposeful use of boundary transgression, the same provider's decision to accept a small holiday gift from a different patient turned out, upon further exploration, to be an unintentionally corrective and helpful role response that also led to additional therapeutic discoveries. Afterward, the patient indicated that had the therapist not accepted the small holiday gift, she would have experienced him as both rejecting and controlling, possibly damaging the treatment. (Unappreciated by the therapist at the time was that refusing the gift would have been a complementary identification with sadistic and controlling aspects of parental/object representations.)

Demonstrating Empathy and Validation

Validation and problem solving are the two core strategies in DBT that are also key elements of general management. As noted earlier, Linehan found that therapy that was focused only on change (problem-solving) strategies was too aversive for patients, as evidenced by their response of either withdrawing or attacking the therapist. When acceptance and validation were added, therapy was less aversive, and patients were more open to change strategies. The validation strategies that Linehan employed are derived from Zen philosophy and are similar to those employed by Jon Kabat-Zinn (2005) in mindfulness-based stress reduction. The component of mindfulness that forms the basis of validation is the ability to observe oneself and one's environment without judgment. Validation then takes this mindful observing a step further by requiring the therapist to look for what is effective in the behavior, even when the overall impact of the behavior is not particularly effective. Lastly, the therapist communicates this nonjudgmental acceptance of the patient's behaviors to the patient.

Gunderson also suggests that empathy and validation are primary therapeutic techniques during the first year of therapy (Gunderson & Links, 2008). The literature on empathy is broad, diverse, and divided—especially within the psychoanalytic/psychodynamic literature. Some therapists distinguish empathy from sympathy, noting that empathy is an attempt to understand a patient by imaging oneself *as the patient* in his or her shoes, whereas sympathy is imagining *oneself* in the patient's shoes. Most authors consider empathic validation to be a supportive intervention. Beitman and Yue (2004) describe empathy as a person's experience of the feelings of another person and the imagination of what it is like for the other person. For Beitman and Yue, empathic validation was reflecting feelings to convey empathy. We can therefore see how empathic validation not only supports the therapeutic alliance but also helps patients to identify feelings. When a therapist says to a patient "you feel angry and abandoned when your boyfriend doesn't call when he stays out later than expected," the therapist is not only validating the patient's perception but also helping the patient identify the feelings or affects that she or he may not fully recognize. This is similar to what Fonagy and Target (2003) describe when they write about the development of the capacity for mentalization and the need for marked and contingent mirroring.

In most therapies, empathy and validation imply approaching the patient and his or her behaviors, feelings, and thoughts as if they are necessary and adaptive in one sense and destructive and maladaptive in another. It means helping the patient to understand why he or she behaves or feels in a certain way, accepting the purpose for such behaviors while not reinforcing the unrealistic aspects of the experience or resultant behaviors. One can empathize by understanding how complicated sets of established object relations (based on past and fantasized ones) create difficulty in the here and now. Such examples are not restricted to only transference repetitions. When a patient rages about her father's failure to protect her from the abuse of her stepmother, an empathic response would not join with the patient in demonizing the father (or stepmother). This process is characterized by the therapist's accurately reflecting the patient's affect while also demonstrating an ability to cope with the patient's experience. In our example, the therapist would inquire about the relationships (thereby learning more about the patient's experience) and comment on how difficult it must be now to relate to certain people who are identified with the father or mother without becoming enraged.

Paying Attention to the Therapist's Effectiveness and Observing for Negative Transference and Countertransference Issues

When therapy is not working—for instance, in the vignette about M—the therapist is required to develop an understanding with the patient of the problem behavior (in the case of M, investing time and energy into the wish that the therapist would be a friend or parent and not actively seeking supports outside of therapy), the chain of events leading up to the problematic behavior (M's abused childhood, the comfort and soothing that she received from a previous therapist that she had never received in a nontherapeutic relationship, the therapist's reluctance to identify how irritated and anxious it made her feel), and the consequences that follow or reinforce the behavior (M's belief that someone would step in and take care of her problems for her, her resultant decrease in anxiety, the therapist's withdrawal from the therapy, and M's increasing distress at the thought that her therapist no longer wanted to work with her). In addition to approaches to deal with behaviors that threaten therapy, such as behaviors that push therapists' limits, there are also a number of assumptions in DBT and GPM that therapists are asked to work with. These assumptions are not facts but are ways of thinking about therapy and about patients with BPD that help improve the motivation of therapists. One of these assumptions, "patients cannot fail in therapy," suggests that when a patient fails in therapy, it is the therapy or the therapist who has failed, not the patient. Thinking this way increases therapist motivation to look at failure in therapy as a problem of the therapy, not the patient, and increases therapist motivation to figure out, along with the patient, problems that interfere with the success of the therapy. This approach greatly improves the ability to maintain an effective therapeutic alliance because it does not blame patients for therapeutic failures.

Although GPM is a psychodynamically informed treatment, direct interpretations of hostile and aggressive transferences in the here and now are avoided (Gabbard et al., 1994). Patients are understood from a deficit perspective, particularly in emotional processing, rather than from a conflict-oriented perspective. As patients are typically seen for only 12 months, they are not prepared to make use of direct transference interpretations regarding underlying aggressive object relations, and early interpretations often convey a sense of blame to the patient, especially if they are not delivered in a careful manner, cushioned by a stable working relationship. Similar to the intersubjectivity and self-psychology literature and to DBT, expressions of anger or rage in the here and now are reframed in terms of adaptive or maladaptive emotional responses and as a reflection of past empathic failures or traumas contributing to these deficits. This does not mean that negative transferences should be ignored in more time-limited treatments nor that they should not be directly addressed early in treatment. Hostility and negative transferences, with concordant and complementary negative countertransferences (Gabbard & Wilkinson 1994), are to be expected and are common. Negative transference should be addressed early on by the therapist (Gunderson, 2001). It is handled as a maladaptive behavior on the part of the patient but understood as necessary for the patient at that moment, although the patient may not fully understand his or her behavior. Negative countertransferences may be understood as maladaptive counterresponses on the part of the therapist. Although such responses are helpful clues for understanding the patient that are known to contain both realistic and unrealistic components, negative countertransference should be dealt with primarily through supervision or consultation with a colleague. In that setting, providers should present and air their feelings, concerns, and worries about their patients. In order to prevent or lessen enactments, providers discuss how to use these feelings to understand their patients and to create more empathic interventions that facilitate the understanding of patients' (mal)adaptive maneuvers. In this sense, and using terms acquired from Bion (1984) and Winnicott (1965), the provider is responsible for helping the treatment dyad contain the negative feelings aroused. Weekly supervision plays an integral role by helping providers tolerate the hostility.

Case Example

A therapist arrives at supervision reporting to the team that if her patient is not discussed within the very near future, her postsession retail therapy will be putting her in the poorhouse. She informs the team that retail therapy (making purchases after her sessions) is a new behavior for her and that it is concerning in that it is occurring weekly and directly after her session with her male patient, who is "wearing her down." She said that he is refusing (or unable) to move beyond storytelling in his sessions—graphic stories of horrific abuses perpetrated against him and stories of heroism on his part. He has told her (a social worker) that his only experiences of social workers have been as abusers. He has stated to her that he will likely not be able to work with her for very long because (1) he has never gone beyond five sessions with anybody and (2) he doesn't know where her head is at and "for all I know, you've been abused and I'm triggering you." She commented that she feels helpless and does not know what to do with him. If she asks him questions or identifies a potential feeling that she is hearing in the story he is telling, he informs her that she is wrong. She has come to the supervision group stating that she is fearful of saying anything to him and has come to believe that her skill set is useless in the context of this patient and that she will never be able to help him. The supervision group listens attentively and empathizes with the therapist's helplessness and feelings of being worn down. In the supervision, the patient's identification with the aggressor is discussed as his means to protect himself against his vulnerability. The therapist feels less helpless, and the supervision group, expecting benefits from the advice, recommends that she bake instead of shop to recover from his sessions.

In the last 6 weeks of therapy, the patient was able to tolerate hearing that his stories of heroism were directly paralleled to feelings of vulnerability in the here and now, based on the emotional memories of maltreatment during his youth. He stated that although he had many reservations about therapy in the beginning, he would like to continue with therapy, asking when this therapist would be able to work with him. He was able to describe himself as "better than a year ago" and still "a work in progress," The therapist concurred with his assessment of himself.

Supervision and Consultation

A significant component of therapy is ongoing supervision. For example, some type of supervision is important when treating patients with personality disorders, even if the therapist is experienced, and the importance of others' input is acknowledged as critical to maintaining an effective therapeutic stance. Well-structured supervision allows the clinician to attend to countertransference feelings and to creatively adapt input from the supervision to understanding the patient.

Careful attention to countertransference feelings and setting a low threshold for seeking consultation or ongoing supervision are seen as important principles in establishing a therapeutic alliance with these patients. The purpose of the supervision is to support the therapist, to offer alternative perspectives to problem-solve clinical dilemmas, to anchor therapy to the theoretical model being used in the therapy, and to assist the therapist in maintaining a benevolent, caring, and curious attitude toward the patient's vicissitudes (Gunderson & Links, 2008).

How does a therapist decide whether a supervision arrangement is working or if he or she is being an effective supervisor? Supervision should provide a safe place for therapists to reveal themselves. Similar to Adler's (1994) description of a "transitional space" in therapy, supervision should be a place that allows the baring of uncertainty and the avoidance of "pathological" certainty. Supervision should foster the containment of projections placed on the therapist and allow the therapist to reflect rather than react to and act out (or enact) the projections. Supervision that is effective should be creative and fun. The playful atmosphere allows the therapist to look for novelty and perceive how interventions might be adapted to move patients slightly off balance but a little ahead of where they were in the previous session. This procedure is taken from Vygotsky's (1986) idea of making suggestions that are in the patient's zone of proximal development and involves making an intervention or providing insight that matches where the patient is or is just a small step ahead of the patient. Therefore, supervision that is fun and feels safe will usually be effective. Principally, a clinician is unwise to undertake ongoing psychotherapy with patients with personality disorders if adequate consultation or peer supervision with trusted colleagues is not readily available.

The following vignette provides an example of how a supervision group reminded the therapist about the principles of interrelatedness and wholeness. The patient with BPD can be experienced both as being irrational and driven by dysregulated emotions and as an individual who is very expressive but functions quite normally. Taking either of these two positions in isolation results in only a piece of the whole and will limit therapeutic effectiveness.

Case Example

M (the woman referred to earlier) struggled with a severe learning disability all her life. Despite this, and the fact that the learning disability was not addressed throughout her schooling, she managed to complete high school. However, she was very fearful of situations that would expose her learning disability and explained to her therapist that "they will know that I am stupid." This feeling had a significant impact on what types of jobs she felt she could apply for when she looked for work. Her employer had an affirmative action program that would accommodate her disability, but she refused to let them know about the disability because of her fear that "they will all know that I am stupid." This stance greatly limited her options for returning to work, which she had identified as an important goal in building a life worth living. On the other hand, her therapist knew that she was highly skilled in her work with children.

In one session, M was extremely dysregulated as a result of fear and indecision regarding her return to work. She kept saying over and over "I am stupid," using her learning disability as proof of this statement. Her therapist, feeling considerable frustration because she felt this way of thinking was stalling the development of a plan for returning to work and also because it was simply not true, kept insisting that M was "smart" and used her effectiveness with children as "proof." The session was painful and ended with M being dysregulated and the therapist both frustrated and anxious about M's risk of self-harm or suicide.

The therapist discussed the situation in the next consultation team meeting. The team leader encouraged the therapist to describe her emotional responses to the situation. She then pointed out that the therapist was engaging in nondialectical thinking; that is, she was trying to use logic to overrule M's position. However, intuitively M's position did make sense. The therapist was able to acknowledge that both positions were important and part of the understanding of the whole. At the next session, the therapist brought up the previous session and her own emotional responses (frustration and anxiety) and stressed that, in fact, both positions were important. The therapist and M were then able to come up with a synthesis of both positions—that M was in fact good with children and that her learning disability did limit employment opportunities and would require some effort to overcome. The impact of thinking this way was assessed. M and her therapist were more hopeful but recognized that it was going to be more difficult than either of them would like to help M find work that she felt was consistent with a life worth living. Both noted that they were resigned to this reality and willing to move forward with this work.

CONCLUDING COMMENTS

In this chapter, we have drawn from two diverse evidence-based psychotherapies for patients with personality disorders: DBT and GPM. Summarizing across these therapies demonstrated that the theoretical rationale provided by each model of therapy is not the necessary ingredient in establishing a treatment framework and therapeutic alliance. However, the strategies directly arising from the therapeutic interactions are necessary for establishing and maintaining the therapeutic framework and alliance. As discussed, the therapist has to take the lead in engaging the patient, being consistent, and being the boundary keeper while also demonstrating empathy and validation. Success is enhanced by ready access to consultation and supervision. The final message to therapists must be that therapy with patients with personality disorders is manageable and rewarding and requires the integration of various theoretical perspectives.

REFERENCES

Adler, G. (1994). Transference, countertransference and abuse in psychotherapy. *Harvard Review of Psychiatry, 3,* 151–159.

American Psychiatric Association. (2001). Practice guideline for the treatment of patients with borderline personality disorder. *American Journal of Psychiatry, 158,* 1–52.

Bateman, A. W., & Fonagy, P. (2000). Effectiveness of psychotherapeutic treatment of personality disorder. *British Journal of Psychiatry, 177,* 138–143.

Beitman, B. D., & Yue, D. (2004). *Learning psychotherapy: A time-efficient, research-based, and outcome-measured psychotherapy training program.* New York: Norton.

Bender, D. S. (2005). The therapeutic alliance in the treatment of personality disorders. *Journal of Psychiatric Practice, 11,* 73–87.

Bennett, D., Parry, G., & Ryle, A. (2006). Resolving threats to the therapeutic alliance in cognitive analytic therapy of borderline personality disorder: A task analysis. *Psychology and Psychotherapy: Theory, Research and Practice, 79,* 395–418.

Bion, W. R. (1984). *Second thoughts: Selected papers on psycho-analysis.* New York: Aronson.

Bordin, E. S. (1979). The generalizability of the psychoanalytic concept of the working alliance. *Psychotherapy: Theory, Research and Practice, 16,* 252–260.

Fonagy, P., & Target, M. (2003). *Psychoanalytic theories: Perspectives from developmental psychopathology.* New York: Brunner Routledge.

Gabbard, G. O., Horwitz, L., Allen, J. G., Frieswyk, S., Newsom, G., Colson, D. B., et al.. (1994). Transference interpretation in the psychotherapy of borderline patients: A high-risk, high-gain phenomenon. *Harvard Review of Psychiatry, 2*, 59–69.

Gabbard, G. O., & Lester, E. P. (1996). *Boundaries and boundary violations in psychoanalysis*. New York: Basic Books.

Gabbard, G. O., & Wilkinson, S. M. (1994). *Management of countertransference with borderline patients*. Washington, DC: American Psychiatric Press.

Goin, M. K. (2001). Borderline personality disorder: The importance of establishing a treatment framework. *Psychiatric Services, 52*, 167–168.

Gunderson, J. G. (2001). *Borderline personality disorder: A clinical guide*. Washington, DC: American Psychiatric Publishing.

Gunderson, J. G., Frank, A. F., Ronningstam, E. F., Wachter, S., Lynch, V. J., & Wolf, P. J. (1989). Early discontinuance of borderline patients from psychotherapy. *Journal of Nervous and Mental Disease, 177*, 38–42.

Gunderson, J. G., & Links, P. S. (2008). *Borderline personality disorder: A clinical guide* (2nd ed.). Washington, DC: American Psychiatric Publishing.

Gutheil, T. G., & Havens, L. (1979). The therapeutic alliance: Contemporary meanings and confusion. *International Review of Psycho-Analysis, 6*, 467–481.

Kabat-Zinn, J. (2005). *Full catastrophe living: Using the wisdom of your body and mind to face stress, pain, and illness* (15th anniversary ed.). New York: Delta Trade Paperback/Bantam Dell.

Kernberg, O. F., Selzer, M. A., Koenigsberg, H. W., Carr, A. C., & Appelbaum, A. H. (1989). *Psychodynamic psychotherapy of borderline patients*. New York: Basic Books.

Lewis, J. M. (2000). Repairing the bond in important relationships: A dynamic for personality maturation. *American Journal of Psychiatry, 157*, 1375–1378.

Linehan, M. M. (1993a). *Cognitive-behavioral treatment of borderline personality disorder*. New York: Guilford Press

Linehan, M. M. (1993b). *Skills training manual for treating borderline personality disorder*. New York: Guilford Press.

Linehan, M., M. (2007). Foreword. In L. A. Dimeff & K. Koerner (Eds.), *Dialectical behavior therapy in clinical practice: Applications across disorders and settings* (p. xi). New York: Guilford Press.

Linehan, M. M., Armstrong, H. E., Suarez, A., Allmon, D., & Heard, H. L. (1991). Cognitive-behavioral treatment of chronically parasuicidal borderline patients. *Archives of General Psychiatry, 48*, 1060–1064.

Links, P. S., Heslegrave, R. J., Mitton, J. E., van Reekum, R., & Patrick, J. (1995). Borderline personality disorder and substance abuse: Consequences of comorbidity. *Canadian Journal of Psychiatry, 40*, 9–14.

McMain, S. F., Links, P. S., Gnam, W. H., Guimond, T., Cardish, R. J., Korman, L., et al. (2009). A randomized controlled trial of dialectical behavior therapy versus general psychiatry management for borderline personality disorder. *American Journal of Psychiatry, 166*, 1365–1374.

Oldham, J. M. (2005). *Guideline watch: Practice guideline for the treatment of patients with borderline personality disorder*. Arlington, VA: American Psychiatric Association. Available at *www.psych.org/psych_pract/treatg/pg/prac_guide.cfm*.

Skodol, A. E., Buckley, P., & Charles, E. (1983). Is there a characteristic pattern to the treatment history of clinic outpatients with borderline personality? *Journal of Nervous and Mental Disease, 171*, 405–410.

Vygotsky, L. (1986). *Thought and language*. Cambridge, MA: MIT Press.

Winnicott, D. W. (1965). *The maturational process and the facilitating environment: Studies in the theory of emotional development*. New York: International Universities Press.

Yeomans, F. E., Gutfreund, J., Selzer, M. A., Clarkin, J. F., Hull, J. W., & Smith, T. E. (1994). Factors related to drop-outs by borderline patients: Treatment contract and therapeutic alliance. *Journal of Psychotherapy Practice and Research, 3*, 16–21.

Zanarini, M. C., Frankenburg, F. R., Hennen, J., Reich, D. B., & Silk, K. R. (2005). The McLean Study of Adult Development (MSAD): Overview and implications of the first six years of prospective follow-up. *Journal of Personality Disorders, 19*, 505–523.

part three

GENERAL CHANGE PRINCIPLES AND MECHANISMS

chapter 6

A Relational Approach to Personality Disorder and Alliance Rupture

Sumru Tufekcioglu and J. Christopher Muran

It is agreed by clinicians from diverse orientations as the cognitive (Pretzer & Beck, 2005), interpersonal (Benjamin, 2005), attachment (Levy, 2005), and object relations (Clarkin, Yeomans, & Kernberg, 2006) perspectives that clients with personality disorders encounter difficulties with self or identity and interpersonal functioning. In fact, more often than not, it is an interpersonal problem in the social or work environment that brings clients with personality disorders into treatment. As such, interpersonal functioning is a major focus of treatment with this group of clients.

Although they are taken from different theoretical orientations, many different treatments have been proven to be effective in treating personality disorders, suggesting that it might be the common elements in these various approaches rather than the modalities of treatments that are responsible for change. One such common element contributing to successful treatment of personality disorders has been shown to be the interpersonal component in therapy (Clarkin, Levy, & Ellison, 2011). In fact, it can be posited that each successful treatment for personality disorder is "a carefully considered, well-structured and coherent interpersonal endeavour" (Bateman & Fonagy, 2000, p. 142). It follows, then, that an integrative approach to treating personality disorders would have to focus on the interpersonal component of therapy; that is, the therapeutic relationship.

In this chapter we examine, with a relational approach to personality and the psychotherapy process, the therapeutic relationship with clients with personality disorders. First, we present a relational view of the self. Next, we discuss how this "self in relation to the other" emerges in the therapeutic relationship and how the therapeutic relationship is used as a mechanism of change. We also present the challenges that are encountered in the therapeutic relationship, namely, ruptures, especially with individuals with personality disorders. We examine how ruptures are resolved in the therapeutic relationship, provide a view of ruptures as change events, and illustrate this notion with clinical examples. Finally, we discuss the training implications of this approach. Our perspective has been informed by our research on rupture resolution (Safran & Muran, 1996) and in turn has informed the development of a treatment model and training regimen with some empirical support (e.g., Muran, Safran, Samstag, & Winston, 2005; Safran et al., 2014).

A RELATIONAL THEORY OF PERSON AND PERSONALITY DISORDER

Muran and Safran have written about the person as a relational phenomenon (Muran, 2001; Safran, 1998; Safran & Muran 2000), describing the continuous interplay among the various processes and structures of the self. The processes refer to the various cognitive and interpersonal operations that establish and protect the representational structures of the self. This refers to the self in relation to others, as well as to itself. The structures refer to memory stores of multiple discrete experiences of the self in relation to significant others. These are relational schemas that are abstracted on the basis of interactions with attachment figures (and others of interpersonal significance) to increase the likelihood of maintaining a relationship with those figures. They contain specific procedural information regarding expectancies and strategies for negotiating the dialectically opposing needs for agency or self-definition and for relatedness or communion (see Safran & Muran, 2000, for elaboration). They are also considered emotional structures that include innate expressive-motor responses that develop from birth into subtle and idiosyncratic variations and that serve a communicative function in that they continually orient the person to the environment and the environment to the person.

We have also described the emergence of a corresponding experience, a particular state of mind or *self-state,* with the activation of a particular relational schema. Self-states are the experiential products of the various processes and structures of the self, the crystallization in subjective experience of an underlying relational schema. Different self-states can activate different relational schemas, resulting in a cycling through different states of mind. The transition points or boundaries among the various self-states that each person experiences vary in terms of seamlessness. They are naturally smoothed over, creating the illusory sense of continuity and singular identity, through the process of dissociation. The more conspicuous and abrupt the transitions between self-states are, however, the more problematic the dissociative process is. It is useful to distinguish between dissociation as a healthy process of selectively focusing attention and dissociation as an unhealthy process resulting from traumatic overload and resulting in severing connections between relational schemas.

Finally, a central tenet of our relational perspective is the recognition that there is an ongoing reciprocal relationship between the self-states of one person and those of the other in a dyadic interaction. This refers to the ways in which self-states are interpersonally communicated and mutually regulated in a dyadic encounter. As individuals cycle through various self-states in an interpersonal encounter, they should both influence and be influenced by the various self-states of the other. In such encounters, one is always embedded in a *relational matrix* (Mitchell, 1988) that is shaped moment by moment by the various states and implicit desires of the two individuals.

As noted earlier, relational schemas shape the person's perceptions of the world, leading to cognitive processes and interpersonal behaviors that in turn shape the environment in a way that confirms the representational content of the schemas. To the extent that they are limited in the scope of internalized interpersonal experiences, they will restrict the range of interpersonal behaviors, which pull for similar responses from a range of different people, resulting in redundant patterns of interaction and limiting the possibility of new information in the form of new interpersonal experiences. For example, an individual who generally expects others to be essentially hostile and attacking might tend to act in a defensively hostile and aggressive manner, which would invariably provoke the response from others that is expected—a frequent pattern seen in individuals with personality disorders.

THE THERAPEUTIC ALLIANCE

We have found a conceptualization of the therapeutic alliance along the lines that Bordin (1979) suggested to be useful in our work (see, e.g., Safran & Muran, 2000). Bordin defined the alliance as comprising three interdependent factors of the agreement between client and therapist: on (1) the *tasks* and (2) the *goals* of treatment and (3) the *affective bond* between client and therapist. This definition highlights the interdependence of relational and technical factors: It suggests that the meaning of technical factors can be understood only in the relational context in which they are applied. It also highlights the importance of negotiation between client and therapist on the tasks and goals of therapy, which is consistent with an increasingly influential way of conceptualizing the psychotherapy process as one involving the negotiation between the client's desires or needs and those of the therapist (see Mitchell & Aron, 1999). As such, in our relational approach, the therapeutic relationship is the vehicle for change, and one major component of the therapeutic relationship that leads to change is the inevitable failures in relatedness between the client and the therapist, that is, the ruptures.

RUPTURES IN THE THERAPEUTIC ALLIANCE

Clients and therapists are always embedded in a *relational matrix* (Mitchell, 1988) that is shaped, moment to moment, by their implicit needs and desires. Ruptures in the therapeutic alliance mark points at which there is a tension between the client's and the therapist's respective desires (see Safran & Muran, 2000). Ruptures indicate vicious cycles or enactments that can be unduly driven by one participant's dysfunctional *relational schemas* described earlier. Ruptures also invariably involve the unwitting participation of the other member of the dyad. Ruptures are inevitable events and are viewed not as obstacles to overcome but as opportunities for therapeutic change. They can be understood as windows into the relational worlds of both the client and the therapist and thus as opportunities for expanded awareness and new relational experiences. Alliance ruptures have received increasing attention over the past 25 years in the research literature, with growing evidence that they are common events (e.g., they are reported by patients in as much as 50% of sessions; they are observed by third-party raters in 70% of sessions); they predict premature termination and negative outcome, but when resolved they predict good outcomes (Eubanks-Carter, Muran, Safran, 2010; Safran, Muran & Eubanks-Carter, 2011; Samstag, Batchelder, Muran, Safran, & Winston, 1998).

In a self-report and observer-based study of ruptures, Sommerfeld, Orbach, Zim, and Mikulincer (2008) found that sessions in which both patient and observer saw a rupture were rated as having greater depth by the patient. As ruptures that are identified by both self-report and observer report are likely ones that are explicitly discussed in the session, this finding suggests that patients find therapy more helpful when therapists are sensitive to subtle indications of ruptures and encourage patients to explore them. Sommerfeld and colleagues (2008) also found a significant association between the occurrence of ruptures and the appearance of dysfunctional interpersonal schemas involving the therapist, identified by using the core conflictual relationship theme (CCRT) method (Luborsky & Crits-Christoph, 1998). This finding suggests that when ruptures occur, dysfunctional schemas are likely to be active; thus ruptures provide critical opportunities to identify, explore, and change patients' self-defeating patterns of thought and behavior.

Ruptures can be organized into two main subtypes: (1) *withdrawal ruptures* and (2) *confrontation ruptures* (Harper, 1989a, 1989b). In withdrawal ruptures, clients withdraw from the therapist (e.g., through long silences) or from their own experience (e.g., by denying their emotions or by being overly deferential to the therapist's wishes). In confrontation ruptures, clients move against the therapist, either by expressing anger or dissatisfaction (e.g., complaining about the therapist or the treatment) or by trying to control the therapist (e.g., telling the therapist what to do). These markers can be understood as reflecting different ways of coping with the dialectical tension between the need for self-definition and the need for relatedness: Withdrawal ruptures mark the pursuit of relatedness at the expense of the need for self-definition; confrontation ruptures mark the expression of self-definition at the expense of relatedness.

RUPTURES AND PERSONALITY DISORDER

As noted earlier, relational schemas shape how a person views the world, leading to interpersonal behaviors that in turn lead to experiences with other people similar to the original relational schema, thus confirming and perpetuating a pattern of relating to others. To the extent one's relational schemas are limited in terms of interpersonal experiences, they will restrict the range of behaviors he or she is able to exhibit in relations with others. This will pull for similar responses from others, resulting in a repetition of a particular relational pattern, and will limit possibilities for new information and new experiences.

Clients with personality disorders, who invariably have a restricted range of interpersonal behaviors that lead to significant interpersonal problems, might have more difficulty developing a good alliance with the therapist in our interpersonally focused treatment. In particular, as Muran, Segal, Samstag, and Crawford (1994) found in their study of short-term cognitive therapy, clients with a tendency toward hostile, dominant interpersonal behaviors, which are characteristic of DSM Cluster B personality disorders (American Psychiatric Association, 1994), might have difficulty establishing a good alliance. Further, outcome research has shown that patients with personality disorders are especially challenging and resistant to treatment, resulting in more negative process, higher attrition rates, and greater treatment length (Benjamin & Karpiak, 2002; Clarkin & Levy, 2004; Westen & Morrison, 2001). This is particularly significant given that patients diagnosed with personality disorders in clinics and practices make up as many as 45% of the total of patients seen (Zimmerman, Chelminski, & Young, 2008).

In examining the therapeutic alliance and the inevitable ruptures therein with clients with personality disorders, a particular issue arises that requires further consideration and poses challenges to the therapists: that the characteristics that pertain to personality disorders in general seem to be multidimensional (Dimaggio et al., 2012). As noted earlier, patients with personality disorders are observed, regardless of the particular type of disorder, to present with constricted and inhibited personality traits such as (1) poor metacognition (Bateman & Fonagy, 2004, and Chapter 7, this volume; Dimaggio, Popolo, Carcione, & Salvatore, Chapter 8, this volume; Dimaggio, Semerari, Carcione, Nicolò, & Procacci, 2007); (2) dysfunctional constructions of self-with-other relationships, such as seeing oneself as not lovable, unworthy, guilty, omnipotent, and betrayed and the other as rejecting, abusing, and so forth (Benjamin, 1996); and (3) emotion and impulse dysregulation (Linehan, Armstrong, Suarez, Allmon, & Heard, 1991) or overregulation. For example, a patient might have poor metacognition while also presenting with negative constructions of self with others. This multidimensional aspect of personality disorder makes it more complicated for therapeutic intervention and requires treatment of all of the elements involved, each with specific techniques. This calls for an integrated approach possibly combining therapeutic components from different models (Clarkin, Levy, Lenzenweger, & Kernberg, 2007; Dimaggio et al., 2012; Livesley, 2003). Furthermore, this multidimensional and complex picture of patients with personality disorder lends itself to a layer-by-layer unfolding of the therapy process, and it is observed that different aspects of the disorder might surface at different stages of therapy. This necessitates specific interventions at different stages of treatment based on the particular elements of the pathology that emerge at that point in therapy (Dimaggio et al., 2012). Moreover, patients with personality disorder are observed to have a negative view of themselves, and the more they become aware, in therapy, of the features they find unacceptable, the more they feel angry. This will aggravate any alliance ruptures, and any aspects of the patient that emerge need constant validation from the therapist (Dimaggio, Carcione, Salvatore, Semerari, & Nicolò, 2010).

A further complication in working with clients with personality disorders is that each type of personality disorder produces its own type of interpersonal challenge. In her consideration of the therapeutic alliance with respect to DSM personality disorders, Bender (2005) suggests that each type of personality disorder poses different challenges to forming a working alliance in psychotherapy and outlines specific challenges for each of the following types of personality disorders.

Cluster A: Eccentric

Cluster A personality disorders—the so-called odd/eccentric cluster—involve a profound impairment in interpersonal relationships, often with paranoid characteristics. In negotiating the therapeutic alliance, this group of clients pose challenges to their therapists that are characteristic of this type of personality, such as suspiciousness of the therapist's intentions, profound interpersonal discomfort with the therapist, emotional aloofness, and hypersensitivity to perceived criticism.

Schizotypal

Although it is often assumed that clients with schizotypal personality disorder have no desire to become involved in relationships, it is demonstrated by Bender and colleagues (2003) that clients with schizotypal personality disorder had the highest involvement with therapy outside the session. These clients reported wishing to be friends with and missing their therapists, while also having aggressive and negative feelings. For many such clients, it is a matter of being extremely uncomfortable around people rather than not having a desire for connection. The discomfort that schizotypal clients often experience may not be readily apparent, so being attentive to clues about what is not being said may be required for alliance building.

Schizoid

This is a relatively rare disorder, so we mostly refer here to people with schizoid traits appearing in the context of other (e.g., avoidant) personality disorders. Schizoid traits are mostly associated with keeping people at a safe emotional distance. Clients with schizoid features may also present with affective coldness, dullness, lack of conflict, and emotional detachment. However, underlying this detachment, many of these clients feel an intense neediness for others and have some capacity of interpersonal responsiveness with a few selected people (Aktar, 1992). Thus many clients with schizoid traits can form an alliance in therapy, although this would require, from the therapist, special attention tailored specifically to these clients' characteristics.

Paranoid

Individuals with paranoia obviously pose challenges for alliance building, as they are usually vigilantly looking out for signs to get suspicious and find offense in the most benign of circumstances (Bender, 2005). However, it has also been suggested that behind their defensive paranoid presentation, these individuals have an extremely fragile self-concept and that thus it may be possible to build alliance with them in time with a sensitive affirmative approach and tactful handing of the ruptures (Benjamin, 1993).

Cluster B: Dramatic

Cluster B personality disorders—the "dramatic" cluster—is associated with pushing the limits and poses challenges to the therapeutic alliance, such as extremely demanding behavior, unstable emotional states, proneness to acting out, and need for constant approval (Bender, 2005).

Borderline

Clients with borderline personality frequently exhibit emotional instability, self-destructive acting out, and anger and aggression, and they tend to perceive their therapist in ways that alternate between idealization and devaluation. Thus it can expected that the therapy process with these clients will be rocky and challenging and will require special attention to the repairing of the many ruptures that will inevitably occur. For example, Horwitz and colleagues (1996), studying the therapeutic alliance in the treatment of borderline personality disorder, observed that "the repair of moment-to-moment disruptions in the alliance often was the key factor in maintaining the viability of the psychotherapy" (p. 173). This finding underscores the importance not only of alliance building but also of moment-to-moment attention from the therapist to the ruptures in the therapeutic relationship with these clients.

Narcissistic

Narcissistic personality is associated with intense grandiosity and a need to maintain self-esteem through omnipotent fantasies and defeating others. As such, these clients pose significant challenges to therapists in alliance building. These clients will likely "know best" and not allow the therapist to express an alternative view to theirs for a long time in treatment. Although this interpersonal dynamic might be very difficult to tolerate for therapists, it might be possible to establish alliance with this group of clients by a consistent respect for their vulnerability and their need not to trust, as this may in time allow for a lessening of their defensive needs (Bender, 2005; Meissner, 1996).

Histrionic

Histrionic personality is associated with a need to be the center of attention, little tolerance for frustration, and demands for immediate gratification. As such, building alliance with individuals with histrionic personality requires the therapist to have the necessary skills to manage escalating demands, dramatic acting out, and the related ruptures that will inevitably emerge in the relationship with such clients.

Cluster C: Anxious

Clients with Cluster C personality disorders are observed to be emotionally inhibited and averse to interpersonal conflict. Although building alliance with these clients is seemingly easier than it is with clients with Cluster A and B disorders, it may involve the following certain specific challenges.

Dependent

Clients with dependent personality have been noted to be passive and submissive and fearful of offending others. In therapy, they are easily engaged but will often withhold information and refrain from being assertive from fear of offending the therapist in some way. Thus more withdrawal types of ruptures will likely occur in therapy. Moreover, the therapist may become more frustrated as time passes by and the client is not taking full responsibility for actions aimed at breaking patterns. The therapist can then become critical or judgmental (Dimaggio et al., 2007).

Avoidant

Avoidant individuals are extremely sensitive to criticism and fearful of saying something foolish or humiliating. This sensitivity poses challenges in building alliance with avoidant clients and keeping them in therapy. The therapists need to be mindful of how their comments will be experienced by the clients and will need to be able to attend to the moment-by-moment withdrawal ruptures that will not be readily apparent.

Obsessive–Compulsive

Obsessive–compulsive personality is associated with rigidity and maintaining control over internal experience and the external environment. In the context of therapy, these clients tend to be controlling and stubborn, but they also try to be "good patients," which likely enables the building of a constructive alliance (Bender, 2005). Their restricted expression of positive affects may evoke in the therapist feelings of boredom, distance, and mild irritation at the moralistic attitudes these patients sometimes endorse (Dimaggio et al., 2010).

Therapeutic Alliance and Personality Disorder

Considering the aforementioned characteristic ways of interpersonal relating that clients with Cluster A and B disorders most likely demonstrate in therapy, it can be posited that in working with such clients, a therapeutic alliance will be harder to establish and a higher frequency of alliance ruptures (especially confrontation ruptures) will likely be observed. Cluster C personality disorders, on the other hand, are characterized by being "anxious/fearful," emotionally inhibited, and averse to interpersonal conflict. These clients tend to be prone to shame and humiliation, perfectionistic toward themselves and others, conscientious, friendly, and compliant. They tend to internalize blame and take responsibility for their issues and will readily engage with the therapist to sort out their problems. This characteristic way of relating is very different from that of clients with Cluster A and B disorders, which in fact often facilitates alliance building (Bender, 2005). Considering the characteristic ways of relating that clients with Cluster C disorders typically demonstrate, a more positive therapy process and a higher frequency of withdrawal ruptures will likely be observed. In fact, a recent study examining the therapy process with 145 patients who received two different time-limited treatments compared patients with pretreatment diagnoses of Cluster C personality disorders with patients who did not receive personality disorder diagnoses found that patients with Cluster C personality disorders reported a significantly more positive therapy experience in a number of alliance measures. Further, the study found that there were no significant differences between the two groups of patients in terms of dropout rates (Tufekcioglu, Muran, Safran, & Winston, 2013).

The dynamics that emerge in the relationship with these clients can be specific to each disorder (Bender, 2005). It should be noted, however, that these challenges become more complicated when one faces patients comorbid with multiple personality disorders or diagnosed with personality disorder—not otherwise specified according to DSM, in which features of personality disorders from different clusters are in evidence. In addition, considering the multidimensional nature of personality disorder, including poor metacognition (Bateman & Fonagy, 2004; Dimaggio et al., 2007), dysfunctional constructions of self-with-other relationships (Benjamin, 1996), and emotion and impulse dysregulation or overregulation, it follows that in successfully building and maintaining alliance with clients with personality disorders, an approach that is tailor-made not only to each type of disorder but also to each particular patient and to the particular stage in therapy is needed. This brings to the forefront the importance of the therapist's being attentive to the moment-by-moment shifts and ruptures in the relationship, which is the central tenet of our approach to resolving ruptures. We discuss this approach and illustrate it with clinical examples in the following sections.

RUPTURE RESOLUTION AS CHANGE EVENT

Psychotherapy change is essentially understood as involving the two parallel processes of (1) increasing immediate awareness of self and other and (2) providing a new interpersonal experience. Increasing immediate awareness begins with attending more closely to the details of experience at a molecular level. The client starts to develop a sense of the choices he or she is making on a moment-by-moment basis. With greater awareness of how he or she constructs his or her experience, the client develops an increased sense of responsibility and agency. This change process does not simply suggest a correction of a distorted interpersonal schema; instead, increasing the client's immediate awareness of the processes that mediate a dysfunctional interpersonal pattern leads to an elaboration and clarification of the client's self—in other words, expanded awareness of who one is in a particular interpersonal transaction. The clarification of the client's self invariably involves greater clarification of the therapist's self as well. Following our relational understanding of the role of increased immediate awareness in the change process, we have identified a specific mechanism of change: *decentering*, which consists of inviting the client to observe his or her contribution to a rupture or enactment in the relational matrix of the therapeutic relationship. We find the notion of mindfulness to be particularly useful in this regard. A primary task for therapists is to direct clients' attention to various aspects of their inner and outer worlds as they are occurring. This attention promotes the type of awareness discussed earlier that deautomates habitual patterns and helps clients experience themselves as agents in the process of constructing reality rather than as passive victims of circumstances. We also believe that the principle of metacommunication captures the spirit of this type of collaborative exploration and the essence of what we mean by *decentering*. Metacommunication involves an attempt to disembed from the interpersonal claim that is being enacted by taking the current interaction as the focus of communication. It is an attempt to bring awareness to bear on the relational matrix as it unfolds. It is also important to recognize that the psychotherapeutic process is not only discovery oriented but also constructive (Mitchell, 1993). Operating in parallel with the process of increasing immediate awareness, the constructive process of psychotherapy helps to bring about change by providing the client with a new interpersonal experience. In this regard, we have identified another specific mechanism of change: the *disconfirmation* of the client's maladaptive relational schema through the new interpersonal experience in the therapeutic interaction.

As noted earlier, our relational approach conceptualizes change as occurring through the process of decentering, or increasing awareness, and the process of disconfirmation, whereby the client has a new interpersonal experience with the therapist that challenges the client's existing interpersonal schemas. The method for achieving these changes is to draw the client's attention to aspects of his or her experience that he or she is avoiding or disowning while maintaining a validating and empathic stance that provides a corrective emotional experience for the client. In particular, the therapist pays close attention to ruptures in the alliance, highlighting them when they occur and encouraging the client to explore them. The therapist draws on his or her own experience of the relationship and his or her sense of being connected to or disconnected from the client as a guide for identifying therapeutic impasses. When the therapist feels disconnected, this is a sign that the client may be withdrawing from the interaction or may not be in contact with his or her own inner experience.

One particular area that requires further consideration when working with personality disorders is that the process of decentering needs to be managed carefully based on the client's ability, at any particular point in therapy, to tolerate awareness of aspects of him- or herself that may be viewed as negative by the client. As clients with personality disorders often have a negative view of themselves, becoming aware of the characteristics that they find unacceptable often makes them angry. This leads to alliance ruptures; therefore, exquisite attunement and constant validation from the therapist are required as the process unfolds (Dimaggio et al., 2010, 2012).

RUPTURE RESOLUTION INTERVENTIONS

A number of interventions can be applied to problems related to the tasks and goals of therapy and the affective bond between client and therapist. In this section, we present a taxonomy of rupture resolution interventions. The strategies in the taxonomy are organized according to whether they address the rupture in a direct manner or whether they take an indirect approach to resolving the rupture. We begin with interventions that operate at a more surface level and then proceed to interventions, including metacommunication, that focus in more depth at the level of underlying meaning.

Surface-Level Strategies: Disagreements on Tasks and Goals

Indirect Resolution Strategy: Change or Reframe Tasks and Goals

The therapist may respond to the client's dissatisfaction with therapy tasks and goals by changing or reframing them, or the therapist may reframe the meaning of therapy tasks or goals by describing them in a way that is more appealing to the client. It is important that this intervention not be delivered in a manipulative way. The therapist must believe that the reframing is another valid way of understanding the task or goal rather than a "white lie."

Direct Resolution Strategy: Clarify Rationale and Tasks

The therapist also can outline or reiterate a rationale for treatment, or he or she can illustrate a therapy task.

Surface-Level Strategies: Problems Associated with the Affective Bond

Indirect Resolution Strategy: Ally with the Resistance

With indirect resolution strategies the therapist does not challenge the client's defensive behaviors but rather validates the ways in which they are adaptive and understandable. Allying with, rather than challenging, the resistance can help clients access aspects of their experience that they have been avoiding.

Direct Resolution Strategy: Clarify Misunderstandings

In an open, nondefensive manner, the therapist directly addresses misunderstandings that have led to tension or strain in the relationship with the client.

Depth-Level Strategies

Indirect Resolution Strategy: Provide a New Relational Experience

With this indirect strategy, the therapist addresses problems in the bond by behaving in a way that disconfirms the client's maladaptive relational schema. It is important to note that the surface strategies described earlier can also serve to provide a new relational experience and thus disconfirm a patient's schema.

Direct Resolution Strategy: Explore Core Relational Themes

Exploring strains in the bond can lead to exploration of the client's characteristic ways of experiencing and engaging in interpersonal relationships. It is important to note, however, that premature attempts to explore relational themes via transference interpretations can elicit client defensiveness and obstruct further exploration.

Although we outline different types of rupture resolution interventions as surface versus depth and direct versus indirect, it should be noted that the ways ruptures unfold in a therapy session and their resolution is a complex process in that surface interventions can simultaneously lead to depth interventions. For example, an intervention aiming at clarifying goals and tasks can also lead to a new relational experience. In other words, by attending to a surface-level rupture, the therapist also brings change at the depth level. Likewise, indirect interventions can lead to direct interventions. For example, allying with the resistance can lead to exploring core relational themes. In fact, in the course of a session, the therapist often employs surface and depth, as well as indirect and direct strategies, and sometimes surface and indirect interventions can have the function of preparing the patient for depth and direct interventions. In the following clinical illustrations, we demonstrate the outlined rupture resolution strategies and show how complex this process can be with patients with personality disorder.

Case Example 1

Jim is a 42-year-old patient who has borderline personality characteristics and a history of multiple suicide attempts, most recently a few weeks before he started therapy after being discharged from the hospital. At the beginning of his first psychotherapy session, when the clinician asked him if this was his first therapy experience, he said, "Yes, and I'm skeptical about it."

THERAPIST: In what ways are you feeling skeptical about it?

JIM: I don't think it can be helpful. How can talking be helpful with anything! I'm on medications and they help, otherwise I feel depressed and try to kill myself. So, how is talking going to help?

THERAPIST: Good question. And it's natural to feel this way when you don't have previous experience with therapy. I would have felt the same way, too. I would think how can talking be helpful!

JIM: Yeah!

THERAPIST: OK, so then let me try to explain to you how it can help. And I'm glad you're bringing this up. It's important to talk about it at the beginning. So, the thinking is that medications help you with the symptoms of depression, which is important. And what we do in therapy is to get to know you better in terms of your current experiences that seem to trigger negative feelings. We also talk about your past experiences and explore together how they might have impacted you. A better, more detailed understanding of how you think and feel, and greater self-awareness, can help you deal with

> life's challenges more effectively, and maybe not engage so automatically in habits that defeat you and leave you depressed.

In the preceding example, the clinician, by attending to Jim's skepticism about therapy in a nondefensive manner, validating his concern, and clarifying the rationale for therapy (a direct and surface-level strategy) helped resolve this rupture and made it possible for Jim to feel more comfortable. A few sessions later, he told the therapist that, coming to his first session, he was expecting to find a therapist who would pressure him to change his behavior and be critical of him but that he was happy to see that, instead, he found an understanding and flexible approach and that he enjoyed talking with the therapist. Thus the therapist's intervention in this session, while starting with a direct surface-level resolution strategy by clarifying rationale for therapy, also provided a new relational experience for Jim (an indirect depth-level strategy) that challenged an underlying schema.

Resolution of Withdrawal Ruptures

As noted earlier, in withdrawal ruptures the client withdraws from the therapist (withdrawal from other) or from his or her own experience (withdrawal from self). A withdrawal rupture can be very subtle; for example, the client may seem to be complying with the therapist with respect to a therapy task but behaves in an overly deferential way that suggests that the client is not in contact with his or her true feelings about the task. This kind of appeasement is indicative of a pseudo-alliance rather than a truly genuine and collaborative interaction. When clients withdraw, they are prioritizing their need for relatedness at the expense of their need for agency. The process of resolving withdrawal ruptures involves exploring the interpersonal fears, expectations, and internalized criticisms that are hindering the client from directly expressing his or her feelings, especially negative ones. The goal is to help clients assert their true feelings and underlying wishes. For example, Jim sometimes would go silent in sessions. In one instance, the therapist invited him and was able to get him to talk about what he was experiencing. She found that Jim was afraid to ask her if they could extend the length of the session or schedule another that week for fear that she would reject the request. This revelation set the stage for an exploration of Jim's feelings of isolation and his wish to be connected to another: in this case, the therapist. It also resulted in the clarification of what he could realistically expect in his relationship with the therapist.

Resolution of Confrontation Ruptures

In a confrontation rupture, the client moves against the therapist. Confrontation ruptures can be very difficult for therapists to endure because they may arouse feelings of anger, impotence, and even despair. The client may express anger or dissatisfaction by complaining about the therapist's competence or about different aspects of the therapy. In a confrontation, the client favors the need for agency over the need for relatedness. The resolution process for confrontation ruptures involves exploring the fears and self-criticisms that are interfering with the client's expression of underlying needs and helping the client to express more vulnerable feelings. Sometimes confrontations are mixed with withdrawal, and in such instances the resolution process begins much like the withdrawal resolution process, whereby the therapist's task is to get the client to stand by his or her anger. For example, later in treatment, Jim angrily confronted his therapist: He said that he had been noticing, in many of his sessions, that the therapist vividly remembered the details of their previous sessions and of what Jim had told her, which made him feel very happy at the time. However, after his last session, while walking home, it suddenly occurred to him that the therapist was most likely taking notes after sessions to look at before the following session to remember the details of what Jim had said. He complained: "You tricked me! How stupid of me! How could I think that you really cared and that I was more than just a patient on paper!" An exploration of Jim's feelings led to an expression of more vulnerable feelings, including his wish to be special in the eyes of the therapist. This added a further dimension to his understanding of his underlying need for connection.

Resolution via Metacommunication

Metacommunication is the critical technical principle for exploring core relational themes and resolution of ruptures. First introduced to the psychotherapeutic situation by Kiesler (1996), the principle of metacommunication is an approach that fits the relational formulations presented earlier especially well. In very simple terms, *metacommunication* means communicating about the communication. It is predicated on the idea that we are in constant communication—that all behavior in an interpersonal situation has message value and thus involves communication. Metacommunication describes an attempt to increase awareness of each person's role in an interaction by stepping out of the interaction and communicating directly about what is taking place between the client and therapist (Safran & Muran, 2000). Efforts at metacommunication attempt to minimize the degree of inference and are grounded as much as possible in the therapist's immediate experience of some aspect of the therapeutic relationship—either the therapist's own feelings or an immediate perception of some aspect of the client's actions.

Ruptures not only are the result of a collaborative effort but also can only be understood or resolved by a collaboration of both patient and therapist (Safran & Muran, 2000). Therapists are not seen as being in a privileged position of knowing; rather, their understanding of themselves and their clients is always partial, evolving, and embedded in the complex, interactive, patient–therapist matrix (Hoffman, 1998; Mitchell, 1993; Stern, 1997). Metacommunication is the effort to look back at a recently unfolded relational process from a different vantage point; however, "because we are always caught in the grip of the field, the upshot for clinical purposes is that we face the endless task of trying to see the field and climb out of it—and into another one, for there is nowhere else to go" (Stern, 1997, p. 158). The following list includes some basic principles that we have found useful in our efforts to metacommunicate with clients. (For more detailed descriptions of these and other principles, see Safran & Muran, 2000.)

- *Invite a collaborative inquiry and establish a climate of shared dilemma.* Clients often feel alone during a rupture. Frame the impasse as a shared dilemma that you and the client will explore collaboratively; acknowledge that "we are stuck together." Communicate observations in a tentative, exploratory manner that signals your openness to client input. In this way, instead of being yet one more in an endless succession of figures who do not understand the client's struggle, you can become an ally who joins him or her.
- *Keep the focus on the immediate, and privilege awareness over change.* The focus should be on the here and now of the therapeutic relationship rather than on events in prior sessions or even earlier in the same session. In addition, keep the focus on the concrete and specific rather than abstract, intellectualized speculation. A specific, immediate focus helps clients become more mindful of their own experience. The goal is not to change the client's experience but to increase the client's awareness of his or her experience because awareness is the necessary precursor to lasting change.
- *Emphasize your own subjectivity and be open to exploring your own contribution.* All metacommunications should emphasize the subjectivity of the therapist's perception. This helps establish a collaborative, egalitarian environment in which the client feels free to decide how to make use of the therapist's observation. In addition, therapists should be open to exploring their contributions to the interaction with the client in a nondefensive manner. This process can help clients become more aware of feelings that they have but are unable to clearly articulate, in part because they fear the therapist's response. Accepting responsibility for one's contributions can validate clients' experience of the interaction and help them to trust their own judgment. Increasing clients' confidence in their judgment helps to decrease their need for defensiveness, which facilitates their exploration and acknowledgment of their own contribution to the interaction.

Metacommunication is a valuable principle for exploring core relational themes. The process of metacommunication can begin with questions or observations that focus the client's attention on different aspects of the client–therapist interaction. The therapist might start by focusing the client's attention on his or her own experience with a direct question, such as "What are you feeling right now?" or with an observation about the client's self-state, such as "You seem anxious to me right now. Am I reading you right?" To direct attention to the interpersonal field, the therapist might ask "What's going on here between us?" or offer an observation about the interaction, such as "It seems like we're in some kind of dance. Does that fit with your sense?" A third potential avenue for metacommunication is to focus on the therapist's experience by asking a question that encourages the client to be curious about the therapist's self-state: "Do you have any thoughts about what might be going on for me right now?" Alternatively, the therapist could make a self-disclosure about his or her internal experience, such as "I'm aware of feeling defensive right now." It is important to bear in mind that these three foci represent parallel dimensions.

Although the preceding outlined principles can be applied fairly successfully with most clients, it can be much more challenging in the presence of personality disorders. Attempts at metacommunication can be responded to with resistance, and escalation of the rupture can be observed in the session. As noted earlier, clients with personality disorders have a restricted range of interpersonal behaviors and, more often than not, can feel threatened by the therapist's attempts at metacommunication. What follows is a clinical illustration of a rupture resolution that involves both withdrawal and confrontation and the use of metacommunication.

Case Example 2

Jean is a 44-year-old patient who had a childhood sexual abuse history and borderline personality characteristics. Jean had abusive and critical parents who put the blame on her for their own failures at parenthood. For example, when Jean's mother was unavailable and neglectful when Jean needed her help, her mother would tell Jean that her own incompetence made her need her mother and that Jean should be able to take care of herself. In the following exchange, the therapist tries to employ metacommunication to collaboratively explore a rupture in the session:

THERAPIST: Jean, I'm getting a sense that something is different today. It seems like you don't want to talk. Am I reading you right?

JEAN: Yes, I don't feel like talking today.

THERAPIST: OK, do you have any thoughts about why that might be?

JEAN: I don't know. Maybe it's because you don't want to talk today.

THERAPIST: What do you mean?

JEAN: Just what I said. You don't seem engaged with me today, and so I don't feel like talking with you, either.

Here, the client moves against the therapist in a confrontation rupture. In what follows, the therapist tries to explore the fears that are interfering with the client's expression of underlying needs and to help the client express more vulnerable feelings:

THERAPIST: What made you think that I wasn't engaged with you today?

JEAN: See, this is what I don't like. You always do this! It's always my fault when I think something about you. It's never that I'm right that you don't want to talk today; it's always "in my head," and not the reality!

THERAPIST: Oh, OK. I didn't know you felt that way.

JEAN: Yes, you're like my mother. She always made it about me. When I complained about something that she did, she always said it was in my head.

THERAPIST: OK, I understand. Sorry for making you feel that way. Let me think. Do I not feel like talking with you today? Well, I agree I'm not feeling fully present today. I do have a lot on my mind. . . .

As demonstrated in the preceding conversation, the therapist's attempts at metacommunication were leading to an escalation of the rupture with Jean. It did not seem possible to invite her to a collaborative inquiry until the therapist openly explored her own contribution and validated Jean's point of view. This opened the way to a conversation in which Jean was able to expand her awareness of her expectations, based on a core relational theme of neglect and blame, which ultimately led to an examination of how Jean meets her needs in negotiations with those of another. This is a case that involves withdrawal mixed with confrontation, as the client initially was withdrawing from the therapist by not talking much. As much as it was important for the client to assert herself with the therapist, it was also important for her to recognize her expectation that the therapist will be like her mother. This is a good example of how ruptures can come in both types in a single case and how the resolution process can help a client negotiate the dialectic between the need for agency and the need for relatedness. Learning to negotiate this dialectic more adaptively is essential to rupture resolution, especially with clients with personality disorders. This example also involves exploration of core relational themes (a direct depth-level strategy), demonstrating the complexity of the rupture resolution process and the need for the therapist to be attuned to the moment-by-moment shifts in the alliance over the course of a session in order to be able to make effective rupture resolution interventions.

IMPLICATIONS FOR TRAINING

Elsewhere, we have provided a detailed description of our training regimen (Muran, Safran, & Eubanks-Carter, 2010). Here we provide a brief overview. Recently, with another grant from the National Institute of Mental Health (MH071768: Principal Investigator, J. Christopher Muran), we have been examining the additive impact of this training to a cognitive-behavioral therapy for personality disorders and have found some preliminary support for its benefit to the interpersonal process between patient and therapist (Safran et al., 2014).

Basic Therapist Skills

Research has consistently demonstrated that therapists' individual differences strongly predict alliance quality and treatment success (Baldwin, Wampold, & Imel, 2007; Luborsky et al., 1986). Some therapists are consistently more helpful than others and are better able to facilitate the development of the therapeutic alliance, thus underlining the importance of an alliance-focused approach to the training of therapists. Based on our relational approach to psychotherapy, the training of psychotherapists concentrates on the development of therapists' abilities to recognize ruptures and to resolve them. With regard to rupture recognition, our training targets three specific skills—*self-awareness*, *affect regulation*, and *interpersonal sensitivity*—which we see as interdependent and as critical to establishing an optimal observational stance. By self-awareness, we refer to developing therapists' immediate awareness and bare attention to their internal experience. Our aim here is to increase therapists' attunement to their emotions so that they may use them as a compass to understand their interactions with their patients. By affect regulation, we refer to developing therapists' abilities to manage negative emotions and tolerate distress, their own as well as their patients.' In other words, we try to facilitate their abilities to resist the natural reaction to anxiety—to turn one's attention away or to avoid dealing with it in some way, which means not attending to or exploring a rupture. By interpersonal sensitivity, we refer to increasing therapists' empathy to their patient's experience and their awareness of the interpersonal process they engage in with their patients. In this regard, we try to balance therapists' attention to what they or their patients say with an increased sensitivity to how statements are communicated, the impact of expressions, and the nature of their interactions with patients. The training also attempts to teach the various rupture resolution strategies from direct to indirect and from surface to depth, but with special attention to the technical principle of metacommunication, which, as discussed earlier, we have found useful for exploring core relational themes.

Fundamental Training Principles

In this section, we outline some of the fundamental principles that guide our alliance-focused approach to training.

- *Recognizing the relational context.* The relational context is of utmost importance in training as in therapy. It is impossible for the supervisor to convey information to the trainee that has meaning independent of the relational context in which it is conveyed. Supervision thus needs to be tailored to the specific needs and development of the trainee. Supervisors need to recognize and support trainees' needs to maintain their self-esteem and must calibrate the extent to which they need support versus new information or confrontation in a given moment. It is also critical for supervisors to monitor the quality of the supervisory alliance in an ongoing fashion that parallels the ongoing monitoring of the quality of the alliance in therapy. When strains or tensions emerge, the exploration of the supervisory relationship should assume priority over other concerns.

- *Establishing an experiential focus.* For many trainees, the process of establishing an experiential focus involves a partial unlearning of things that they have already learned about doing therapy. Often the training of therapists emphasizes the conceptual at the expense of the experiential. Trainees study the formulations of different psychotherapy theorists and learn to apply the ideas they are learning to their clinical experience. Although this type of knowledge is essential, it can also serve a defensive function. It can help them to manage the anxiety that inevitably arises as a result of confronting the inherent ambiguity and chaos of lived experience but can lead to premature formulations that foreclose experience. It can also help them to avoid dealing with the painful and frightening conflicting feelings that inevitably emerge for both patients and therapists. In some respects, this conceptual knowledge can be useful in navigating one's anxieties and therapeutic impasses; in others, it can serve to tighten deadlocks.

- *Emphasizing self-exploration.* Although there are times when specific suggestions about ways of conceptualizing a case or intervening are useful, there is an overarching emphasis in our approach on helping therapists to find their own unique solutions to their struggles with patients. The particular therapeutic interaction that is the focus of supervision is unique to a particular therapist–patient dyad. Therapists will thus have their own unique feelings in response to particular patients, and the particular solution they formulate to their dilemma must emerge in the context of their own unique reactions. An important aim of training, therefore, is to help therapists to develop a way to dialogue with their patients about what is going on in the moment that is unique to the moment and their experience of it. Suggestions about what to say provided by supervisors or fellow trainees may look appropriate in the context of a videotape being viewed but may not be appropriate to the context of the next session. The supervisor's task is thus to help trainees develop the ability to attend to their own experience and use it as a basis for intervening.

Training Strategies and Tools

Our training program makes use of various strategies to develop therapist abilities and essential skills to recognize and resolve ruptures. The main training strategies we use include:

- *Manualization.* In this regard, we use our book *Negotiating the Therapeutic Alliance: A Relational Guide* (Safran & Muran, 2000) as a training manual. It provides background and justification for our relational approach to practice and training. Probably the most important benefit of this book is that it presents various clinical principles and models, including our own empirically derived rupture resolution model, which can serve to help therapists organize their experience, regulate their affect, and manage their anxiety in the face of a very difficult treatment process (see Aron, 1999, for more on this point).

- *Process coding.* We provide a brief orientation to various research measures of psychotherapy process, such as those that focus on vocal quality, emotional involvement, and interpersonal behavior, in order to sensitize trainees to the psychotherapy process. This can be very important to the development of one's clinical ear, namely how to observe and listen to process (and not just content). Trainees may even be asked to track one of their sessions with a particular coding scheme in mind. The use of such measures (in addition to the rupture resolution model) is a good example of how research can influence practice.
- *Videotape analysis.* We also conduct intensive analysis of videotaped psychotherapy sessions. This provides a view of a treatment process unfiltered by the trainees' reconstructions and an opportunity to step outside their participation and to view their interactions as a third-party observer. It facilitates an orientation to interpersonal process. There are a variety of useful ways to use videotape, including as a prompt for accessing and defining a trainee's internal experience and to provide the trainee with subjective feedback about the impact of the patient on others, which can be validating when it corresponds but also illustrative of the uniqueness of interactions when it differs.
- *Mindfulness training.* We introduce mindfulness meditation to our trainees, which we consider a systematic strategy for developing an optimal observational stance toward internal experience. Often trainees have difficulty at first distinguishing between their experience and their ideas about their experience, and it is useful to use structured mindfulness exercises to help them grasp this distinction and develop openness to their experience. Such exercises also help trainees sharpen their abilities to become participant-observers. We also appreciate the benefits of this training in developing affect regulation and interpersonal sensitivity. We incorporate mindfulness in supervision sessions but also encourage trainees to establish personal practices.
- *Awareness exercises.* We make extensive use of awareness-oriented exercises, including the use of role plays and two-chair techniques to practice metacommunication. For example, trainees might be asked to alternate between playing their patients and then themselves in a difficult enactment observed on video with the aim of exploring their experience (especially their fears and expectations regarding the patient) and experimenting with different ways of trying metacommunication. These exercises are at the heart of the training model. They are valuable for grounding training at the experiential level and promoting self-awareness and empathy.

CONCLUDING COMMENTS

One of the most consistent findings emerging from psychotherapy research is that the quality of the therapeutic alliance is a robust predictor of outcome across a range of different treatments and that, conversely, weakened alliances are correlated with unilateral termination by the patient (e.g., Horvath, Del Re, Flückiger, & Symonds, 2011; Tryon & Kane, 1995). Patients with personality disorders that are associated with serious impairment in interpersonal relationships pose significant challenges to therapists, especially in building and maintaining the therapeutic alliance. Furthermore, as noted earlier, each type of personality disorder produces different challenges to forming a working alliance in psychotherapy, suggesting the necessity of a customized approach to working with personality disorders.

One such tailored approach to enhancing the therapeutic relationship involves the negotiation of the ruptures that inevitably take place in every therapy relationship. In the last two decades, a "second generation" of alliance research has emerged, attempting to clarify the factors leading to the development of the alliance, as well as those processes involved in repairing ruptures in the alliance when they occur (Safran, Muran, Samstag, & Stevens, 2002). Ruptures and their resolutions take on added importance when working with patients with personality disorders, as this group of patients is associated with difficulties in interpersonal relationships. Thus a therapist's attunement to subtle indications of alliance ruptures and ability to resolve ruptures becomes one of the most critical factors in the therapy process with personality disorders. In our relational approach to personality disorder and alliance ruptures, training of psychotherapists focuses on developing therapists' abilities in effective rupture resolution. We believe that training therapists in more effective negotiation of the therapeutic alliance, in a more attuned and responsive approach to their patients' characteristic ways of interpersonal relating, and in the specific challenges they experience in the therapeutic alliance represents the next frontier.

REFERENCES

Aktar, S. (1992). *Broken structures: Severe personality disorders and their treatment.* Northvale, NJ: Jason Aronson.

American Psychiatric Association. (1994). *Diagnostic and statistical manual of mental disorders* (4th ed.). Washington, DC: Author.

Aron, L. (1999). Clinical choices and the relational matrix. *Psychoanalytic Dialogues, 9*(1), 1–29.

Baldwin, S. A., Wampold, B. E., & Imel, Z. E. (2007). Untangling the alliance–outcome correlation: Exploring the relative importance of therapist and patient variability in the alliance. *Journal of Consulting and Clinical Psychology, 75*(6), 842–852.

Bateman, A., & Fonagy. P. (2004). *Psychotherapy for borderline personality disorder: Mentalization-based treatment.* Oxford, UK: Oxford University Press.

Bateman, A. W., & Fonagy, P. (2000). Effectiveness of psychotherapeutic treatment of personality disorder. *British Journal of Psychiatry, 177*, 138–143.

Bender, D. S. (2005). The therapeutic alliance in the treatment of personality disorders. *Journal of Psychiatric Practice, 11*, 73–87.

Bender, D. S., Farber, B. A., Sanislow, C. A., Dyck, I. R., Geller, J. D., & Skodol, A. E. (2003). Representations of therapists by patients with personality disorders. *American Journal of Psychotherapy, 57*, 219–236.

Benjamin, L. S. (1993). *Interpersonal diagnosis and treatment of personality disorders*. New York: Guilford Press.

Benjamin, L. S. (1996). *Interpersonal diagnosis and treatment of personality disorders* (2nd ed.). New York: Guilford Press.

Benjamin, L. S. (2005). Interpersonal theory of personality disorders: The structural analysis of social behavior and interpersonal reconstructive therapy. In M. F. Lenzenweger & J. F. Clarkin (Eds.), *Major theories of personality disorder* (2nd ed., pp. 157–230). New York: Guilford Press.

Benjamin, L. S., & Karpiak, C. P. (2002). Personality disorders. In J. C. Norcross (Ed.), *Psychotherapy relationships that work: Therapist contributions and responsiveness to patients* (pp. 423–438). New York: Oxford University Press.

Bordin, E. (1979). The generalizability of the psychoanalytic concept of the working alliance. *Psychotherapy: Theory, Research, and Practice, 16*, 252–260.

Clarkin, J. F., & Levy, K. N. (2004). The influence of client variables in psychotherapy. In M. J. Lambert (Ed.), *Bergin and Garfield's handbook of psychotherapy and behavior change* (5th ed., pp. 194–226). New York: Wiley.

Clarkin, J. F., Levy, K. N., & Ellison, W. D. (2011). Personality disorders. In L. M. Horowitz & S. Strack (Eds.), *Handbook of interpersonal psychology: Theory, research, assessment, and therapeutic interventions* (pp. 383–403). Hoboken, NJ: Wiley.

Clarkin, J. F., Levy, K. N., Lenzenweger, M. F., & Kernberg, O. F. (2007). Evaluating three treatments for borderline personality disorder: A multiwave study. *American Journal of Psychiatry, 164*(6), 922–928.

Clarkin, J. F., Yeomans, F., & Kernberg, O. F. (2006). *Psychotherapy of borderline personality: Focusing on object relations*. Washington, DC: American Psychiatric Publishing.

Dimaggio, G., Carcione, A., Salvatore, G., Semerari, A., & Nicolò, G. (2010). A rational model for maximizing the effect of regulating therapy relationship in personality disorders. *Psychology and Psychotherapy: Theory, Research, and Practice, 83*, 363–384.

Dimaggio, G., Salvatore, G., Fiore, D., Carcione, A., Nicolo, G., & Semerari, A. (2012). General principles for treating personality disorder with a prominent inhibitedness trait: Towards an operationalizing integrated technique. *Journal of Personality Disorders, 26*(1), 63–83.

Dimaggio, G., Semerari, A., Carcione, A., Nicolò, & Procacci, M. (2007). *Psychotherapy of personality disorders: Metacognition, states of mind and interpersonal cycles*. London: Routledge.

Eubanks-Carter, C., Muran, J. C., & Safran, J. D. (2010). Alliance ruptures and resolution. In J. C. Muran & J. P. Barber (Eds.), *The therapeutic alliance: An evidence-based guide to practice* (pp. 74–94). New York: Guilford Press.

Harper, H. (1989a). *Coding guide: I. Identification of confrontation challenges in exploratory therapy*. Unpublished manuscript, University of Sheffield, Sheffield, UK.

Harper, H. (1989b). *Coding guide: II. Identification of withdrawal challenges in exploratory therapy.* Unpublished manuscript, University of Sheffield, Sheffield, UK.
Hoffman, I. Z. (1998). *Ritual and spontaneity in the psychoanalytic process: A dialectical- constructivist view.* Hillsdale, NJ: Analytic Press.
Horvath, A. O., Del Re, A. C., Flückiger, C., & Symonds, D. (2011). Alliance in individual psychotherapy. *Psychotherapy, 48*(1), 9–16.
Horwitz, I., Gabbard, G. O., Allen, J. G., Frieswyk, S. H., Colson, D. B., & Newsom, G. E. (Eds.). (1996). *Borderline personality disorder. Tailoring the psychotherapy to the patient.* Washington, DC: American Psychiatric Press.
Kiesler, D. J. (1996). *Contemporary interpersonal theory and research: Personality, psychopathology, and psychotherapy.* New York: Wiley.
Levy, K. N. (2005). The implications of attachment theory and research for understanding borderline personality disorder. *Development and Psychopathology, 17*(4), 959–986.
Linehan, M. M., Armstrong, H. E., Suarez, A., Allmon, D., & Heard, H. L. (1991). Cognitive-behavioral treatment of chronically parasuicidal borderline patients. *Archives of General Psychiatry, 48*(12), 1060–1064.
Livesley, W. J. (2003). Personality disorder: Evidence of changing perspectives? [Review of the book *Personality Disorders Over Time: Precursors, Course, and Outcome* by J. Paris]. *Journal of Nervous and Mental Disease, 191*(12), 767–770.
Luborsky, L., Crits-Christoph, P., McLellan, A. T., Woody, G., Piper, W., Liberman, B., et al. (1986). Do therapists vary much in their success?: Findings from four outcome studies. *American Journal of Orthopsychiatry, 56*(4), 501–512.
Luborsky, L., & Crits-Christoph, P. (1998). *Understanding transference: The core conflictual relationship theme method* (2nd ed.). Washington, DC: American Psychological Association.
Meissner, W. W. (1996). *The therapeutic alliance.* New Haven, CT: Yale University Press.
Mitchell, S. A. (1988). *Relational concepts in psychoanalysis.* Cambridge, MA: Harvard University Press.
Mitchell, S. A. (1993). *Hope and dread in psychoanalysis.* New York: Basic Books.
Mitchell, S. A., & Aron, L. (1999). *Relational psychoanalysis: The emergence of a tradition.* Hillsdale, NJ: Analytic Press.
Muran, J. C. (2001). Meditations on "both/and." In J. C. Muran (Ed.), *Self-relations in psychotherapy process* (pp. 347–372). Washington, DC: American Psychological Association.
Muran, J. C., Safran, J., Samstag, L., & Winston, A. (2005). Evaluating an alliance-focused treatment for personality disorders. *Psychotherapy: Theory, Research, Practice, Training, 42*, 532–545.
Muran, J. C., Safran, J. D., & Eubanks-Carter, C. (2010). Developing therapist abilities to negotiate alliance ruptures. In C. J. Muran & J. P. Barber (Eds.), *The therapeutic alliance: An evidence-based guide to practice* (pp. 320–340). New York: Guilford Press.
Pretzer, J. L., & Beck, A. T. (2005). A cognitive theory of personality disorders. In M. F. Lenzenweger & J. F. Clarkin (Eds.), *Major theories of personality disorder* (2nd ed., pp. 43–113). New York: Guilford Press.
Safran, J. D. (1998). *Widening the scope of cognitive therapy.* Northvale, NJ: Jason Aronson.

Safran, J. D., & Muran, J. C. (1996). The resolution of ruptures in the therapeutic alliance. *Journal of Consulting and Clinical Psychology, 64*(3), 447–458.

Safran, J. D., & Muran, J. C. (2000). *Negotiating the therapeutic alliance: A relational treatment guide.* New York: Guilford Press.

Safran, J. D., Muran, J. C., Demaria, A., Boutwell, C., Eubanks-Carter, C., & Winston, A. (2014). Investigating the impact of alliance-focused training on interpersonal process and therapists' capacity for experiential reflection. *Psychotherapy Research, 24,* 269–285.

Safran, J. D., Muran, J. C., & Eubanks-Carter, C. (2011). Repairing alliance ruptures. *Psychotherapy, 48*(1), 80–87.

Safran, J. D., Muran, J. C., Samstag, L. W., & Stevens, C. (2002). Repairing alliance ruptures. In J. C. Norcross (Ed.), *Psychotherapy relationships that work: Therapist contributions and responsiveness to patients* (pp. 235–254). New York: Oxford University Press.

Samstag, L. W., Batchelder, S., Muran, J. C., Safran, J. D., & Winston, A. (1998). Predicting treatment failure from in-session interpersonal variables. *Journal of Psychotherapy Practice and Research, 5,* 126–143.

Sommerfeld, E., Orbach, I., Zim, S., & Mikulincer, M. (2008). An in-session exploration of ruptures in working alliance and their associations with clients' core conflictual relationship themes, alliance-related discourse, and clients' postsession evaluations. *Psychotherapy Research, 18*(4), 377–388.

Stern, D. B. (1997). *Unformulated experience: From dissociation to imagination in psychoanalysis.* Mahwah, NJ: Analytic Press.

Tufekcioglu, S., Muran, J. C., Safran, J. D., & Winston, A. (2013). Personality disorder and early psychotherapy process in two time-limited therapies. *Psychotherapy Research, 23,* 646–657.

Tryon, G. S., & Kane, A. S. (1995). Client involvement, working alliance, and type of therapy termination. *Psychotherapy Research, 5,* 189–198.

Westen, D., & Morrison, K. (2001). A multidimensional meta-analysis of treatments for depression, panic, and generalized anxiety disorder: An empirical examination of the status of empirically supported therapies. *Journal of Consulting and Clinical Psychology, 69*(6), 875–899.

Zimmerman, M., Chelminski, I., & Young, D. (2008). The frequency of personality disorders in psychiatric patients. *Psychiatric Clinics of North America, 31*(3), 405–420.

chapter 7

The Role of Mentalization in Treatments for Personality Disorder

Anthony W. Bateman and Peter Fonagy

This chapter proposes that borderline personality disorder (BPD) and perhaps other personality disorders may be conceptualized as a problem of mentalizing, that treatments for BPD are not as distinctive as they sound, and that their effectiveness may be underpinned by an ability to effect change in mentalizing processes. BPD is a complex and serious mental disorder characterized by a pervasive pattern of difficulties with emotion regulation, impulse control, and instability, both in relationships and in self-image, with a mortality rate, associated with suicide, that is 50 times that of the general population (Skodol et al., 2002). Fortunately, over the past decade progress has been made in developing a range of effective treatments. At first sight the treatments seem distinct. Some are behaviorally oriented, whereas others are psychodynamically focused; some target schemas and cognitions, whereas others have more general aims. Yet all of them have shown an ability to effect positive outcomes for patients with BPD.

The acute symptoms of the disorder respond best to treatment—that is, the marked emotional dysregulation, suicidality, self-harm, and impulsivity, long believed to be chronic in nature. These symptoms have also been shown to remit naturally without treatment, with patients experiencing substantial reductions far earlier than previously assumed (Gunderson et al., 2011).

Around a 50% remission rate of the acute symptoms occurs by 4 years from the time of first diagnosis to the extent that patients do not meet diagnostic criteria even though significant problems may remain. The remission in terms of diagnostic criteria is steady (10–15% per year), with 78–99% of patients showing remission at 16-year follow-up. Recurrences are rare, perhaps no more than 10% over 6 years and less over 10 years (Zanarini, Frankenburg, Reich, & Fitzmaurice, 2010, 2012). However, it is apparent that, even though people may not meet criteria for BPD, debilitating symptoms in social and interpersonal functioning do not easily respond to treatment, and patients are left with disabling functional impairment.

The remission of the acute symptoms of BPD appears to be independent of treatment and is in contrast to the pessimistic outcomes reported in the earlier literature (Stone, 1990). Given the unavailability of the newly developed effective treatments in health services and the fact that most patients are treated in general psychiatric services, the ostensible change in prognosis possibly occurs because general psychiatric treatment has improved, first by progressively being influenced by the theories and interventions of the specialist treatments and second by increasingly avoiding harmful interactions (Fonagy & Bateman, 2006b). This is significant. We suggest that the recent findings that general psychiatric treatment is as effective as specialist treatment in reducing the acute symptoms of BPD indicates that there may be a common underlying mechanism of change that is not dependent on particular therapy interventions.

SPECIALIST TREATMENTS FOR BPD

Despite the finding that patients with BPD may improve without treatment, it has been assumed over the past two decades that they needed a specialist intervention rather than general psychiatric treatment to bring forward this natural change. This view is now being challenged.

Dialectical behavior therapy (DBT) was the first specialist treatment to challenge the atmosphere of therapeutic nihilism and remains the best studied. Studies of DBT for BPD suggest that treatment had powerful effects on the management of behavioral problems associated with impulsivity, although its effects on mood state and interpersonal functioning appeared more limited (Linehan, Armstrong, Suarez, Allmon, & Heard, 1991; Linehan, Heard, & Armstrong, 1993; Linehan et al., 2006).

It is notable that most trials of DBT showing superiority over treatment as usual or treatment by expert took place in the United States, used highly trained practitioners, and were undertaken at a time when treatment as usual, and even treatment by expert, was poorly organized and lacked coordination to the extent that therapy was independent of other services offered to the patient, such as crisis intervention, and when clinicians in treatment as usual had no obvious support and supervision systems specific to treatment of

BPD. Trials of outpatient DBT in other health systems have not produced such positive results, possibly suggesting either that general psychiatric treatment elsewhere is better organized and more effective for patients with BPD than in the United States or that DBT is not easily transportable, for example, in the Netherlands (Verheul et al., 2002) and in the United Kingdom (Feigenbaum et al., 2011). Finally, a recent well-conducted trial in Canada comparing DBT with general psychiatric treatment showed no differential effects between treatments (McMain et al., 2009). Both groups showed equal improvement on all measures over the treatment period, and the gains in both groups were maintained over a 2-year follow-up (McMain, Guimond, Cardish, Streiner, & Links, 2012).

The increasing finding of equivalence of outcomes among well-organized treatments for BPD may not be particular to DBT. In recent years, every time a named specialist treatment for BPD has been compared with an alternative well-structured general psychiatric intervention, organized around and specific to the supposed underlying pathology of BPD, differences in outcomes have been either nonexistent or, at best, only moderate (Bateman & Fonagy, 2009; Chanen et al., 2008; Clarkin, Levy, Lenzenweger, & Kernberg, 2007; Doering et al., 2010).

NONSPECIALIST TREATMENTS FOR BPD

It seems possible that, if a disparate group of specialist and general treatments are all effective in treatment of BPD, there is considerable overlap between them, that "many roads lead to Rome"—that is, that the pathways to helping a patient manage acute symptoms of BPD are many and varied, or that there is a common mechanism underlying the process of change. Indeed, comparing the operationalized, effective comparator treatments used in the research trials of general psychiatric management (GPM; Gunderson, 2011), supportive psychotherapy (SP; Clarkin, Levy, Lenzenweger, & Kernberg, 2004), good clinical care (GCC; Chanen et al., 2008), and structured clinical management (SCM; Bateman & Krawitz, 2013), it is striking how similar they are.

GPM consisted of psychodynamically informed psychotherapy, case management, and symptom-targeted medication as adjunct using the American Psychiatric Association algorithm. This psychodynamic approach was drawn from the work of John Gunderson (Gunderson, 2008) and emphasizes early attachment as an important theoretical perspective and disturbed attachment processes as a primary target for therapy. In the trial, therapy was provided by clinicians with "expertise, aptitude and interest" (McMain et al., 2009) in the treatment of BPD (66% were psychiatrists). Frequency of sessions was 1 hour weekly with crisis meetings if necessary. In SP there was also a strong emphasis on attachment, and the therapist focused on establishing and maintaining a comfortable, relaxed therapy relationship. There was minimal use of interpretation so that the clinician could provide emotional support and advice on the daily problems facing the patients without the use of interpretation to differentiate it from the specialist treatment (transference-focused psychotherapy; Clarkin et al., 2007). The fundamental vehicle of change was seen as the client identifying with the clinician's consistent attitudes of benevolence, interest, kindness, and nonjudgmental acceptance toward him or her (Appelbaum, 2006).

Superficially, GCC and SCM look dissimilar to GPM and SP, as they both utilize cognitive-behaviorally informed techniques using a problem-solving paradigm as the core treatment intervention, with high value placed on effective organizational structures, rather than being psychodynamically informed. But again, in both interventions the relationship is considered to be of central importance. In GCC cognitive-behaviorally trained clinical psychologists provided both the therapy and case management; all clients had access to a psychiatrist and were discussed weekly in team meetings. Therapy sessions were flexible in time and number, and flexible case management sessions were organized on a "need" basis. Importantly, clinicians were instructed that intervention involves more than just formal psychotherapy and that the therapeutic alliance is key to effective treatment. SCM also emphasizes the relationship alliance, using a counseling model close to that of SP and exhorts the clinician to use nonjudgmental acceptance, warmth, and supportive techniques within case management work (Bateman & Fonagy, 2009).

In sum, the nonspecialist treatments used in general psychiatric services are organized around the development of an attachment relationship with the patient, a focus on the therapeutic alliance and repair of ruptures, and the offer of basic psychological techniques that have a chance of helping the patient with their symptoms. Importantly, all of them are delivered according to a carefully constructed protocol, which informs the clinician about how to manage common clinical situations.

EFFECTING CHANGE

Over a decade ago (Bateman & Fonagy, 2000), we suggested that part of the benefit that individuals with personality disorder derive from treatment comes through the experience of being involved in a carefully considered, well-structured, and coherent interpersonal endeavor. What may be helpful is the internalization of a thoughtfully developed structure, the understanding of the interrelationship of different reliably identifiable components, the causal interdependence of specific ideas and actions, the constructive interactions of professionals, and, above all, the experience of being the subject of reliable, coherent and rational thinking. Social and personal experiences such as these are not specific to any treatment modality but, rather, are correlates of the level of seriousness and the degree of commitment with which teams of professionals approach the problem of caring for this group, who may be argued on empirical grounds to have been deprived of exactly such consideration and commitment during their early development and quite frequently throughout their later lives.

There is no doubt that the nonspecialist and the specialist treatments we have just described meet all these requirements; all are well structured and offer an experience of a coherent interpersonal endeavor with identification of a clear pathway to improvement. However, the question arises about how these general experiences can effect personal change in the patient. Certainly the creation of a well-constructed protocol outlining a coherent theory of the condition and identifying clinical interventions in a range of common clinical situations emboldens and "grounds" the clinician. This is a start and may account for some of the success of the general treatments; the protocols used for these comparator treatments in research trials have been much more carefully developed in recent years, and studies no longer rely on uncoordinated treatment as usual as a comparison. The mind of the clinician is less likely to be disrupted by inappropriate demands; he or she will be able to maintain a focus on task, not lose direction, and intervene judiciously rather than because of his or her own anxiety. It seems that the development of agreed protocols shared between a group of clinicians is key to the treatment of people with BPD and that the problem with treatment as usual in the past was that clinicians reacted with uncoordinated provision of service, much of which was at best harmless and at worse detrimental.

What Effects Change?

None of the randomized controlled trials testing specialist treatments tell us which patients got better or how they improved. Indeed, a number of patients in the trials deteriorated or remained the same, whereas others did extremely well. We have very limited knowledge about moderators and mechanisms of change in psychotherapy itself, let alone in the complex psychosocial treatments for BPD. Neacsiu, Rizvi, and Linehan (2010) examined the role of DBT skills in improving treatment clinical outcomes. Unsurprisingly, participants treated with DBT reported using three times more behavioral skills by the end of treatment compared with those assigned to a control treatment. But use of DBT skills mediated the decrease in suicide attempts and depression and the increase in control of anger and partially mediated the decrease in nonsuicidal self-injury over time, suggesting that skills acquisition and practice may be an important mechanism of change in DBT. This creates an illusion of an explanation, which fails when we generalize and ask how patients treated with GPM change equally without receiving any skills training.

So, returning to our question: What makes people with BPD change given that so many disparate treatments using apparently contrasting interventions achieve similar outcomes? Do all these treatments have something in common alongside the fact that they are carefully organized interpersonal endeavors delivered according to a structured protocol? We have suggested that all therapies for BPD show certain characteristics (Bateman, 2012), along with the generic features of well-constructed treatment protocols identified previously. These elements, rather than the specific techniques of treatment, may be responsible for their effectiveness. They (1) provide a structure, through their manuals, that supports the clinician and provides recommendations for common clinical problems; (2) are structured so that they encourage increased activity, proactivity, and self-agency for the patients; (3) focus on emotion processing, particularly on creating robust connections between acts and feeling; (4) increase cognitive coherence in relation to subjective experience in the early phase of treatments by the inclusion of a model of pathology that is carefully explained to the patient; and (5) encourage an active clinician stance which invariably includes an explicit intent to validate and demonstrate empathy and generate a strong attachment relationship to create a foundation of alliance. But even these features do not inform us about the process of change. So we argue that what makes therapies for BPD effective is the extent of their ability to stimulate an increasingly robust mentalizing process in the patient while avoiding iatrogenic harm.

MENTALIZING

Concepts such as insight, empathy, the observing ego, and even introspection have been around throughout the "psychotherapeutic century" (Allen & Fonagy, 2002; Allen, Fonagy, & Bateman, 2008). The concept of mentalization, in our view, crystallizes the biological and relational processes that underpin the phenomena that these venerable clinical concepts denote. There are many constructs that cover more or less the same ground (see Choi-Kain & Gunderson, 2008), such as reflectiveness (Bleiberg, 2001), mindfulness (Brown & Ryan, 2003), coherence of "self-narrative" (Westen & Cohen, 1993), and yet they do not cover exactly the same areas. Mentalizing is the guiding construct of our therapeutic approach; psychotherapy with patients with BPD should focus on the capacity for mentalization, by which we mean the implicit or explicit perception or interpretation of the actions of others or oneself as intentional, that is, mediated by mental states or mental processes (Fonagy, Gergely, Jurist, & Target, 2002). Following its development for people with BPD, this focus for psychotherapy has now been extended to treatment of other personality disorders, for example, antisocial personality disorder, on the basis that if the condition can be understood in terms of mentalizing problems, a focus on those problems may be helpful (see later discussion).

We believe that an important common factor in the psychotherapeutic approaches to personality disorder mentioned in this chapter is their shared potential to recreate an interactional matrix of attachment in which mentalization develops and sometimes flourishes. In the course of normal development, social cognition in general—mentalization in particular—emerges; we use the term *matrix* to evoke the whole panoply of past relationships that have been experienced over the course of development, for example, internal working models, that lead people to anticipate patterns within social situations and endow them with the capacity to navigate them through appropriate affect regulation and interpersonal sensitivity.

The attachment matrix that has to be recreated in treatment consists of a number of elements and is not simply the formation of a therapeutic bond that is primarily related to role investment, empathic resonance, and mutual affirmation. First, the clinician balances facilitation of proximity-seeking attachment behaviors to induce a sense of safety with encouragement of behaviors that increase independence and autonomy. Second, there is a focus on using the treatment itself and the security of the relationship to engage in nonattachment behaviors, for example undertaking social tasks. Finally, all clinicians provide a developmental pathway for change, which involves careful focus on the internal, both cognitive and affective, experience of the patient. In effect, the clinician mentalizes the patient in a way that fosters the patient's mentalizing, which is a key facet of the therapeutic relationship.

In all treatments for personality disorder, the therapist presents his or her construction of a social situation related by the patient, for example, an experience of a humiliation, and may work on the way he or she or others might feel in the same situation while not necessarily behaving in the same way as the patient. Jointly, patient and therapist build a collaborative understanding of the patient's mental states that lead to his or her behavior. In the traditional model of therapy, the patient's mental state as constructed by the therapist is presented to the patient, or the behavioral theoretical framework is used to provide alternative ways of behaving. But contemporary treatments for BPD focus more on the *process* of elaborating mental states than on defining them and understanding their content more explicitly. The difference is therefore not so much in content of treatment but more in how the content is treated. This emphasis on process cannot happen if treatment is delivered in an uncoordinated and variable manner, and equally it cannot happen if the treatment method takes over the patient's mental function rather than expediting its more robust development. Taking over mental function can be done in many ways—for example, by telling the patient what is happening to him or her, by providing insight into his or her past, or by taking an expert stance on what the patient feels or telling him or her what to do. From a mentalizing perspective, the crux of the value of psychotherapy with BPD and probably other personality disorders is the experience of another human being having the patient's mind in mind. Mentalizing-based therapy (MBT) makes this the core of treatment and specifically asks the therapist to focus on the mental states of the patient and to elucidate them in detail within the attachment relationship in a structured way. This is in contradistinction to "teaching" a patient how to manage emotions and behaviors.

It should be clear from this discussion that we consider the *process* of therapy, rather than the *content* of the therapy or the nonspecific supportive aspects of therapy, to be at the heart of the treatment and at the core of effecting change (Bateman & Fonagy, 2004). The explicit content of interpreting, defining schemas, or delivering skills is merely the vehicle for the implicit process, which has therapeutic value. This is a bold claim. As we suggested earlier, these explicit interventions provide a developmental experience for the individual of being the subject of reliable, coherent and rational thinking, which is something that people with personality disorder have hitherto been denied. In other words, the effect of all these interventions is to increase the individual's mentalizing capacity, which is the very process that is required for successful and mutually constructive social and personal interaction. Once more robust mentalizing is established, it will allow the individual to take advantage of felicitous social and interpersonal events that had hitherto not been able to be used to effect positive change.

Mentalizing and Personality Disorder

Initially the breadth of the concept of mentalizing encouraged us to see mentalizing as one of many common factors in psychotherapy. Positive changes in mentalizing, stimulated as a by-product of interventions, act as a catalyst for further change in cognitions, emotions and behavior, irrespective of the therapeutic target—mentalizing begets mentalizing and healthier psychological functioning. This is to suggest that a perspective of having a patient's mind in mind makes any therapeutic effort more efficient. This is not a radical suggestion; if a patient feels his or her subjective states of mind are understood, he or she is more likely to be receptive to therapeutic intervention—that is, techniques themselves need a foundation on which to be applied if they are to be maximally helpful. But this catalytic view of mentalizing might be selling the idea short. More radical is the idea that without a change in mentalizing processes over time, there can be no change in the patient with personality disorder as a result of therapy, irrespective of the patient's ability to apply skills or to understand the genesis of his or her dysregulating emotional states. This is an empirical question that needs study—for example, do mentalizing changes precede behavioral changes, and do those patients who show change in mentalizing show greater rehabilitative changes over time than those who do not?

Personality disorder has been conceptualized as a serious impairment in interpersonal relationships, intimacy, identity, and self-direction (Skodol et al., 2011). In its broadest sense, mentalization is a psychological self-narrative that maintains an agentive sense of self (Fonagy & Target, 1997). Unlike a simple historical autobiographical account, mentalizing is a psychological self-narrative that concerns the history of experiences that are held together by the individual's self-involvement. Remembering oneself in a particular situation normally entails remembering one's state of mind in that situation. This creates a continuity that ultimately adds up to having a sense of self because memories are held together by the thoughts, feelings, wishes, and desires that one has had across a range of situations over time. In effect, there is not necessarily a genuine coherence across situations in how we behave, but remembering the experiences of thoughts and feelings in those situations creates the thread. If we lose the capacity to mentalize, then we lose the thread because we lose the continuity of thoughts and feelings over time, and in doing so we lose that sense of selfhood. It is remembering a thought as we see or experience something that provides a subjective experience that adds up to feeling that we are a person with presence. Here we are considering self not as a representation but rather as a process with specific qualities that are closely related to the notion of autonomy, a consciously accessible sense of regulating one's own behavior and person rather than being the way one is seen by others. This does not depend on self-reflection; it is an accumulation of an infinite number of implicit mentalizing experiences. In effect, in poor mentalizing, experiences are not connected, so there are fragments of self-experience rather than a coherent narrative.

The failure of self-narrativization creates characteristic gaps or discontinuities in self-experience. Although our emphasis is on the process of self rather than its representation, changes in the phenomenology of the self are invariably associated with the temporary failure of mentalization. In the face of negative affect, patients may feel unable to experience themselves as authors of their actions, leading not only to a sense of temporally diffused identity (Kernberg, 1983) but also to experiences of inauthenticity or painful incoherence, feelings of emptiness and inability to make commitment, disturbances of body image, and gender dysphoria (Akhtar, 1992). This is borne out by factor-analytic studies of data from clinically experienced informants for adult and adolescent patients (Betan, Heim, Zittel Conklin, & Westen, 2005). Ultimately, failure of mentalization is marked by a tendency to misread minds, both one's own and those of others. Individuals with this difficulty—and we have made a case that people with BPD and other personality disorders show this problem (Fonagy & Bateman, 2008b)—consequently perform dramatically badly in social contexts, not only upsetting people whom they wish to recruit to be helpful (King-Casas et al., 2008) but frequently exhibiting deficits in social problem solving. When mentalization fails, prementalistic modes of organizing subjectivity emerge that have the power to disorganize interpersonal relationships and destroy the coherence of self-experience that the narrative provided by normal mentalization generates. It is that this point, we suggest, that a personality disorder becomes apparent. It is this process that leads to the symptoms of BPD, namely problems with emotion regulation and impulse control and instability both in relationships and in self-image.

Dimensions of Mentalizing

The concept of mentalization has been appropriately criticized as a marker of a specific form of psychopathology such as BPD because in its original formulation the theory offered a construct that was too broad and multifaceted to be operationalized (Choi-Kain & Gunderson, 2008). It is essential to realize that mentalization is not a static and unitary skill or trait. Rather, it is a dynamic capacity that is influenced by stress and arousal, particularly in the context of specific attachment relationships (Allen et al., 2008). Moreover, mentalization is a multifaceted capacity (Bateman & Fonagy, 2012; Luyten et al., 2013). Multiple polarities underlie mentalizing, and patients may show impairments in some of these polarities but not necessarily in others. One of these components is the implicit and explicit nature of the process. But other components of mentalizing have been clarified over the past few years and are relevant to the understanding of change in psychotherapeutic process. These include poles of self- and other mentalizing, external and internal focus of mentalizing, and cognitive and affective mentalizing. Each of these dimensions possibly relates to a different neurobiological system, and the interested reader is referred to Fonagy and Bateman (2006a) for further discussion of this. But although separating out the different dimensions of mentalizing may help clarity, the key to successful mentalizing is the integration of all the dimensions into a coherent whole.

Implicit (Automatic) and Explicit (Controlled) Mentalizing

Mentalization can be both implicit and explicit. Implicit mentalization is a nonconscious, unreflective, procedural function. As Simon Baron-Cohen (1995) put it, "We mind-read all the time, effortlessly, automatically and mostly unconsciously" (p. 3). Explicit mentalization is only likely to happen when we hit an interactive snag (Allen et al., 2008). Explicit mentalization, particularly when it is of a higher order, can be the apparent substance of psychological therapy; for example, Person A can reflect upon his awareness of what Person B thinks about Person A's feelings or thoughts. Elsewhere we have pointed out that such explicit mentalization (metacognition) can only be considered genuine and productive when the link between these cognitions and emotional experience are strong. We have referred to this as *mentalized affectivity* (Fonagy et al., 2002; Jurist, 2005). Others have approached this metaphorically in talking about "making a feeling felt" (Siegel, 1999, p. 149). In fact, the dissociation between implicit and explicit mentalization in the course of development may be a defining criterion of psychological disturbance.

Self- and Other Mentalizing

Impairments and imbalances in the capacity to reflect about oneself and others are common, and it is only when they become more extreme that they begin to cause problems. Some people become experts at reading other people's minds, and if they misuse this ability or exploit it for their own gain, we tend to think they have antisocial characteristics; others focus on themselves and their own internal states and become experts in what others can do for them to meet their requirements, and we then suggest that they are narcissistic. Thus excessive concentration on either the self or other leads to one-sided relationships and distortions in social interaction. Inevitably this will be reflected in how patients present for treatment and interact with their clinicians. Patients with BPD may be oversensitive, carefully monitoring the clinician's mind at the expense of their own needs and being what they think the clinician wants them to be. They may even take on the mind of the clinician and make it their own. Clinicians should be wary of patients who eagerly comply with everything said to them. Such compliance may alternate with a tendency to become preoccupied and overly concerned about internal states of mind, leaving the clinician feeling left out of the relationship and unable to participate effectively.

External and Internal Mentalizing

Internal mentalizing refers to a focus on one's own or others' internal states, that is, thoughts, feelings, and desires; external mentalizing implies a reliance on external features such as facial expression and behavior. This is not the same as the self–other dimension, which relates to the actual object of focus. Mentalization focused on a psychological interior may be self- or other-oriented. Patients with BPD have a problem with internal mentalizing, but they also have difficulties with externally focused mentalizing. Inevitably both components of mentalizing inform each other, so patients with BPD are doubly disadvantaged. The difficulty is not so much that patients with BPD necessarily misinterpret facial expressions, although they might sometimes do so, but more that they are highly sensitive to facial expressions and so tend to react rapidly and without warning (Lynch et al., 2006; Wagner & Linehan, 1999). Any movement of the clinician's might trigger a response. Glancing out of the window, for example, might lead to a statement that the clinician is obviously not listening and so the patient might feel compelled to leave; a nonreactive face is equally disturbing, as patients continuously attempt to deduce the clinician's internal state using information derived from external monitoring. Anything that disrupts this process will create anxiety, which leads to a loss of mentalizing and the reemergence of developmentally earlier ways of relating to the world.

Cognitive and Affective Mentalizing

The final dimension to consider relates to cognitive and emotional processing: belief, reasoning, and perspective taking on the one hand, and emotional empathy, subjective self-experience, and mentalized affectivity on the other

(Jurist, 2005). A high level of mentalizing requires integration of both cognitive and affective processes. But some people are able to manage one aspect to a greater degree than the other. Patients with BPD are overwhelmed by affective processes and cannot integrate them with their cognitive understanding. They may understand why they do something but feel unable to use their understanding to manage their feelings; they are compelled to act because they cannot form representations integrating emotional and cognitive processes. Others, such as people with antisocial personality disorder, invest considerable time in cognitive understanding of mental states to the detriment of affective experience (Bateman & Fonagy, 2008).

Mentalizing as a Core Component of the Psychotherapeutic Process

So what are the strong arguments in favor of mentalization as a key aspect of effective psychotherapeutic process and a mediator of change for people with BPD treated effectively with specialist and general treatments? First, the foundation of any therapeutic work must by definition be implicit mentalization. Without social engagement and interpersonal interaction, there can be no psychological therapy, and without mentalization there can be no constructive social engagement and interpersonal interaction. In our daily interactions, mentalization is predominantly implicit and automatic because in most interpersonal situations we rely on automatic and unreflective assumptions about ourselves, others, and ourselves in relation to others. When things go smoothly, particularly within secure attachment relationships, relying on automatic mentalization appears to be normal because there is no need for more reflective processing (Fonagy & Bateman, 2006a). Indeed, given the speed with which most interpersonal encounters unfold, controlled mentalization may actually hamper interactions. Yet, if needed, we can flexibly switch to controlled mentalization, and this adaptive flexibility (Allen, 2008) is the hallmark of good mentalizing.

Controlled and explicit mentalizing is a core aspect of all therapies. The clinician actively focuses the mind of the patient on aspects of his or her behavior, asks him or her to consider what happened that led to the action, and provides ideas from the clinician's own understanding about how to manage the behavior. In addition, the clinician identifies unsubstantiated automatic assumptions because mentalizing problems are likely to arise if mentalization relies exclusively on automatic assumptions about the self and others that are distorted or overly simplistic or when it is difficult to make such automatic assumptions accessible to conscious reflection and to challenge them. Arguably, all the psychosocial treatments, regardless of theoretical orientation, involve challenging such automatic distorted and/or simplistic assumptions about the self and/or others, making them conscious and inviting the patient to enter into a joint process of reflecting on the assumptions in the context of a therapeutic relationship. Certainly the specialist and general therapies all ask the therapist to focus more explicitly on the patient's implicit assumptions about others, to identify inaccurate or distorted cognitions, and to explore the nonconscious triggers for their behaviors.

Second, since the work of John Bowlby (1988), it has generally been agreed that psychotherapy invariably activates the attachment system and, as a component, generates secure-base experience. In our view, this is important because the attachment context of psychotherapy is essential to establishing the virtuous cycle of synergy between the recovery of mentalization and secure-base experience. In developmental terms, when the attachment system is activated by threat and fear, exploration is inhibited, and the infant seeks proximity. By contrast, if the child feels secure (a secure-base experience), the inhibition of exploration is lifted and natural curiosity can thrive. In therapy the development of a secure-base experience from which the patient can explore him- or herself and his or her current life is necessary for change. The experience of being understood generates an experience of security, which in turn facilitates "mental exploration," the exploration of the mind of the other to find oneself. Mild activation of the attachment system appears to facilitate mentalizing and thus helps the clinician encourage the patient to adopt a controlled, internally focused, self–other differentiated stance toward his or her mental state. In DBT, for example, the clinician engages the patient in a carefully crafted interpersonal interaction and insists on undertaking a functional analysis with the patient about the pathway leading to destructive behaviors (Linehan, 1993). This is a process of shared attention in which the implicit is made explicit in the context of the attachment relationship. In MBT the clinician focuses on the changes in the patient's mental states that lead to the destructive behaviors and how the inability of the patient to be aware of and attend to them early leads inexorably to a destructive behaviors (Bateman & Fonagy, 2006).

However, for reasons that may carry selective advantage from an evolutionary perspective, the intense activation of the brain networks underpinning attachment feelings and experiences also appears to inhibit the intensity of cognitive and emotional scrutiny over mental contents (Fonagy & Bateman, 2008a). In BPD this may be more than a simple relationship between arousal and performance. People with BPD are aroused in social situations in which the attachment system is activated. There is limited evidence that arousal independent of interpersonal stress affects them in the same way in terms of their mentalizing. This emphasis on interpersonal sensitivity is the domain of inquiry begun by Gunderson (Gunderson & Lyons-Ruth, 2008) in which it is suggested that interpersonal hypersensitivity links to high arousal in attachment contexts and is mainly restricted to that area. Nevertheless, it remains possible that the converse is the case; people with BPD may be sensitive to loss of mentalizing in the context of a wide range of stressors due to attachment disorganization in their past histories or because mentalizing processes are not well established because of genetic predisposition. Collapse of mentalizing then makes the individual sensitive to interpersonal situations. Of course, this is the chicken-and-egg dilemma, and whether it is poor mentalization that leads to interpersonal sensitivity in the social situation and increased stress or interpersonal sensitivity that makes people more susceptible to stress and therefore to lose mentalizing more easily is uncertain. What is certain is that all feed back to each other, and a cycle of problems ensues. In either case the interpersonal problems are embedded within a disorganized attachment history. So managing the attachment relationship is of paramount importance if harmful interaction is to be avoided.

In general, in psychotherapy, by activating attachment we inevitably activate memories; negative and traumatic memories come to the fore—for example, a thought and feeling that a person's father hates him or her and always did. These memories generate fear, which activates the attachment system. Our suggestion is that this inhibits mentalizing to some degree, along with some memory function. As a result, in those whose negative experiences are not overwhelming—that is, those who maintain some mentalizing capacity while memories are triggered—there is a window of opportunity in therapy to reorganize their experience in a meaningful way. For patients with BPD who are susceptible to loss of mentalizing in these circumstances, this system can work negatively because presenting negative experiences leads to distress and activation of the attachment system. The reduction in mentalizing means that the person cannot think clearly and create a coherent model of his or her experience. The psychotherapeutic interaction increases the person's distress, which intensifies his or her attachment and clinging and dependency on therapeutic process but does not necessarily allow a window in which the experiences can be reorganized. We can speculate that, because the attachment system to some degree disrupts mentalizing, overactivation will create problems. Yet, by balancing the activation of the attachment system, including affective down-regulation, with the presentation of negative mental contents, the clinician is able to present new mental contents to the patient without evoking mental resistance against the incorporation of new ways of experiencing the world into existing cognitive-emotional schemas.

Attachment activation loosens associative connections by temporarily disabling mentalizing, allowing new ways of experiencing the same event. Yet the same process in BPD does not produce a momentary loss of mentalizing that allows a new way of thinking but a more substantial experience of confusion from which patients do not recover. This makes them dependent on the mind of the therapist to hold them together. Hence the importance in all the psychotherapies for BPD of a focus on supporting the clinician to maintain mental stability and treatment focus; in DBT there is a consultation system, in MBT a supervision process focusing on the therapist's mentalizing in relation to the patient.

The psychotherapeutic process is compromised for people with BPD and perhaps some other personality disorders by the hyperactivation of the attachment system. This is predictable given what we know about the attachment system and psychotherapy. When therapy itself gives rise to distress and fear, perhaps because material emerges that frightens the patient, and the clinician is unable or unwilling to offer reassurance, the patient's attachment system will inevitably be activated. Seeking proximity to a clinician who lacks the capacity to soothe or whose interventions are designed to create additional anxiety at these moments will risk causing further panic and fail to help to create a secure base. This state of affairs is, of course, most likely to occur with individuals, such as those with BPD, who have had exceptionally adverse attachment experiences. When such experiences are reactivated by the process of the therapy, this can lead to distress in the context of the therapeutic relationship. In these instances the balance of mentalizing and attachment needs to be redressed before meaningful therapeutic work can begin to take place. It is our view that all specialist therapies for BPD are organized to prevent overstimulation of the attachment system—for example, all require clinician supervision or consultation with the express aim of preventing clinician overinvolvement with the patient. In contrast, the treatments as usual that are used as comparators in early studies failed to do this and so are likely to have generated iatrogenic effects that undermined mentalizing. More recent general psychiatric interventions are more carefully structured, with clinicians, as we have mentioned, being more "grounded," using a shared theoretical base, and following clear instructions as to how to manage common clinical situations. In addition, more recently supervision and clinician support have been embedded within the framework of general psychiatric treatment.

The third argument in favor of mentalization as a key aspect is that clinicians, with all patients but particularly with those who experience their mental world as diffuse and confusing, will continually construct and reconstruct in their own minds an image of the patient's mind. They label feelings, they explain cognitions, and they spell out implicit beliefs. Techniques for doing these activities are spelled out in all the treatment manuals. Importantly, clinicians engage in a mirroring process, highlighting the marked character of their verbal or nonverbal mirroring displays; that is, showing their mind states while differentiating them from their representations of the patients' mind states. They offer alternative perspectives on shared experience, asking the patients, for example, to consider what is happening in therapy while giving their own understanding of it. So, for example, if a patient believes that the therapist is bored with him because she looked at her watch, the therapist, while validating the patient's experience, may offer an alternative, authentic perspective of what was in her mind, such as worrying about how long they had left in the session to deal with the problem being discussed. Their training and experience further hones their capacity to show that their reactions are related to the patients' states of mind rather than their own. This process stimulates awareness of self and other mentalizing.

Fourth, mentalizing in psychological therapies is prototypically a process of shared, joint attention, in which the interests of patient and clinician intersect in the mental state of the patient. The shared attentional processes entailed by all psychological therapies in our view serve to strengthen the interpersonal integrative function (Fonagy, 2003a). It is not simply what is focused on that we consider therapeutic from this point of view, but the fact that patient and clinician can jointly focus on a shared content of subjectivity and experience.

Fifth, the explicit content of the clinician's intervention will be mentalistic regardless of orientation, whether the clinician is principally concerned with transference reactions, automatic negative thoughts, reciprocal roles, linear thinking, schematic representation, or interpersonal skills development. We suggest that all approaches entail explicit mentalization insofar as they attempt to enhance coherent representations of desires and beliefs even if they aim to help the patient to organize his or her mind through the acquisition of skills. That this is the case is supported by the common experience that such efforts at explicit mentalization will not be successful unless the clinician succeeds in drawing the patient in as an active collaborator in any explication. One may view psychotherapy for individuals with BPD as an integrative process in which implicit and explicit mentalization are brought together in an act of "representational redescription," the term Annette Karmiloff-Smith (1992) used to refer to the process by which "implicit information in the mind subsequently becomes explicit knowledge to the mind" (p. 18).

Sixth and finally, the dyadic nature of therapy inherently fosters the patient's capacity to generate multiple perspectives. For example, the interpretation of the transference may be seen as presenting an alternative perspective on the patient's subjective experience. The identification of primary and secondary emotions allows the patient to reflect more on the complexity of his or her emotional states; the patient begins to recognize that it is not his or her emotion of rage that is the main difficulty, although it might be disproportionate to a current problem, but that his or her reaction of shame about the rage creates interpersonal withdrawal. We view this process as optimally freeing the patient from being restricted to the reality of "one view," experiencing the internal world in a mode of absolutes. This process also becomes accessible through engagement in group psychotherapy. In either individual or group psychotherapy, mental states are necessarily represented at the secondary level and are therefore more likely to be recognized as such, as mental representations. It should be remembered that this will only be helpful if implicit and explicit mentalization have not been dissociated and feelings are genuinely felt rather than just talked about.

In sum, it is our belief that the relatively safe (secure-base) attachment relationship with the clinician provides a relational context in which it is safe to explore the mind of the other in order to find one's own mind within it. Although it is quite likely that this is an adaptation of a mechanism provided to us probably by evolution to "recalibrate" our experience of our own subjectivity through social interaction, it is a unique experience for individuals with BPD because their pathology serves to distort the subjective experience of the other to a point where they have little hope of finding themselves in the relationship. The engagement in a psychotherapeutic context, either individually or in groups, thus does far more than provide nurturance, warmth, or acceptance. The clinician, in holding on to his or her view of the patient and overcoming the patient's uncertainty of him- or herself, fosters mentalizing and a secure attachment experience. Feeling recognized creates a secure-base feeling that in turn promotes the patient's freedom to explore her- or himself in the mind of the clinician. The increased sense of security in the attachment relationship with the clinician, as well as in other attachment relationships, possibly fostered by the therapeutic process, reinforces a secure internal working model and through this, as Bowlby (1988) pointed out, a coherent sense of the self. Simultaneously the patient is increasingly able to allocate mental space to the process of scrutinizing the feelings and thoughts of others, perhaps bringing about improvements in the fundamental competence of the patient's mind-interpreting functions, which in turn may generate a far more benign interpersonal environment. In short, the patient is able to operate flexibly around the different dimensions of mentalizing in an increasingly wider range of contexts.

Mentalizing as a Focus for Effecting Change in Other Personality Disorders

If our focus on mentalizing as a key problem in some personality disorders has traction, it suggests that other personality disorders may be usefully reconsidered in terms of mentalizing problems. More recently we have considered people with antisocial and other personality disorders in terms of the areas of their mentalizing problems and have developed treatments to address these areas.

As we have suggested, people without disorders lose mentalizing at times, and the process itself fluctuates naturally, for example, with context and mood. It follows that personality pathology does not simply arise because of a loss of mentalizing. It occurs for a number of reasons. First, it matters how easily we lose our capacity to mentalize: Some individuals, such as those with BPD, are sensitive and reactive, rapidly moving to nonmentalizing modes in a wide range of contexts. Second, it matters how quickly we regain mentalizing once it has been lost. We have suggested in this chapter and elsewhere that frequent, rapid, and easily provoked losses of mentalizing within interpersonal relationships combined with associated difficulties in regaining mentalizing and the consequent lengthy exposure to nonmentalizing modes of experience is characteristic of BPD (Bateman & Fonagy, 2004). Third, mentalizing can become rigid, lacking flexibility. People with paranoid disorder, for example, often show rigid hypermentalization with regard to their own internal mental states and lack any real understanding of others (Dimaggio, Lysaker, Carcione, Nicolò, & Semerari, 2008a; Nicolò & Nobile, 2007). At best they are suspicious of motives and at worst they see people as having specific malign motives and cannot be persuaded otherwise. The mental processes of people with antisocial personality disorder (ASPD) are less rigid than those found in people with paranoia. Finally, the balance of the components of mentalizing can be distorted. Patients with narcissistic personality have a well-developed self-focus but a very limited understanding of others (Dimaggio et al., 2008b). In contrast, patients with ASPD are experts at reading the inner states of others from a cognitive perspective while being unable to identify affectively or empathically with their states; that is, they demonstrate reasonable other-cognitive mentalizing but lack aspects of other-affective mentalizing. In addition, they misuse their cognitive-other mentalizing abilities to coerce or manipulate others. It is also likely that they avoid self-affective states and so fail to develop any real understanding of their own inner world and their motives (Bateman & Fonagy, 2008). Finally, people with ASPD lack the ability to read certain emotions, or perhaps even a range of emotions, accurately. This is the externally based focus of mentalizing. Although this formulation of the mentalizing problems in ASPD is speculative, it forms the basis for further research and is supported to some degree by our current knowledge.

The link between ASPD and the affective and external components of mentalizing is well established, both developmentally and in adults. Marsh and Blair (2008), in a meta-analysis of 20 studies, showed a robust link between antisocial behavior and specific deficits in recognizing fearful expressions, an external component of mentalizing. This impairment was not attributed solely to task difficulty. Failure to recognize fearful faces implies dysfunction in neural structures such as the amygdala that subserve fearful expression processing. Youths with conduct problems have been shown to have hypoactivation of their amygdalas in response to pictures normally considered emotionally arousing, particularly those in which a potentially painful aggressive act was depicted (Jones, Laurens, Herba, Barker, & Viding, 2009). Amygdala hyporesponsiveness may indicate a dysfunction in limbic structures, leading to reduced responsiveness of the amygdala to fearful faces and consequent impairment in recognizing distress cues in others and thus a lack of empathy and deficient control of aggressive behavior that would normally be inhibited by observation and empathic identification of distress in another (affective-other mentalizing). Alternatively, we may see these abnormalities as reduced sensitivity to stimuli indicating threat (fearlessness). Developmentally it is likely that preferential amygdala responses to fearful faces are reserved for the modulation of vigilance primarily in threatening situations rather than subserving recognition of social cues in everyday situations. However, constitutional fearlessness would stop infants from regularly seeking their attachment figures when experiencing distress; this intersubjective experience of relating in an attachment context is critical for the normal development of mentalizing and social cognition (Fonagy, 2003b). Mentalizing inhibits unwarranted aggression. So there may be a complex interaction between constitutional fearfulness and its effect on the development of the normal mentalizing inhibitory factors that protect against antisocial interaction.

More recently, other researchers (e.g., Dadds, Jambrak, Pasalich, Hawes, & Brennan, 2011) have suggested that antisocial actions and psychopathy may be associated with abnormal attention to socially relevant cues, such as scanning the eyes, and that dysfunction in attentional mechanisms underlies emotion recognition deficits (Dadds, El Masry, Wimalaweera, & Guastella, 2008; Dadds et al., 2006). Lack of attention to the eyes implies a more general problem with the external component of mentalizing and loss of association and interest in links to internal mental states. This suggests there may be an extensive reduction in ability to recognize emotions in others rather than a specific diminution in ability to recognize fear. If deficits in processing emotion cues are pervasive, which would be consistent with the idea of reduced external mentalizing, there are likely to be widespread difficulties in those social and interpersonal interactions requiring empathic and emotional responsiveness. Misreading emotion cues, or more likely not even registering them, will make it more difficult to understand the subtleties of others' perspectives. Certainly the internal affective state, which is a key component of empathy and mentalizing of the other person, will remain a mystery. Examining the role of empathy, the ability to understand and care about the emotions of others, in individuals who are antisocial, Baron-Cohen (2005) found that lack of care for others led to antisocial and destructive behaviors, possibly due to a partial but fundamental impairment of mentalizing, "mindreading without empathizing." So, although not recognizing others' distress cues may be important (Blair, 1995, 2006), additional, more wide-ranging problems related to social and emotional functioning may contribute to the problems facing people with ASPD. This formulation has important clinical implications.

If MBT is beneficial for patients whose BPD is embedded in other personality problems, could it be adapted appropriately for patients with different mentalizing problems, such as those outlined for ASPD? As we have discussed, mentalizing is a key component of self-identity and a central aspect of interpersonal relationships and social functioning, and if personality disorder is conceptualized as a serious impairment in interpersonal relationships, intimacy, identity, and self-direction (Skodol et al., 2011), enhancing mentalizing might benefit personality disorder as a whole, regardless of subtype. This remains to be seen and is the subject of current research. But given the mentalizing understanding of ASPD, MBT for people with ASPD focuses on:

1. Understanding emotional cues—external mentalizing and its link to internal states.
2. Recognition of emotions in others—other-affective mentalizing.
3. Exploration of sensitivity to hierarchy and authority—self-cognitive mentalizing.
4. Generation of an interpersonal process to understand subtleties of others' experience in relation to one's own—self-other mentalizing.

5. Explication of threats to loss of mentalizing that lead to teleological understanding of motivation—self-other mentalizing and self-affective mentalizing.

Mentalizing group therapy is the core mode of treatment. Individual sessions with the group clinician are offered monthly to process problems experienced in the group. This treatment format has been outlined elsewhere (Bateman & Fonagy, 2008). Group work is essential for people with ASPD. Many people with ASPD live within a subculture of barely restrained violence and implicit threats; in this regard they are more likely to be influenced by their peer group than by clinicians, whom they see as unlikely to understand the sociocultural context in which they live. More important, group work stimulates a hierarchical process within a peer group, which can be harnessed *in vivo* by the clinician to explore the participant's sensitivity to hierarchy and authority and his or her mentalizing distortions.

CONCLUDING COMMENTS

Placing mentalization as central to therapy with patients with BPD and other people with personality disorder may unify numerous effective approaches to the treatment of this challenging group of patients. Although it provides a common understanding of why a range of disparate approaches all "work," the implication of this formulation is not that all approaches are equally effective and the best approach is a judicious combination of existing techniques. The way forward cannot be a mix-and-match system, using techniques as and when the clinician thinks it is appropriate. This would deliver unstructured treatments without coherence. It is to generate an increasingly coherent theory of the disorder, underpinned by an understanding of mechanisms of change, and to translate this into a carefully crafted therapeutic package. Only then is it likely that people with BPD and other personality disorders will have a better chance of functional improvement. Our argument presented here suggests that treatments must (1) meet certain organizational requirements, (2) have particular characteristics in the way that the different components are knitted together, (3) emphasize the importance of managing carefully the patient–therapist interaction, and (4) use techniques that directly or indirectly increase the robustness of the patient's mentalizing capacity. Such qualities as these are not specific to any one psychotherapy. Indeed, if we are correct, general mental health clinicians should be able to offer patients with personality disorders safe intervention in community psychiatric services without receiving extensive additional training. Recent evidence suggests that this is the case, with specialist treatments showing less advantage than hitherto. The widespread availability of a general treatment meeting these basic criteria would improve the experience and outcomes of this neglected group of patients beyond recognition. The question now is not so much which specialist treatment is better than another but which patients with personality disorder, if any, require a specialist treatment.

REFERENCES

Akhtar, S. (1992). *Broken structures: Severe personality disorders and their treatment.* Northvale, NJ: Aronson.

Allen, J., & Fonagy, P. (2002). *The development of mentalizing and its role in psychopathology and psychotherapy* (Technical Report No. 02-0048). Topeka, KS: Menninger Clinic, Research Department.

Allen, J. G., Fonagy, P., & Bateman, A. (2008). *Mentalizing in clinical practice.* Washington, DC: American Psychiatric Publishing.

Appelbaum, A. H. (2006). Supportive psychoanalytic psychotherapy for borderline patients: An empirical approach. *American Journal of Psychoanalysis, 66,* 317–332.

Baron-Cohen, S. (1995). *Mindblindness: An essay on autism and theory of mind.* Cambridge, MA: MIT Press.

Baron-Cohen, S. (2005). Autism. In B. Hopkins with R. Barr, G. Michel, & P. Rochat (Eds.), *The Cambridge encyclopedia of child development* (pp. 398–401). Cambridge, UK: Cambridge University Press.

Bateman, A. (2012). Treating borderline personality disorder in clinical practice. *American Journal of Psychiatry, 169,* 1–4.

Bateman, A., & Fonagy, P. (2000). Effectiveness of psychotherapeutic treatment of personality disorder. *British Journal of Psychiatry, 177,* 138–143.

Bateman, A., & Fonagy, P. (2004). *Psychotherapy for borderline personality disorder: Mentalisation-based treatment.* Oxford, UK: Oxford University Press.

Bateman, A., & Fonagy, P. (2006). *Mentalization-based treatment: A practical guide.* Oxford, UK: Oxford University Press.

Bateman, A., & Fonagy, P. (2008). Comorbid antisocial and borderline personality disorders: Mentalization-based treatment. *Journal of Clinical Psychology: In Session, 64,* 1–14.

Bateman, A., & Fonagy, P. (2009). Randomized controlled trial of outpatient mentalization-based treatment versus structured clinical management for borderline personality disorder. *American Journal of Psychiatry, 166,* 1355–1364.

Bateman, A., & Fonagy, P. (2012). *Handbook of mentalizing in mental health practice.* Washington, DC: American Psychiatric Publishing.

Bateman, A., & Krawitz, R. (2013). *Borderline personality disorder: An evidence-based guide for generalist mental health professionals.* Oxford, UK: Oxford University Press.

Betan, E., Heim, A. K., Zittel Conklin, C., & Westen, D. (2005). Countertransference phenomena and personality pathology in clinical practice: An empirical investigation. *American Journal of Psychiatry, 162*(5), 890–898.

Blair, R. J. R. (1995). A cognitive developmental approach to morality: Investigating the psychopath. *Cognition, 57,* 1–29.

Blair, R. J. R. (2006). The emergence of psychopathy: Implications for the neuropsychological approach to developmental disorders. *Cognition, 101,* 414–442.

Bleiberg, E. (2001). *Treating personality disorders in children and adolescents: A relational approach.* New York: Guilford Press.

Bowlby, J. (1988). *A secure base: Clinical applications of attachment theory*. London: Routledge.

Brown, K. W., & Ryan, R. M. (2003). The benefits of being present: Mindfulness and its role in psychological well-being. *Journal of Personality and Social Psychology, 84,* 822–848.

Chanen, A. M., Jackson, H. J., McCutcheon, L. K., Jovev, M., Dudgeon, P., Yuen, H. P., et al. (2008). Early intervention for adolescents with borderline personality disorder using cognitive analytic therapy: Randomised controlled trial. *British Journal of Psychiatry, 193*(6), 477–484.

Choi-Kain, L. W., & Gunderson, J. G. (2008). Mentalization: Ontogeny, assessment, and application in the treatment of borderline personality disorder. *American Journal of Psychiatry, 165*(9), 1127–1135.

Clarkin, J. F., Levy, K. N., Lenzenweger, M. F., & Kernberg, O. (2004). The Personality Disorders Institute/Borderline Personality Disorder Research Foundation randomised controlled trial for borderline personality disorder: Rationale, methods, and patient characteristics. *Journal of Personality Disorders, 18,* 52–72.

Clarkin, J. F., Levy, K. N., Lenzenweger, M. F., & Kernberg, O. (2007). Evaluating three treatments for borderline personality disorder. *American Journal of Psychiatry, 164,* 922–928.

Dadds, M. R., El Masry, Y., Wimalaweera, S., & Guastella, A. J. (2008). Reduced eye gaze explains fear blindness in childhood psychopathic traits. *Journal of the American Academy of Child and Adolescent Psychiatry, 47,* 455–463.

Dadds, M. R., Jambrak, J., Pasalich, D., Hawes, D. J., & Brennan, J. (2011). Impaired attention to the eyes of attachment figures and the developmental origins of psychopathy. *Journal of Child Psychology and Psychiatry and Allied Disciplines, 52,* 238–245.

Dadds, M. R., Perry, Y., Hawes, D. J., Merz, S., Riddell, A. C., Haines, D. J., et al. (2006). Attention to the eyes and fear-recognition deficits in child psychopathy. *British Journal of Psychiatry: The Journal of Mental Science, 189,* 280–281.

Dimaggio, G., Lysaker, P. H., Carcione, A., Nicolò, G., & Semerari, A. (2008). Know yourself and you shall know the other . . . to a certain extent: Multiple paths of influence of self-reflection on mindreading. *Consciousness and Cognition, 17*(3), 778–789.

Dimaggio, G., Nicolò, G., Fiore, D., Centenero, E., Semerari, A., Carcione, A., et al. (2008). States of minds in narcissistic personality disorder: Three psychotherapies analyzed using the grid of problematic states. *Psychotherapy Research, 18*(4), 466–480.

Doering, S., Hörz, S., Rentrop, M., Fischer-Kern, M., Schuster, P., & Benecke, C. (2010). Transference-focused psychotherapy v. treatment by community psychotherapists for borderline personality disorder: Randomised controlled trial. *British Journal of Psychiatry, 196,* 389–395.

Feigenbaum, J. D., Fonagy, P., Pilling, S., Jones, A., Wildgoose, A., & Bebbington, P. E. (2011). A real-world study of the effectiveness of DBT in the UK National Health Service. *British Journal of Clinical Psychology, 51*(2), 121–141.

Fonagy, P. (2003a). The development of psychopathology from infancy to adulthood. *Infant Mental Health Journal, 24,* 212–239.

Fonagy, P. (2003b). Towards a developmental understanding of violence. *British Journal of Psychiatry, 183,* 190–192.

Fonagy, P., & Bateman, A. (2006a). Mechanisms of change in mentalization-based therapy of borderline personality disorder. *Journal of Clinical Psychology, 62*, 411–430.

Fonagy, P., & Bateman, A. (2006b). Progress in the treatment of borderline personality disorder. *British Journal of Psychiatry, 188*, 1–3.

Fonagy, P., & Bateman, A. (2008a). Attachment, mentalisation, and borderline personality disorder. *European Psychotherapy, 8*, 35–47.

Fonagy, P., & Bateman, A. (2008b). The development of borderline personality disorder: A mentalizing model. *Journal of Personality Disorders, 22*(1), 4–21.

Fonagy, P., Gergely, G., Jurist, E. L., & Target, M. (2002). *Affect regulation, mentalisation and the development of the self.* New York: Other Press.

Fonagy. P., & Target, M. (1997). Attachment and reflective function: Their role in self-organization. *Development and Psychopathology, 9*, 679–700.

Gunderson, J. G. (2008). *Borderline personality disorder: A clinical guide.* Washington, DC: American Psychiatric Publishing.

Gunderson, J. G. (2011). Clinical practice: Borderline personality disorder. *New England Journal of Medicine, 364*(21), 2037–2042.

Gunderson, J. G., & Lyons-Ruth, K. (2008). BPD's interpersonal hypersensitivity phenotype: A gene–environment–developmental model. *Journal of Personality Disorders, 22*, 22–41.

Gunderson, J. G., Stout, R. L., McGlashan, T. H., Shea, M. T,, Morey, L. C., Grilo, C. M., et al. (2011). Ten-year course of borderline personality disorder: Psychopathology and function from the Collaborative Longitudinal Personality Disorders Study. *Archives of General Psychiatry, 68*, 827–837.

Jones, A. P., Laurens, K. R., Herba, C. M., Barker, G. J., & Viding, E. (2009). Amygdala hypoactivity to fearful faces in boys with conduct problems and callous-unemotional traits. *American Journal of Psychiatry, 166*, 95–102.

Jurist, E. J. (2005). Mentalized affectivity. *Psychoanalytic Psychology, 22*, 426–444.

Karmiloff-Smith, A. (1992). *Beyond modularity: A developmental perspective on cognitive science.* Cambridge, MA: MIT Press.

Kernberg, O. F. (1983). Object relations theory and character analysis. *Journal of the American Psychoanalytic Association, 31*, 247–271.

King-Casas, B., Sharp, C., Lomax-Bream, L., Lohrenz, T., Fonagy, P., & Read Montague, P. (2008). The rupture and repair of cooperation in borderline personality disorder. *Science, 321*, 806–810.

Linehan, M. M. (1993). *Cognitive-behavioral treatment of borderline personality disorder.* New York: Guilford Press.

Linehan, M. M., Armstrong, H., Suarez, A., Allmon, D., & Heard, H. (1991). Cognitive-behavioural treatment of chronically parasuicidal borderline patients. *Archives of General Psychiatry, 48*, 1060–1064.

Linehan, M. M., Comtois, K. A., Murray, A. M., Brown, M. Z., Gallop, R. J., Heard, H. L., et al. (2006). Two-year randomized controlled trial and follow-up of dialectical behavior therapy vs. therapy by experts for suicidal behaviors and borderline personality disorder. *Archives of General Psychiatry, 63*(7), 757–766.

Linehan, M. M., Heard, H. L., & Armstrong, H. E. (1993). Naturalistic follow-up of a behavioral treatment for chronically parasuicidal borderline patients. *Archives of General Psychiatry, 50*, 971–974.

Luyten, P., Fonagy, P., Mayes, L. C., Vermote, R., Lowyck, B., & Bateman, A. (2013). *Broadening the scope of the mentalization based approach to psychopathology: mentalization as a multi-dimensional construct.* Manuscript submitted for publication.

Lynch, T. R., Rosenthal, M. Z., Kosson, D. S., Cheavens, J. S., Lejuez, C. W., & Blair, R. J. (2006). Heightened sensitivity to facial expressions of emotion in borderline personality disorder. *Emotion, 6*(4), 647–655.

Marsh, A. A., & Blair, R. J. (2008). Deficits in facial affect recognition among antisocial populations: A meta-analysis. *Neuroscience and Biobehavioral Reviews, 32,* 454–465.

McMain, S., Guimond, T., Cardish, R., Streiner, D., & Links, P. (2012). Clinical outcomes and functioning post-treatment: A two-year follow-up of dialectical behavior therapy versus general psychiatric management for borderline personality disorder. *American Journal of Psychiatry, 169,* 650–661.

McMain, S., Links, P., Gnam, W., Guimond, T., Cardish, R., Korman, L., et al. (2009). A randomized controlled trial of dialectical behaviour therapy versus general psychiatric management for borderline personality disorder. *American Journal of Psychiatry, 166,* 1365–1374.

Neacsiu, A. D., Rizvi, S. L., & Linehan, M. M. (2010). Dialectical behavior therapy skills use as a mediator and outcome of treatment for borderline personality disorder. *Behaviour Research and Therapy, 48*(9), 832–839.

Nicolò, G., & Nobile, M. (2007). Paranoid personality disorder: Model and treatment. In G. Dimaggio & A. Semerari (Eds.), *Psychotherapy of personality disorders* (pp. 188–220). Hove, UK: Routledge.

Siegel, D. J. (1999). *The developing mind: Toward a neurobiology of interpersonal experience.* New York: Guilford Press.

Skodol, A. E., Clark, L. A., Bender, D., Krueger, R. F., Morey, L. C., Verheul, R., et al. (2011). Proposed changes in personality and personality disorder assessment and diagnosis for DSM-5: Part I. Description and rationale. *Personality Disorders: Theory, Research, and Treatment, 2,* 4–22.

Skodol, A. E., Gunderson, J. G., Pfohl, B., Widiger, T. A., Livesley, W. J., & Siever, L. J. (2002). The borderline diagnosis: I. Psychopathology, comorbidity, and personality structure. *Biological Psychiatry, 51*(12), 936–950.

Stone, M. H. (1990). *The fate of borderline patients: Successful outcome and psychiatric practice.* New York: Guilford Press.

Verheul, R., Van Den Bosch, L. M., Koeter, M. W., De Ridder, M. A., Stijnen, T., & Van Den Brink, W. (2003). Dialectical behaviour therapy for women with borderline personality disorder: 12-month, randomised clinical trial in The Netherlands. *British Journal of Psychiatry, 182,* 135–140.

Wagner, A. W., & Linehan, M. M. (1999). Facial expression recognition ability among women with borderline personality disorder: Implications for emotion regulation? *Journal of Personality Disorders, 13*(4), 329–344.

Westen, D., & Cohen, R. P. (1993). The self in borderline personality disorder: A psychodynamic perspective. In Z. V. Segal & S. J. Blatt (Eds.), *The self in emotional distress: Cognitive and psychodynamic perspectives* (pp. 334–360). New York and London: Guilford Press.

Zanarini, M. C., Frankenburg, F. R., Reich, D. B., & Fitzmaurice, G. (2010). The 10-year course of psychosocial functioning among patients with borderline personality disorder and Axis II comparison subjects. *Acta Psychiatrica Scandinavica, 122*(2), 103–109.

Zanarini, M., Frankenburg, F. R., Reich, D., & Fitzmaurice, G. (2012). Attainment and stability of sustained symptomatic remission and recovery among patients with borderline personality disorder and Axis II comparison subjects: A 16-year prospective follow-up study. *American Journal of Psychiatry, 169*, 476–483.

chapter 8

Improving Metacognition by Accessing Autobiographical Memories

Giancarlo Dimaggio, Raffaele Popolo, Antonino Carcione, and Giampaolo Salvatore

Clinicians dealing with personality disorders need to overcome two prominent barriers to treatment: poor metacognition, or difficulty understanding the mental states of oneself and others, and impoverished self-narratives, that is, the inability to provide rich and nuanced autobiographical memories conveying the correlates of subjective experience. An impoverished self-narrative and limited self-knowledge and self-understanding are formidable obstacles to treatment because they result in both clinicians and patients being unclear about the problems contributing to distress, especially the cognitive–affective processes underlying impaired interpersonal functioning and affect regulation. Hence, without an enriched self-narrative and increased awareness of the psychological mechanisms underlying symptoms and social dysfunctions, it is difficult to delineate targets for change.

A patient with avoidant and obsessive–compulsive features, with problems at work where he feels overwhelmed, may describe himself as prey to panic attacks and general tension and distress but is unable to elaborate on what he thinks and feels and what the "tension" and "distress" mean. He may also feel socially alienated, lonely, and depressed but unable to provide anything more than intellectualized statements about the reasons for his suffering and alienation, such as "Doing one's duty is very important in modern society" or "People should be more responsible, and I am different from other, more callous, people." Faced with such a limited self-understanding, a therapist can offer only simple behavioral strategies for dealing with anxiety or prescribe medication, but it is unlikely that the processes underlying the personality dysfunction will respond to these interventions. Promoting autobiographical memory and improving metacognition or self-awareness may, after a few sessions, yield more reflective self-descriptions, such as: "When the boss told me he had no time to talk with me, I thought he was unhappy with my performance and that he would give me a negative evaluation and I'd get fired. I returned to my desk and worked doggedly all day trying to fill the gaps. Once I got home, I started to sweat, my legs were trembling, and I was convinced I was about to faint."

With such an episode, the cognitive–affective processes underlying the panic attacks are clearer, as are the interpersonal expectations underpinning the suffering: The patient fears social criticism, tends to interpret others' behavior as signs of criticism and rejection, and copes by becoming perfectionistic, and there is always the underlying fear of impending failure. Such a case formulation is a good basis for creating a therapy plan aimed first at improving self-understanding and then at changing the cognitive–affective processes underlying personality pathology.

In this chapter, we briefly outline the pathologies involving impaired self-narratives and metacognition and describe how they hinder treatment and the establishment of a good therapeutic relationship. Subsequently, we provide formalized step-by-step procedures (Dimaggio, Salvatore, Nicolò, Fiore, & Procacci, 2010; Dimaggio et al., 2011, 2012) for enriching patients' narratives and promoting metacognition until they begin to see their descriptions of interpersonal relationships as internalized patterns and not mere reflections of reality. The overarching goal of this chapter is to provide the clinician with a strategy for working with the patient to build the psychological knowledge and understanding needed to change impaired emotional regulation and interpersonal functioning. We consider this to be a general strategy that is a central part of therapy for all patients with personality disorders.

NARRATIVE IMPOVERISHMENT

Many patients suffering from personality disorders find it difficult to describe why they suffer and what causes their problems. Many describe the reasons for their problems in intellectualized ways or theorize about why relationships go awry without providing supporting evidence from relational episodes (Dimaggio, Semerari, et al., 2007; Spinhoven, Bamelis, Molendijk, Haringsma, & Arntz, 2009). For example, they may note that the atmosphere at work is tense or that marital relationships are a source of distress for everyone in the Western world, but when their clinicians ask for specific autobiographical episodes exemplifying what happens in their lives, they are scarcely able to provide any. They also tend to externalize responsibility for their difficulties by blaming others without providing any clear account of what others and they themselves actually did, thought, or felt during a specific moment when problems arose. Statements such as "I've always kept my girlfriends at a distance because I want to preserve my freedom," "My relationships always head south because men are unreliable" convey little knowledge and fail to provide the clinician with the information needed to understand the patient.

To develop a case formulation and plan treatment, the clinician needs to understand and describe the cognitive–emotional structures and processes guiding actions that may be identified from the examination of specific autobiographical episodes. These processes are like maps that show how (1) the person needs to act in order to fulfill his or her motives; (2) others might respond; and (3) the self typically reacts in order to cope with problems and setbacks. Note that these processes are consistent with the idea of problematic interpersonal schemas and Luborsky's and Crits-Christoph's (1990) formulation of the core conflictual relationship theme. The maps include (4) strategies for avoiding suffering and compromise solutions for accomplishing a wish after negative reactions from relevant others.

Narrative episodes are the most productive way to access the elements of subjective experience—emotions, beliefs, plans, and forecasts—needed to construct a shared understanding of a patient's mentalistic world and craft a joint plan for achieving wellness.

METACOGNITIVE DYSFUNCTIONS

Personality disorders feature difficulties in reasoning about mental states, that is, individuals' metacognitive capacities are reduced (Dimaggio & Lysaker, 2010; Dimaggio, Semerari, Carcione, Nicolò, & Procacci, 2007; Semerari, Dimaggio, Nicolò, Procacci, & Carcione, 2007). Examples of dysfunctional metacognitive acts include difficulty describing inner states, such as labeling different forms of emotional arousal; problems understanding the interpersonal events that elicited an emotion, such as anger triggered by impending rejection; difficulty inferring emotions from facial expression, posture, and prosody; and difficulty inferring the intent behind others' overt behaviors.

Another key element in metacognitive dysfunction is a lack of awareness that one's opinion about oneself and the other is just a point of view, which can change when things are seen from a different angle. This problem is termed *poor differentiation* or *lack of critical distance*—a failure to differentiate between one's ideas and reality (see Bateman & Fonagy, 2004; also Chapter 7, this volume). When this occurs, patients are guided by stereotyped expectations about how to behave in order to accomplish their goals, about how others will typically react, and what the fate of their innermost desires will be. They are unaware of these patterns and thus consider their beliefs to mirror the truth. They are unable to question their beliefs by adopting a third-party observer's perspective.

For example, a patient looking for appreciation from her boss might describe him as spiteful and favoring other, less talented colleagues, and she will continue to insist that this perception is true. In treatment, she may need to be helped to form a metarepresentation in which she acknowledges that this may be partially true but that also reflects her schema in which she feels constantly undervalued, a schema grounded on memories of reference figures who were contemptuous and unfair. In short, patients with personality disorder take their schemas or interpretations of events as fixed, concrete realities, rather than one of several possible constructions of the same events, and they do not recognize that others may see the same events differently.

Although metacognitive or mentalistic dysfunction has long been hypothesized to be a typical feature of personality disorder (Fonagy, 1991), it is only recently that empirical support has emerged. Current knowledge about metacognitive dysfunctions in personality disorder suggest that metacognition has multiple components (Dimaggio & Lysaker, 2010) and that impairments can occur in some forms of metacognition but not others. For example, a patient may have no difficulty describing his or her emotions but be unable to infer mental states of others from facial expressions. Nevertheless, some types of impairment are found in many forms of personality disorder. Thus alexithymia, or poor emotional awareness (Taylor, Bagby, & Parker, 1997), occurs in patients with avoidant, dependent, passive–aggressive, schizoid, borderline, or depressive personality disorders (Grabe, Spitzer, & Freyberger, 2004; Nicolò et al., 2011) and in women with eating disorders and narcissism (Lawson, Waller, Sines, & Meyer, 2008). A consistent finding is that avoidant personality disorder features alexithymia more than do other disorders (Nicolò et al., 2011). Clinical observation also suggests that persons with more severe personality pathology tend to have widespread metacognitive impairments (Colle, d'Angerio, Popolo, & Dimaggio, 2010). Overall, research suggests that metacognitive difficulties are indeed a feature of personality disorders. They include difficulties in guessing others' emotions from faces (Domes et al., 2008); forming complex and nuanced representations of the self with others (Semerari et al., 2005); and taking the other's perspective (Dimaggio et al., 2009). As the empirical evidence of a metacognitive disorder in personality disorder grows, it becomes increasingly apparent that improving metacognition or mentalizing is a key element in any personality disorder therapy. The more clinicians are informed about the actual dysfunctions they will find in personality disorder, the more they can tailor treatment accordingly (Allen, Fonagy, & Bateman, 2008; Dimaggio & Lysaker, 2010). Case formulation requires an assessment of the metacognitive problems detected and the need to adjust therapy operations accordingly, and examining these needs is one of the goals of this chapter.

POOR SELF-NARRATIVES AND IMPAIRED METACOGNITION AS BARRIERS TO TREATMENT

Poor self-narrative and dysfunctional metacognition hinder therapy. One reason is that these impairments, especially limited capacity for autobiographical thinking, force many patients to use intellectualizations to explain their suffering and relationship problems rather than using more detailed accounts of their experience. Intellectualizations and general statements such as "too many persons are self-centered, which is why I and other sensitive people suffer" are often hard to address in therapy because patients firmly hold these beliefs to be true and any attempt to challenge them leads to deterioration in the therapeutic alliance, with minimal increase in self-awareness. Moreover, such intellectualizations limit self-understanding by glossing over the details of specific experiences about what happened, how one felt, and how one behaved—the very details that the therapist and patient need to understand to promote change. Hence the promotion of emotional awareness is essential because emotions are the driving force behind maladaptive actions and decisions. Actually, emotionally laden autobiographical episodes provide reliable knowledge about what a person truly felt and thought at a specific moment and what the cognitive–affective processes taking control of their behavior were. Put simply, one person might describe himself as a devoted father, but, when invited to recall specific episodes, he might talk only about punishing his little daughter for misbehaving without displaying any verbal or nonverbal sign of warmth and playfulness.

Poor metacognition also hinders treatment. For example, when a patient with narcissistic personality disorder describes his experience as "tension" or "discomfort," a therapist can see that the patient is trying to communicate his distress but is unable to make sense of its contents. At this level, one potentially suitable intervention is to try to empathize with the distress and solicit involvement in shared attempts at further exploring the underlying states of mind. Moreover, knowing that the patient has difficulties in accessing his own emotions and putting them in words helps a clinician overcome the negative reactions that patients with emotional unawareness typically elicit (Ogrodniczuk, Piper, & Joyce, 2011; Vanheule, Verhaeghe, & Desmet, 2011).

Another metacognitive dysfunction that hinders treatment occurs when patients have difficulty understanding what event elicited a thought and emotion or what emotion led to a specific behavior. Patients may describe an affect but not be able to say what fueled it. They may mention their coping behaviors, for example, avoidance, but be unable to say why they avoid a particular situation or why sometimes they even fear it. Later we make suggestions about how to promote awareness of emotions, their triggers, and their role in activating behaviors.

Another metacognitive dysfunction is difficulty in questioning one's own ideas and understanding that they do not necessarily mirror reality, a phenomenon referred to earlier as poor differentiation. A recent study, for example, showed that patients with borderline personality disorder (BPD) were similar to healthy controls in understanding the emotions in targets' eyes but were overconfident in their judgments (Schilling et al., 2012). This suggests that once patients with BPD form an impression, they have difficulty revising their impression and recognizing the subjective element to their conclusion. A patient with obsessive–compulsive and dependent traits may say her spouse or boss controls her life and that she is unable to do anything about it because the other is domineering and she feels inadequate and subjugated. We argue that there is little point at this stage in trying to push the patient toward considering such a representation to be a maladaptive schema-driven belief and to consider alternative interpretations because the patient is likely to stick to her interpretation. Therefore, promoting differentiation too early is likely to lead to conflict, so one goal of this chapter is to provide clinicians with procedures that will minimize any potential conflicts by promoting differentiation and the understanding that attributions are often schema-driven or that schemas dictate overreacting to cues that have been carefully appraised but that the patient cannot let go. Moreover, with narcissistic or paranoid patterns, when others are considered to deserve humiliation or to be threatened, thus justifying preventive aggression, there is no point arguing or promoting a more compassionate view of the others. A therapist risks taking side with the others described in the episode and entering a battle with the patient, who eventually includes the therapist in the negative pattern.

In summary, poor or disorganized self-narratives hinder treatment because patients do not use autobiographical memories to describe their self-experience. This leaves the therapist unclear about what actually triggered their thoughts, emotions, and behaviors during relational episodes so that it is difficult to link events with emotional and cognitive reactions. Also, such patients have problems understanding the emotional significance of events and seeing the role of emotions in the chain of events. Note that many therapies for personality disorder insist that looking for such chain-effect links at very specific moments in space and time (i.e., autobiographical memories) is the key starting point for understanding the psychological processes causing dysfunctional behaviors and maladaptation (Bateman & Fonagy, 2004; Dimaggio, Semerari, et al., 2007; Linehan, 1993). Another metacognitive dysfunction is difficulty differentiating representations from reality, which limits patients' perception of options and hinders treatment because patients cling to existing conceptions or representations. Metacognitive problems easily fuel countertransference problems because therapists can get bored or frustrated by the patients' difficulties describing their emotions and their tendency to stick to their convictions.

There are other impairments in the metacognitive system that we do not describe here for space reasons—for example, difficulties in perspective taking and in using psychological knowledge of self and others to solve conflicts, negotiate goals, and empathize with others and problems in forming an integrated picture of one's various self–other representations, such as "I am a loving father" or "I am a harsh teacher," that allow development of coherence and a stable sense of identity. We deal with such problems in other chapters of this book (Dimaggio, Popolo, Carcione, Salvatore, & Stiles, Chapter 17; Salvatore, Popolo, & Dimaggio, Chapter 19). Here we focus on manualized procedures for eliciting and using autobiographical memories to explore mental states and construct more nuanced self-representations.

STEP-BY-STEP PROCEDURES FOR ENRICHING SELF-NARRATIVES AND FOSTERING METACOGNITION

This section outlines a series of step-by-step procedures to enrich autobiographical episodes and explore the correlates of subjective experience in order to promote metacognition (Dimaggio et al., 2010, 2012). Patients' increased metacognitive awareness of the reasons for their suffering can then be used to change personality structures and maladaptive behavioral patterns. We focus on eliciting the details of autobiographical episodes and promoting metacognition using the following steps: (1) fostering awareness of emotions and dominant beliefs; (2) understanding psychological causality, such as how others' actions evoke a belief that in turn triggers an emotion and how that emotion leads to actions; (3) evoking a series of associated episodes to promote awareness of stable patterns and subsequently reformulate schemas; and (4) achieving metacognitive differentiation, or a critical distance, from internalized meaning-making patterns. We suggest that other procedures, such as treating symptoms (see Links & Bergmans, Chapter 9, this volume), changing maladaptive relational patterns (see Cain & Pincus, Chapter 14, this volume) or creating new self-narratives (see Dimaggio et al., Chapter 17, this volume), are more easily achieved after these steps have been completed and the patient and therapist possess a sophisticated knowledge of the cognitive–affective processes leading to suffering and malfunctioning.

Eliciting the Details of Autobiographical Episodes

The more self-presentation relies on autobiographical memories instead of intellectualizations, the easier it is to formulate a collaborative understanding of the causes of a patient's problems. We outline a series of techniques to promote a switch from intellectualized to autobiographical memory modes.

The process begins by using patients' intellectualizations as cues to guide investigation. For example, a patient might talk about slights to her or his self-esteem. Therapists should pose focused questions about space and time boundaries. Where did the incident occur? At home? Work? When did it take place? This is then followed by inquiries about the persons involved, the actual dialogue, and associated actions to promote activation of the autobiographical memory mode. For example, "You said your relationship with your husband is frustrating and you have nothing in common. Could you provide a specific example of that? Did you have an argument recently?" If the patient agrees, the therapist could continue by asking, "When did it happen? Where were you? Were you alone, or with friends or family? Could you tell me how the argument went? What did you say, how did he react and what did you then do or say?" (Angus & McLeod, 2004; Hermans & Dimaggio, 2004; Luborsky & Crits-Christoph, 1990; Neimeyer, 2000).

We find that the process is facilitated by explaining the value of exploring specific memories. We explain that providing details about a specific incident makes the event more vivid and may help the patient to recapture how he or she felt. The following example, taken from therapy with a man named Pietro who was suffering from narcissistic personality disorder with obsessive–compulsive, depressive, and passive–aggressive traits, shows how this patient was able to switch from an intellectualizing thinking style to recalling autobiographical memories.

> Pietro, age 36 years, sought therapy for panic attacks and a sense of emptiness. He became depressed when he realized his grandiose expectations about his university career were doomed to failure. He tends to intellectualize, and as a consequence his therapist finds him detached and aloof. In the early sessions, he reported having problems in his romantic life but gave little information about what actually happened with his girlfriend. A typical narrative was: "Perhaps every time I get interested in a girl, I try to adapt to that person without really being myself. I believe it all depends on self-esteem because, if one tries to be recognized by the other, then one tries to understand what the other wants and to adapt to that." The therapist cannot understand what he is feeling and whether he is reacting to something the woman actually does or does not do. Pietro speaks more like the author of a philosophical essay than a suffering person. The therapist avoids questioning his theories and tries instead to elicit an emotionally significant autobiographical episode with focused questions, such as "Pietro, you're talking about issues that are very relevant to you: self-esteem or being accepted by someone you feel attracted to. Can you recall a specific episode in which you felt those issues were at stake?" Pietro is unable to recall a particular narrative episode and continues intellectualizing, although he furnishes an extra element: His life currently revolves around Milena, a former student of his, with whom he has been having an affair for 6 months. The therapist therefore continues asking Pietro for a specific example of the problematic aspects of his relationship with Milena. Pietro continues theorizing: "Perhaps I'm asking myself at this moment in my life what I've been doing up to now. . . . Perhaps I've in general a need for greater concreteness." This points to ongoing difficulty in accessing the autobiographical memory mode, something the therapist needs to highlight and put on the therapeutic blackboard for joint consideration.
>
> The therapist says he has difficulty understanding what Pietro feels, although he is eager to do so: "I realize we're looking at a very important question. I find your arguments shrewd and polished, but I still can't

grasp what you feel. Think of when we're reading a book: There are the theoretical parts, descriptions of landscapes, and then right after that the characters' actions and emotions. They captivate us much more than the rest because we identify with them and we feel we are on stage. This is why I've asked you several times to relate an episode to me, so that I could be there, on stage, with you. I'd like to ask you to make the effort of relating a specific episode in your relationship with Milena—it can be either recent or more in the past—in which you felt that your self-esteem was the main question at stake."

This request—made after gauging the quality of the therapy relationship (see Tufekcioglu & Muran, Chapter 6, this volume) and ensuring that Pietro did not feel criticized—helped him to describe some episodes. This change did not last, and in the next session he returned to intellectualizing; nevertheless, it represented an important step toward improved access to specific autobiographical memories.

Another method for digging deeper into patients' narratives is to note the central problematic theme in the narrative and ask the patient to try during the forthcoming week to identify events associated with the theme. For example, the therapist may note a theme of feeling harshly criticized and ask the patient to pay attention to events in which someone has been spiteful toward him or her. This helps patients to become more self-aware and self-reflective and to train themselves to rely on autobiographical memories and to hold details of these experiences in working memory. Moreover, the telling of an episode easily triggers the embodied reactivation of that experience, making it likely that the person will reexperience the same feelings.

We think it helpful to try to steer patients' attention consistently toward narratives until access to specific memories becomes easier. In our experience, some patients with intellectualizing tendencies start to recognize that they are intellectualizing and using generalized statements and then note ironically that "You do want an episode, don't you?" to which the reply is: "Correct!" In contrast, with patients with more dysregulated features who tend to recall a large number of episodes, the treatment process is a little different. With these patients, the sheer amount of material recalled obscures the details, and thus, after promoting emotional regulation, the goal is to focus on exploring a specific memory in detail. Overall, narrative episodes are a fertile terrain for accessing mental states and thus improving metacognition or mentalization (see Bateman & Fonagy, Chapter 7, this volume), the next step in our procedure.

Promoting Metacognition: Step 1. Awareness of Emotions and Dominant Beliefs

Once a few narrative episodes have been elicited, they can be used to explore inner experience—what the patient actually thought and felt when interacting with others. The first option is to directly ask about the mental states experienced during episodes while adopting an open-minded stance and trying not to influence the patient's response. This is often successful in patients with some personality disorders such as BPD. Focused questions are the first tool for steering patients' attention to subjective experience. Questions need to be anchored to specific moments in an episode: "When your partner was in the kitchen, didn't look you in the eyes, and told you things were finished between you, what did you feel?"

Nevertheless, with many inhibited or emotionally overregulated patients, direct questions often elicit no response or just vague answers, such as "I felt tense." The therapist should then focus on changes in prosody or facial expression to identify signs of the emergence of specific affects or thoughts: "I know it's hard for you to describe what you feel, but, when you mentioned your partner turned her back on you and avoided facing you, your expression changed. Before that you looked angry, but then perhaps I saw a twinge of sadness. Was that the case?" Feedback about such hypotheses should be sought to avoid disparity between the therapist's observations and the patient's experience, and the therapist must gauge carefully whether the patient's acceptance of the therapist's guesses really corresponds to what he or she thought and felt or whether he or she is merely trying to please the therapist. If a patient partially disagrees with the therapist's attributions, the therapist can start a dialogical process in which both try to form more refined hypotheses until the patient is satisfied with the description of her or his inner experience. Therapists should be careful to step back from their initial ideas and adjust their perspectives to the patient's reactions until they are sure the patient feels understood. As the patients' mental states become clearer, new details of the episode emerge and initiate a positive cycle of improved metacognition and enriched narratives.

Initial attempts to promote metacognition can fail if patients become defensive or perceive the therapist as domineering or imposing his or her own ideas on them. If this happens, the focus may strategically shift from states of mind to topics that are easier to talk about until the alliance is restored and inner states can be explored again.

With some patients, the problem is not only poor affect awareness but also low emotional arousal, which makes narratives devoid of inner states and flattens the therapy conversation. In this case, the therapist can enliven the therapeutic relationship with humor or by encouraging patients to talk about matters that vitalize them. Once patients start to access their inner states, the next step is to understand the links among elements of patients' mental states, for example, what event triggered an affect or how cognition, affects, and behaviors are bound to each other.

Promoting Metacognition: Step 2. Understanding Psychological Causality

One key component of the change process is for patients to understand the psychological cause–effect links between events, emotions, thoughts, and subsequent behaviors, and, once this is achieved, to understand how others react to their behavior and how others' responses influence the patients' own reactions. Once a patient develops the ability to describe thoughts and express somatic sensations in emotional language, the time is ripe to develop an understanding of the causal links among different aspects of experience. This development is achieved through iterative exploration of episodes that leads patients to perceive the psychological processes underlying distress that previously seemed inexplicable. Consider the example of a patient with avoidant, obsessive–compulsive personality disorder and depressive traits who experiences bouts of anxiety, stomach pain, and fatigue but is unable to pinpoint when and why these episodes occur, which makes him prone to catastrophic ruminations about health issues. After exploring events preceding the onset of some intense ruminations about having a deadly disease, the patient begins to recognize that these worries rapidly follow events at work in which he feels his colleagues are ridiculing and rejecting him and that he is likely to be fired. Stomach pain then develops, which he interprets catastrophically. The patient was helped to connect health anxieties to interpersonal events by the therapist's shifting from using cognitive interventions aimed at decatastrophizing and postponing worries to focusing on the conflictual relational theme in order to explicate and soothe health anxiety.

In this example, the therapist tried to promote understanding of psychological causality, exploring the links between the details of a specific event at work in terms of what was said or done and how the patient reacted. This is similar to the standard cognitive therapy method of linking events, thoughts, feelings, and behavioral response. The difference is that, whereas cognitive-behavioral therapy is more focused on intrapsychic psychological processes (e.g., from a stomach pain to the catastrophic interpretation that leads to further negative arousal that fosters the catastrophic interpretations in a vicious cycle), here emphasis is given to understanding the links among processes happening within specific interpersonal episodes, including what the patient was expecting from others, the inferences he or she made about others' mental states, how and why he or she formed these inferences, and his or her reactions to the others' anticipated or perceived intentions.

Therapists should probe whether specific thoughts were associated with behaviors or affects. Simple hypotheses may be offered, such as, "You told me that the climate at work has been tense during the last 2 months and that this is when you started not sleeping and having panic attacks. Do you think that you may be worried about losing your job?" Again, it is important to note changes in nonverbal behaviors, particularly facial expressions, that occur when describing the episode. This helps patients to recognize and focus on shifts in their cognitive–affective appraisal of events. For example, a clinician might note that a patient looks scared when talking about criticism from colleagues and try to frame the link between fear of impending criticism and defensive avoidance in psychological terms.

It is important, when framing any hypothesis, for the therapist to have a conceptual framework in mind, that is, a template for how to interpret relationships. This template paves the way for the more complex step of interpersonal schema reconstruction. We suggest clinicians start by trying to understand patients' desires or motives, what the patient thinks she or he needs to do to get a desired response from the other person, and what the other person's actual response is. Lastly, therapists should investigate what the patient's response is in reaction to the other's response (Luborsky & Crits-Christoph, 1990; Ryle & Kerr, 2002). Such a template helps to guide exploration. For example, "I can now see you longed for approval. So how do you think your colleague reacted? Did you feel he was happy about what you did?" This process helps the patient to recognize his or her own thoughts about what the other person was thinking and feeling. In this case, the patient may realize that she felt the colleague was contemptuous. This then encourages the therapist to ask something like, "And when you noted contempt in his face, how did you feel? Was that why you felt ashamed and undeserving?"

This kind of cooperative dialogue, in which patient and therapist are working to understand the underlying cognitive–affective processes, allows the therapist to offer a summary of what happened in an episode. The formulation at this stage is similar to the description of the self–other schema: "So you asked for support when you were anxious about having done your work properly. But when your colleague hastily said you'd made a mistake, you became confused. I can see shame in your face. Is that correct?" If the patient agrees, the therapist can continue, "Could it be that you longed for approval and, when it didn't come, you felt criticized, thought you were worth nothing, and as a result became ashamed and then confused, and started panicking?" The therapy with Pietro gives an example of this step.

> Pietro gradually progressed to being able to provide narrative episodes. A key episode involved receiving good news about his career that led to his telephoning Milena. His therapist invited Pietro to remember the call in detail to understand what he felt immediately after receiving the good news and what desire had driven him to call Milena immediately. Pietro first replied theoretically: "Simply because at such moments what you want is to know that life offers you revenge." With an ironic tone the therapist reminded him of the agreement they had: "Please, Pietro, avoid intellectualizing like the plague." Pietro smiled and, with the therapist asking him to replay the episode as if in slow motion (Guidano, 1987), he gradually realized he had phoned Milena with a feeling of joy and physical vigor and that he saw himself as a genius finally acknowledged by the world. He called Milena not to share his joy but to be admired. When the therapist tried to reconstruct in detail the flow of his mental states during the call, Pietro had difficulty grasping what was behind the shift from one aspect of experience to another: "It's true that at the start of the call I wanted her admiration, but then, a bit later, I was asking myself who at the end of the day this person was. Simply one who's always used me for her own purposes! And at that point I cut the matter short." His therapist was unable to understand what led to the

shift in mental state and remarked that he had the impression that during the call Pietro had progressively lost interest in Milena's admiration and become angry and contemptuous. When Pietro nodded in agreement, the therapist asked whether he remembered something Milena had said or that he had thought that caused his state of mind toward her to change. These comments helped Pietro to recognize that the change in state of mind occurred when he had the impression that Milena was cold in congratulating him on his success. At this point, the therapist had the elements necessary for linking Pietro's mental states with the variables in the relationship. "So, Pietro, and correct me if I'm wrong, it's possible that you felt the need to display a side of yourself, one full of joy and high self-esteem, to Milena to obtain her admiration. Then when you perceived Milena to be cold and not tuned in to this need, you felt disappointed and for this reason felt an anger that drove you to despise her. What's your opinion?" Pietro confirmed that this hypothesis was correct.

An agreement about a summary in which psychological causality is clear creates the opportunity to help the patient to recognize how his or her distress is linked to the schemas used to construe events. We contend that this is best achieved by guiding patients so that they arrive at this understanding themselves. This is achieved by encouraging patients to see similarities across a series of associated episodes.

Promoting Metacognition: Step 3. Fostering Awareness of Regularities through Association of Episodes and Overt Reformulation of Schemas

The primary goal of the procedure outlined here is for patients to understand how their problems and actions are influenced by maladaptive schemas. Schemas are hard to challenge in personality disorder, and it is often better for therapists to help patients to recognize these schemas for themselves by identifying similar themes across different episodes. This involves stimulating the recollection of episodes associated with a core schema. We suggest that, once a summary of an episode has been agreed upon, the therapist ask the patient if he or she can recall similar episodes so that specific cues can be used to start associative chains: "You said you felt angry (frightened, sad), when your partner did not help you. Has this happened with other people at other moments in your life?" In this way, a patient is not forced to accept that something happening in the present is just a mirror of past events but rather free to make any link between past and present and reason about what connects the episode at a psychological level.

Therapists should not make the associations themselves and should keep interpretative work to a minimum, especially early in therapy. Thus we advise against premature evocation of material coming from family history and against linking this to recent episodes because it runs the risk of the patient rejecting the link or feeling criticized or unsupported by a therapist. Moreover, such intellectual interpretative work by the therapist does not necessarily evoke emotionally hot material and deprives the patient of a sense of agency over his or her own associations. Once several connected episodes have been gathered, the next, more complex step is to use such memories to reformulate schemas. As patients see links between episodes by themselves, it is implicit that the patient knows that there is a relation between them, although she or he may not fully understand the nature of the relationship. Therapists can try to form hypotheses about the schemas and associated feelings, thoughts, and reactions and summarize the main theme. This is what happened with Pietro.

> The dominant motive in the narratives with Milena was the search for admiration and the fear of not receiving it. The therapist asked Pietro if he had had other relationships with this same script. Pietro recalled an episode in which he took a woman he wanted to seduce to a conference where he had been asked to lecture. He acknowledged that in this case too his goal was to have his special qualities appreciated. The therapist asked if he had any more distant memories, drawn perhaps from family origins, in which his need for admiration was not fulfilled. Pietro paused for a long time and seemed to be reflecting deeply. Then he replied that since he was small he had always sought confirmation from others that his intelligence was special but had never really felt deeply appreciated and loved. He thought of his father, an esteemed university teacher, whom he had always admired. First, he described him as strong, scornful, detached, and immune from any bursts of affection, a man who had always publicly boasted about his son's forwardness and intellectual gifts but who had never validated Pietro personally. Then he recalled one occasion when he told his father about his excellent results on his high school final exams. He realized that getting his father's admiration would be the only way to feel the latter's affection. His father replied coldly and brusquely: "Well done, but you were just doing your duty!" With the therapist's help, Pietro recalled that at that moment he "saw himself through his father's eyes" and found himself painfully ridiculous in his search for appreciation. He felt unlovable and ashamed for asking for attention he did not feel he deserved. He realized now that he had been hiding these feelings behind that same mask of scornful contempt that he admired as a sign of superiority in his father.

The task of reconstructing mental states in narratives should be coupled with a constant, tactful promotion of a cooperative therapeutic relationship involving a sense of sharing and reciprocal understanding. In fact, not only does the collaborative work needed to generate this understanding require a good relationship, but the success of this work in the form of increased understanding of events that may previously have seemed inexplicable can also be used to enhance the alliance. Therapists should constantly provide support and validation and discuss how a patient is feeling while talking about these issues.

> In this episode the therapist validated Pietro: "I can see you longed for your father's approval. I can see how you loved him and how proud you felt when you told him about your marks. Any son wants this from a father in an important situation like that, and it must have been very distressful for you to be faced with that coldness." Then, on seeing from Pietro's facial expression that he felt understood and validated, the therapist reformulated the schema. "It would appear, therefore, that in various significant relationships in your life, starting with that with your father and now with Milena, you enter the relationship driven by the understandable desire to be appreciated and loved. But you've learned to believe that you can't be loved for how you are but need to possess special qualities for it to happen. These qualities might generate admiration, but if there is none, as often happens, you consider it a confirmation that you're unworthy of love. This causes you an intolerable distress, which you've learned to more or less manage with the same rather scornful detachment you've acquired from your father. Agreed?" Pietro nodded silently, with a sorrowful expression.

Though this is not the focus of this chapter (see Tufekcioglu & Muran, Chapter 6, this volume), the therapeutic relationship is a gold mine of information that may be used to reconstruct schemas. Clinicians should pay attention to regularly occurring features in patients' in-session behavior and try to understand how they may be driven by relational patterns. This usually happens during a joint observation of patients' verbal and nonverbal manifestations. A patient may say she feels awkward, desperate, or mistrustful of the therapist, and the therapist can in turn explore the mental states underlying such feelings. A simultaneous exploration of nonverbal behavior provides useful insight into recurrent themes. Therapists can also inquire whether patients have ever had any disturbing feelings during a session. If a patient has difficulty replying, whereas the therapist can clearly recall episodes in which the patient acted as in his or her everyday self-narratives, the therapist should point out the link: "You told me that you feel ashamed because your friends consider you clumsy. Last time I thought you almost blushed, as if you were afraid of being criticized by me. Was your emotion in the two situations similar?" If both agree that these analogies are plausible, the therapist can point out that at the core of the patient's narratives there is a meaning-making pattern, which can be a target for treatment.

The overall aim of the steps outlined here is to make patients aware that their inner representations of events drive their interpretations of social relations.

Promoting Metacognition: Step 4. Achieving Differentiation between Inner Schemas and External Reality

Once patients recognize a theme across several episodes or scenarios, the next step is differentiation, the recognition that alternative constructions are necessary; that is, that the schema is not absolute but can be restructured. However, it takes time and work for patients to recognize this possibility.

Patients need to understand how their appraisal of events and their attributions of mental states to others are merely hypotheses that do not necessarily mirror reality, and they need to begin questioning these schemas and their associated beliefs and to treat them as subjective states (Bateman & Fonagy, Chapter 7, this volume; Fonagy, Gergely, Jurist, & Target, 2002). For example, if a partner does not answer a phone call, the patient may interpret it as meaning that she or he will be left alone forever, or a boss's angry expression may be interpreted as meaning that he or she is likely to be fired.

Promoting a distinction between internalized expectations and external reality does not initially entail either challenging irrational beliefs or forcing patients to discard any realistic aspects of their appraisal of relationships. Instead, the differentiation-promoting step consists of cautiously moving toward realizing how internalized relationship patterns restrict the appraisal of relationships and limit social action and that they are easily triggered and associated with negative emotions.

Simply put, a woman with dependent personality disorder may initially complain that her father is dictating her life, causing her to feel inhibited in the way she pursues her own goals and guilty about leaving her father alone, and that she feels crushed by the father's anticipated criticism. Initially, as she discusses this problem, the patient may note that her life would be fine if only the demanding father would change his behavior. However, after having recalled multiple associated episodes and identified underlying themes, the patient may come to recognize that it is possible to change her point of view and that it is possible to see things from a different angle.

Differentiation is then achieved by helping the patient recognize how important the parent's voice is in her own mind: "It seems as if your father is so powerful inside you. It is as if he is in your head. I can see you suffer a lot when he denies support for your work plans, but it's like you need his praise to act. There is a source of action inside yourself that is left in the shade as you pay so much attention to the father that is in your head, who seems even more powerful than your actual father." The simplest way of promoting differentiation is to help the patient to understand how her reactions are triggered not just by others' actions but also by her inner echoes to these actions. Another strategy for achieving differentiation without directly challenging patients' perspectives is to wait for the patient to describe episodes in which he or she acted and felt in ways that do not match his or her schemas. For example, it may be possible to have patients enter positive mental states and access healthy aspects of themselves and then observe from that stance their maladaptive schemas. Patients whose lives are dictated by expectations of criticism and social rejection may recall episodes in which they passed a great night with friends at a restaurant, telling jokes and having fun. Therapists can help patients concentrate on such episodes and validate the positive tone and adaptive actions. They can observe how the events were incompatible with the way a patient usually sees him- or herself. The patient should be invited to reflect upon the negative side of her or his personality from the observing stance arising in the positive episode. The therapy with Pietro provides an example of this technique.

> In a session much later in therapy, Pietro said that he was dating a girl. He realized he had sought her admiration several times but managed to control this tendency and in fact to smile about it self-ironically. One evening for the first time, while watching TV with her, he felt that the girl had a "warm" affection and an "authentic" interest in him. The therapist commented, "We agree that in this episode you felt you were lovable whether you were admired or not. This is something you say is not typical of you or, worse, that you usually regret not being at all able to have such interactions with people. I am curious about what the 'Pietro' in the interaction with this girl thinks of the Pietro you say is unlovable and rejected by everyone." Pietro acknowledged that the former statement was an overgeneralization, which he knew did not match what he felt while watching TV with the girl.

We focus on encouraging a distinction between fantasy and reality only with ego-dystonic self-representations. In fact, prematurely challenging ego-syntonic representations, even if they are subjectively positive (e.g., narcissistic grandiosity) or negative (e.g., anger and retaliation in the case of paranoid personality disorder), is unhelpful. Such interventions run the risk of eliciting negative reactions that threaten the alliance. For example, if a patient with narcissistic features asserts that everyone admires him for his exceptional qualities and that his partner loves him and is ready to forgive his unfaithfulness, little is achieved by pointing out that this assumption is unrealistic. Patients often react to such interventions by feeling that their therapists do not believe them or are siding with the other person. Such invalidation leads to withdrawal or anger.

We contend, therefore, that such ego-syntonic convictions should not be challenged until therapy is well advanced. Preliminary operations with patients featuring these ego-syntonic representations should involve turning back and focusing on other details of their self-narratives until pain or suffering emerges. At this point, one can help patients concentrate not on how others caused the pain but on the pain itself and its enduring quality in spite of others' presence: "I sense that you felt very frustrated when your partner asked you for help. You're probably struggling to do your best to accomplish goals at work and don't feel enough trust and support from others, so that any force distracting you from such important objectives can look like an obstacle to you." If the patient agrees, the next step could be to shift the focus from current interactions by eliciting related episodes in which the patient had the same feeling of being not supported or trusted, until he or she is able to realize that these are basic enduring feelings that others might only elicit but not fully cause.

Treating Symptoms in the Context of Enriching Narratives and Promoting Metacognition

The procedures outlined are iterative and need to be repeated until metacognitive functioning improves, as shown by the patient's ability to provide narrative accounts of his or her life consistently, to understand mental states, and to use this knowledge to promote personality change (see Dimaggio et al., Chapter 17, this volume). In focusing on enhancing metacognitive functioning as a general treatment strategy, we are not implying that this is the only important activity of therapy. Rather, we are drawing attention to a core intervention module and attempting to show how impaired metacognitive functioning can be addressed in a systematic way during the course of therapy. Inevitably, when describing significant events and episodes as part of the treatment, patients will describe and manifest the symptoms and problems that caused them to seek treatment. On many occasions, these things will take priority. We suggest that the therapist use interventions and promote coping strategies that are consistent with the patient's level of metacognition. The poorer the level of narrative metacognition, the more these strategies need to be behavioral or minimally cognitive. For example, a patient presenting with anxiety symptoms who has poor narrative and metacognitive abilities should primarily be offered psychoeducation and techniques for self-soothing, such as diverting attention from or reappraising bodily signals. Those with better metacognitive functioning and those for whom treatment has successfully promoted richer narratives and a more sophisticated understanding of mental states, treatment of symptoms, and relational patterns can be guided by mentalistic knowledge. The patient can be soothed by understanding that outbursts of anxiety follow episodes of perceived rejection or that depression follows signals of negative judgment received. Mentalistically based problem-solving strategies, that is, metacognitive mastery (Carcione et al., 2011), can then be promoted.

The clinician can arrive at a formulation such as, "You tend to withdraw, and you did not attend your university exams because you feared rejection. This usually happens after your parents have criticized you. You entered a negative state in which you shut yourself down, believed you were worth nothing, and so decided not to try to pass the exam. You know now how this is just the old image of yourself triggered by what happened at home last night. We now feel that is not the case; that you have achieved a positive image of yourself. Are you going to be able to bear this in mind during the week and take advantage of this positive memory, so that the negative image remains in the background of your consciousness and you can manage to attend the exam?" It is likely that a major part of the strategies for treating symptoms and regulating affects described by many of the authors in this volume can best be applied in the context of such a rationale, with patients progressively describing episodes in which their understanding of self and others becomes more and more mentalistically oriented.

CONCLUDING COMMENTS

Treatment of patients with personality disorders with poor or disorganized narratives and impaired metacognition may benefit from a systematic progression of interventions that develop their use of the autobiographical self-narrative mode and help them progressively foster their knowledge of the mental states that they themselves, and the characters in the narrative episodes, experience. As the narrative scenario becomes richer, awareness of subjective experience is enhanced, which helps clinician and patient to possess a more fine-grained knowledge of the cognitive–affective processes guiding personality malfunctioning, some of which may be used for joint case formulation and treatment planning. A crucial step is collecting evidence of the existence of recurring maladaptive patterns for making sense of self–other interactions. When clinicians are able to make patients realize that their suffering and social problems derive more from those internalized patterns than from the direct impact of external reality, therapy may aim at promoting change. The process begins with further helping patients to discover that alternative explanations of relational events are possible and that new cognitive–affective patterns can be built up. Clinicians help patients construct richer and more flexible life scripts (see Dimaggio et al., Chapter 17, this volume) that guide them to pursue adaptive goals, negotiating conflicts and regulating the symptoms elicited by distressing interpersonal relationships. Work on symptoms can also be guided by an evaluation of the metacognitive abilities a patient has achieved: The lower the degree of metacognitive skills is, the simpler the strategies need to be. The higher the abilities are, the wider the range of strategies is for soothing distress, including an awareness that symptoms can recede once one has understood their relational triggers.

A final consideration is that this procedure is, we hope, adequately manualized, so that session transcripts can be analyzed for an accuracy check verifying whether progress in sessions really mirrors the actuation of the procedures we have devised here. Training clinicians to adopt such procedures is possible irrespective of their preferred school, thus rendering them a potential tool in overall personality disorder psychotherapy.

REFERENCES

Allen, J. G., Fonagy, P., & Bateman, A. W. (2008). *Mentalizing in clinical practice.* Washington, DC: American Psychiatric Publishing.

Angus, L., & McLeod, J. (Eds.). (2004). *Handbook of narrative psychotherapy: Practice, theory and research.* Thousand Oaks, CA: Sage.

Bateman, A., & Fonagy, P. (2004). *Psychotherapy for borderline personality disorder: Mentalization-based treatment.* Oxford, UK: Oxford University Press.

Carcione, A., Semerari, A., Nicolò, G., Pedone, R., Popolo, R., Conti, L., et al. (2011). Metacognitive mastery dysfunctions in personality disorder psychotherapy. *Psychiatry Research, 190,* 60–71.

Colle, L., d'Angerio, S., Popolo, R., & Dimaggio, G. (2010). Different metacognitive dysfunctions in personality disorders. In G. Dimaggio & P. H. Lysaker (Eds.), *Metacognition and severe adult mental disorders: From basic research to treatment* (pp. 177–195). London: Routledge.

Dimaggio, G., Carcione, A., Conti, M. L., Nicolò, G., Fiore, D., Pedone, R., et al. (2009). Impaired decentration in personality disorder: An analysis with the Metacognition Assessment Scale. *Clinical Psychology and Psychotherapy, 16*, 450–462.

Dimaggio, G., Carcione, A., Salvatore., G., Nicolò, G., Sisto, A., & Semerari, A. (2011). Progressively increasing metacognition through a step-by-step procedure in a case of obsessive–compulsive personality disorder treated with metacognitive interpersonal therapy. *Psychology and Psychotherapy: Theory, Research and Practice, 84*, 70–83.

Dimaggio, G., & Lysaker, P. H. (Eds.). (2010). *Metacognition and severe adult mental disorders: From basic research to treatment.* London: Routledge.

Dimaggio, G., Procacci, M., Nicolò, G., Popolo, R., Semerari, A., Carcione, A., et al. (2007). Poor metacognition in narcissistic and avoidant personality disorders: Analysis of four psychotherapy patients. *Clinical Psychology and Psychotherapy, 16*, 386–401.

Dimaggio, G., Salvatore, G., Fiore, D., Carcione, A., Nicolò, G., & Semerari, A. (2012). General principles for treating the overconstricted personality disorder: Toward operationalizing technique. *Journal of Personality Disorders, 26*, 63–83.

Dimaggio, G., Salvatore, G., Nicolò, G., Fiore, D., & Procacci, M. (2010). Enhancing mental state understanding in the over-constricted personality disorder with metacognitive interpersonal therapy. In G. Dimaggio & P. H. Lysaker (Eds.), *Metacognition and severe adult mental disorders: From basic research to treatment* (pp. 247–268). London: Routledge.

Dimaggio, G., Semerari, A., Carcione, A., Nicolò, G., & Procacci, M. (2007). *Psychotherapy of personality disorders: Metacognition, states of mind and interpersonal cycles.* London: Routledge.

Domes, G., Czieschnek, D., Weidler, F., Berger, C., Fast, K., & Herpertz, S. C. (2008). Recognition of facial affect in borderline personality disorder. *Journal of Personality Disorders, 22*, 135–147.

Fonagy, P. (1991). Thinking about thinking: Some clinical and theoretical considerations in the treatment of a borderline patient. *International Journal of Psychoanalysis, 72*, 639–656.

Fonagy, P., Gergely, G., Jurist, E. L., & Target, M. (2002). *Affect regulation, mentalization, and the development of the self.* New York: Other Press.

Grabe, H. J., Spitzer, C., & Freyberger, H. J. (2004). The relationship between alexithymia, personality and psychopathology. *American Journal of Psychiatry, 161*, 1299–1301.

Guidano, V. F. (1987). *Complexity of the self: A developmental approach to psychopathology and therapy.* New York: Guilford Press.

Hermans, H. J. M., & Dimaggio, G. (Eds.). (2004). *The dialogical self in psychotherapy.* London: Routledge.

Lawson, R., Waller, G., Sines, J., & Meyer, C. (2008) Emotional awareness among eating-disordered patients: The role of narcissistic traits. *European Eating Disorders Review, 16*, 44–48.

Linehan, M. M. (1993). *Cognitive-behavioral treatment of borderline personality disorder.* New York: Guilford Press.

Luborsky, L., & Crits-Christoph, P. (Eds.). (1990). *Understanding transference: The CCRT method.* New York: Basic Books.

Neimeyer, R. A. (2000). Narrative disruptions in the construction of self. In R. A. Neimeyer & J. D. Raskin (Eds.), *Constructions of disorder: Meaning making frameworks for psychotherapy* (pp. 207–241). Washington, DC: American Psychological Association.

Nicolò, G., Semerari, A., Lysaker, P. H., Dimaggio, G., Conti, L., d'Angerio, S., et al. (2011). Alexithymia in personality disorders: Correlations with symptoms and interpersonal functioning. *Psychiatry Research, 190*, 37–42.

Ogrodniczuk, J. S., Piper, W. E., & Joyce, A. S. (2011). Effect of alexithymia on the process and outcome of psychotherapy: A programmatic review. *Psychiatry Research, 190*, 43–48.

Ryle, A., & Kerr, I. (2002). *Introducing cognitive analytic therapy: Principles and practice.* Chichester, UK: Wiley.

Schilling, L., Wingenfeld, K., Löwe, B., Moritz, S., Terfehr, K., Köther, U., et al. (2012). Normal mind-reading capacity but higher response confidence in borderline personality disorder patients. *Psychiatry and Clinical Neurosciences, 66*, 322–327.

Semerari, A., Dimaggio, G., Nicolò, G., Pedone, R., Procacci, M., & Carcione, A. (2005). Metarepresentative functions in borderline personality disorders. *Journal of Personality Disorders, 19*, 690–710.

Semerari, A., Dimaggio, G., Nicolò, G., Procacci, M., & Carcione, A. (2007) Understanding minds, different functions and different disorders?: The contribution of psychotherapeutic research. *Psychotherapy Research, 17*, 106–119.

Spinhoven, P., Bamelis, L., Molendijk, M., Haringsma, R., & Arntz, A. (2009). Reduced specificity of autobiographical memory in Cluster C personality disorders and the role of depression, worry, and experiential avoidance. *Journal of Abnormal Psychology, 118*, 520–530.

Taylor, G. J., Bagby, R. M., & Parker, J. D. A. (1997). *Disorders of affect regulation: Alexithymia in medical and psychiatric illness.* Cambridge, UK: Cambridge University Press.

Vanheule, S., Verhaeghe, P., & Desmet, M. (2011). In search of a framework for the treatment of alexithymia. *Psychology and Psychotherapy: Theory, Research and Practice, 84*, 84–97.

part four

TREATING SYMPTOMS AND DYSREGULATED EMOTIONS

chapter 9

Managing Suicidal and Other Crises

Paul S. Links and Yvonne Bergmans

Treatment of patients with personality disorders can be challenging because of the potential for recurrent crises. Although therapists may avoid treating such patients because they feel unskilled in managing crises, recent studies of evidence-based therapies demonstrate that individual psychotherapy is effective in reducing future suicidal behavior (McMain et al., 2009). This chapter discusses therapeutic strategies for dealing with suicidal and other crises that may occur during treatment. We begin by outlining the potential for suicidal and other crises in these patients and then discuss general principles and therapeutic strategies that may reduce risk. The chapter concludes by discussing specific strategies to assist patients in processing the intense emotional episodes that underlie many crisis presentations and how these interventions may be implemented in collaboration with emergency department staff to ensure the best possible coordinated responses to patients who present in crisis.

POTENTIAL FOR SUICIDE AND OTHER CRISES

Several studies have examined the link between personality disorders and suicidal behavior (Zaheer, Links, & Lui, 2008). Although there is some evidence that Cluster A and C, as well as Cluster B, personality disorders are related to suicidal behavior and suicide, the strongest link is with borderline personality disorder (BPD). Hence, we focus our comments primarily on patients with this diagnosis. However, the general principles and strategies discussed also apply to managing crises in other forms of personality disorders. BPD is the only personality disorder for which recurrent suicidal or self-injurious behavior is one of the diagnostic criteria. A history of suicidal behavior is found in 60–78% of patients with BPD, with an even higher percentage engaging in self-injurious behavior. The lifetime risk of suicide for patients with BPD has been reported to be between 3 and 10%. Paris (2004) suggested that a rate of 10% has been confirmed in several cohorts, including a 15-year follow-up from the New York State Psychiatric Institute and a follow-up of patients carried out from 15 to 27 years at a Montreal general hospital. Yoshida, Tonai, and Nagai (2006) also conducted a retrospective review of Japanese patients who received treatment in an inpatient facility from 1973 to 1989 and found that 5 out of 72 patients (6.9%) had committed suicide, in keeping with the lifetime risk found in North American and European studies. Links, Heslegrave, Mitton, van Reekum, and Patrick (1995) followed 130 former inpatients with either the traits or the diagnosis of BPD and found that 6 of 130 (4.6%) died by suicide over 7 years of follow-up. Zanarini, Frankenburg, Hennen, Reich, and Silk (2006), in another prospective study following patients with BPD over 10 years, found a suicide rate of 4%. Perry and colleagues (2009), in their follow-up study of former patients at the Austen Riggs Center, observed that none of their 92 patients with BPD died by suicide over their 7-year follow-up. These lower rates suggest that patients who agreed to follow-up and received regular outpatient treatment may be at much lower risk of dying by suicide and support the need for patients with personality disorders at risk for suicide to receive ongoing contact with mental health services.

When assessing the risk for suicide in a patient with BPD, it is useful to consider a model describing an "acute-on-chronic" risk (Links & Kolla, 2005; Zaheer et al., 2008). This model suggests that acute stressors can increase a patient's baseline level of suicide risk. These patients typically are at a chronically elevated risk of suicide much above that of the general population, and this risk exists primarily because of a history of multiple attempts. A thorough history of the methods and their lethality, the level of intent or planning, and the context of previous attempts can be helpful in estimating a patient's ongoing suicide risk. For example, a patient who has made attempts characterized by high levels of intention and employing highly lethal methods is at a much higher ongoing risk than a patient who has a history of attempts of low lethality and low intent to die. A history of comorbidities, such as substance-use disorders, and a history of sexual abuse can contribute to a patient's chronic level of risk. An acute-on-chronic risk will be present if the patient has comorbid major depression or if the patient is demonstrating high levels of hopelessness or depressive symptoms. In addition, patients with BPD are known to be at risk for suicide around times of hospitalization and discharge. The clinical scenario of a patient presenting in crisis shortly after discharge from an inpatient setting illustrates a time when the risk assessment must be very carefully completed to ensure that a proper disposition is made. This patient is potentially at an acute-on-chronic risk level, and the assessment cannot be truncated because of the recent discharge from the hospital. Proximal substance abuse can increase the suicide risk in a patient with personality disorders. The risk is acutely elevated in patients who have less immediate family support or who have lost or perceive the loss of an important relationship. A careful assessment of a plan for suicide and access to means are of utmost importance in determining the acute risk. Characterizing the patient's ongoing chronic risk for suicide and then determining whether an acute-on-chronic risk exists provides a clear, concise way to formulate and communicate the patient's care to family and other health professionals. Discussing the risk of violence in patients with personality disorders, a recent review by Allen and Links (2012) did not find evidence for a significant increased risk of aggression in patients with BPD when other comorbidities are taken into account. Overall, the research suggests that there is a small subgroup of patients with BPD who are most at risk of repeated aggression and are overrepresented in violent and selected clinical populations. The diagnosis of BPD may be less useful in prediction of violence than one might suspect. Aggressiveness in BPD may not be as strongly determined by impulsivity as is commonly held, and difficulties with emotional processing may be a more important causal factor (Allen & Links, 2012). An individualized assessment of the context of the patient's interpersonal aggression, as well as other risk factors such as antisocial personality disorder and psychopathy, may be more informative to predicting future violence.

STRATEGIES FOR REDUCING AND PREVENTING CRISES

This section describes some general strategies for reducing the frequency of crisis presentations. They were developed in the course of undertaking a large randomized controlled trial involving real-world settings to evaluate the clinical and cost effectiveness of dialectical behavior therapy (DBT) compared with consensus-based best-practice therapy designed to treat the disorder—an approach that we referred to as general psychiatric management (McMain et al., 2009). Previous studies of treatments of suicidal and parasuicidal behavior and associated crises usually used treatment as usual as the control condition. We sought to improve upon earlier research by using a more rigorous, active, and recommended comparison treatment. Consequently, we decided to use general psychiatric management as the control treatment and based this choice on the American Psychiatric Association (2001) practice guidelines for treating BPD because this represented a comprehensive set of evidence-based "best-practice" recommendations for the psychiatric community (Oldham, 2005). The guidelines state that the "primary treatment for BPD is psychotherapy, complemented by symptom-targeted pharmacotherapy."

Consequently, general psychiatric management included both psychotherapy and symptom-targeted pharmacotherapy.

Clinicians providing general management were expected to provide the essential elements of psychotherapy that were described under three broad categories: case management elements, emotion-processing elements, and relational elements. They were also encouraged to oversee or provide symptom-targeted pharmacotherapy. The overall principles of general management included (1) viewing patients as competent adults who were expected to be active participants in all aspects and phases of treatment; (2) encouraging therapists to be flexible within reason regarding patients' preferences for the focus of therapy; and (3) according significant attention to improving patients' role functioning so that progress was always judged partly by their demonstrating some improvement in work, social, or family life (Links, 1996).

Crisis and Safety Monitoring

To reduce future crises, the patient and therapist should develop a method to differentiate nonlethal intention, in which the patient's intent may be to seek a reduction in emotional distress, from "true" suicidal intention, in which the patient's intent is to end his or her life. The therapist must attend to the risk of suicidal behavior, yet must avoid being therapeutically constrained by concerns about the patient's chronic suicidality. To monitor chronic suicidality, the clinician needs to focus on the presence of an acute-on-chronic risk for suicide, as discussed earlier (Gunderson & Links, 2008). Recent studies provide clinicians with objective information on risk factors for suicidal behavior in patients with BPD. These studies suggest that clinicians should not rely on their intuition or "gut" response when seeing a patient in crisis. As discussed, the evidence suggests that acute risk increases when (1) there is worsening of a major depressive episode; (2) there is an increase in substance use; (3) the patient has been recently discharged from a psychiatric inpatient service; (4) recent negative life events, such as loss of immediate family support or legal troubles, have occurred; and (5) there are prominent difficulties with affective instability (Gunderson & Links, 2008; Links & Kolla, 2005).

With each patient, the clinician should work out the "early warning signs" of an acute-on-chronic risk and the actions to be taken as the risk increases (see the discussion on pp. 204–205). As crises appear related to periods of intense negative emotions, the evidence-based therapies focus on enhancing the patient's skills related to emotional awareness, expression, and acceptance. Patients are encouraged to process rather than control emotions. An important strategy is for patients to develop a personal method of scaling their emotional distress to communicate better with their support network about their needs when in crisis. The therapist should help patients to develop these personal scaling methods and to revise and expand them as they learn to understand themselves better.

Dealing with Chronic Suicidal Thoughts: Understanding the Meaning

By tolerating the patient's chronic suicidal thoughts, the clinician can help the patient understand their psychological meaning. If the therapist is able to listen to the patient's reasons for considering suicide as an option, then often the connection of greater understanding is created between the therapist and patient. Therapeutic gains are possible as a patient comes to understand for him- or herself the meaning behind his or her suicidal thoughts.

Case Example

A 46-year-old single mother demonstrated many forms of self-harming behavior but was motivated to rid herself of them because of the impact they had on her teenage children. With her therapist, the patient developed early warning signs to tell when she was at high risk for self-harm with suicidal intent; for example, when she made repeated visits to the drugstore to purchase over-the-counter medications or when she recognized feeling alienated from her family of origin. Observing her many forms of self-harm, she became aware that much of this behavior was an expression of her need to be a "rebellious child." Coming from a large family, she often felt invisible unless she did something dramatic to draw attention to herself. From this observation, she lessened her need to be the "rebellious child" and focused on being an attentive parent with her own children.

Fostering a "Greater Sense of Self-Agency" through the Therapeutic Relationship

In patients with personality disorders, suicide risk may be reduced by helping the patient develop a greater sense of self-agency. Knox (2011) characterized self-agency as the "experience that we can influence our physical and relational environment, that our actions and intentions have an effect on and produce a response from those around us" (p. 7). According to Knox's model, inhibited development of self-agency will be linked to actions such as suicidal behavior, as the person, particularly in the face of intense emotional distress, will be unable to use imagination or symbolic thought as opposed to immediate action. Patients with an inhibited development of self-agency might manifest sudden suicidal behavior, and this combination of poor self-agency and immediate action is particularly found in individuals with narcissistic and borderline personality pathology (Ronningstam, 2009).

Acute suicidal behavior in patients with borderline or narcissistic pathology is often triggered when patients experience intense feelings of shame. Shame-motivated suicide has long been observed (Lester, 1997). Shame that may result from transgressions or failed behaviors is directed inward, altering self-consciousness and leading to reappraisals of self-worth. Shame leads to humiliation, or the "sense of having been exposed and rendered childlike in stature, diminished in power, status, worth, and importance" (Wilson, Drozdek, & Turkovic, 2006, p. 127). Intense shame is accompanied by a disintegration of the dimensions of the self-structure: "the essential vitality of the self feels drained" (p. 134). Wilson and colleagues (2006) elaborate that "the intensity and severity of shame is directly correlated with high suicide potential and fantasies of killing oneself to obliterate the inner experience of shame" (p. 133). Shame also impairs the individual's ability to maintain the dimensions of self, and the self becomes "diminished, lost, dissolved, broken apart" (p. 134). In this state of mind and given the background of impaired development of self-efficacy, patients with narcissistic or borderline personality cannot process the shame emotion nor use imagination or symbolic thought to modify their humiliation, and irrational immediate action is more available than rational safe action. Thus the deficits in self-agency and shame proneness can explain the acute risk of suicide behavior that is observed in patients with narcissistic and borderline personality pathology.

Most of the evidenced-based therapies for BPD include strategies and interventions to increase the patient's sense of self-agency. For example, in DBT, self-agency is fostered by shaping active responses from the patient that promote thought before action, by teaching the patient to manage life problems, and by seeing the patient as capable of doing so (Linehan, 1993). In mentalization-based psychotherapy, the therapist eschews the "expert stance" and participates in the patient's exploration of transference enactments using the perspective of "sitting side-by-side" with the patient (Bateman & Fonagy, 2007). General management emphasizes the principle that patients are competent adults who should be active participants in all parts of therapy.

Specific Strategies for Reducing Crises: Modulating Emotion Processing

Psychotherapy elements that focus on emotion processing include the identification, acceptance, and expression of emotions. Our understanding of the importance of emotions in psychotherapy is partly derived from the work of Greenberg and colleagues (Greenberg, 2002; Warwar, Links, Greenberg, & Bergmans, 2008). Our clinical and research experience revealed that patients in a crisis are often unable to tell care providers what they are experiencing outside of having overwhelming feelings that they desperately need to attenuate by whatever means are available to them. Previous work (Bergmans & Links, 2009) suggested that challenges in emotion processing may be related to alexithymia (Luminet, Vermeulen, Demaret, Taylor, & Bagby, 2006; Warwar et al., 2008)—difficulty identifying or describing emotions. Effective emotional processing requires a degree of "emotional literacy," which has been defined as "the ability to recognize, understand, handle and appropriately express emotions" (Sharp, 2001, as cited in Weare & Gray, 2003). When a patient presents in crisis, it cannot be assumed that the individual at that time is able to identify, describe, understand, or handle his or her emotions.

Identification of Feelings

Work on emotions in patients with personality disorders begins by identifying whether they know the difference between feeling safe and feeling unsafe and what *safe* and *unsafe* look, sound, and feel like. A related differentiation is the important difference between "feeling" versus "being" unsafe.

Case Example

Mr. S was escorting his patient Mr. P to his first group session. Mr. P said that he did not want to walk into the therapy room by himself because he felt unsafe doing so. Mr. S noted that they were in a place where no harm could or would come to Mr. P, noting that the leaders were very well trained with a great deal of experience, that there had never been any incidents in any of the groups, that the room was secure from intruders, and that there were security personnel close by in the event that anything might happen. Mr. P stated that he recognized that Mr. S was focused on the external and visual cues of the environment and discerned that they were safe. However, Mr. P did not "feel" safe internally, an experience which Mr. S could not see. Mr. S agreed to walk into the group room with his patient to make the introductions again, respecting that his patient needed to "feel safe" even though Mr. S believed that he "was safe."

Often people will feel that they are not safe when, in fact, they are working out of their comfort zone and engaging in a situation that is a "risk." The therapist has to help the patient differentiate the experience of taking a "risk" versus "feeling unsafe." Experiencing oneself at risk occurs when (1) the situation is *time-limited*; (2) the individual made the *choice* to engage in a particular activity or interaction; and (3) the person has a degree of *control* in the situation.

Case Example

Ms. M arrives for her appointment stating that she is unable to stay because her anxiety is "over the moon!" She says that she took public transit for the first time in many years, and it was "like being packed in a sardine can! I was soooo scared!" In asking Ms. M what made her decide to take public transit after so many years, she said, "It's time I start being able to do things on my own, and in this city that means taking public transit, especially since I don't drive and I can't afford taxis all the time. Besides, it's only eight subway stops, and I could have gotten off and walked the rest of the way if I had to."

Ms. M took a "risk." She made a *choice* to do something different and something that was beyond her "safe zone." She knew it was *time limited* ("only eight stops"). She was aware that she was able to get off and walk if need be; hence there was still an element of *control*. When this was reflected back to Ms. M as having been an exercise that *felt* unsafe yet contained the elements of choice, time limitation, and control, she was able to recognize that she had indeed been safe. Yet at the time she experienced overwhelming fear, which was reminiscent of previous situations in which she had felt unsafe. Ms. M had not recognized that this situation was time limited, that it was a choice she made, and that she had been in control the entire way. Rather, she was overtaken by the emotional memory of feeling unsafe. She noted that she would now remember the difference between taking "a risk" and being unsafe, given that this experience showed her how these experiences were different. Working with patients to help them understand the differences between feeling unsafe and being at risk and giving names or labels to their experience allows the person to normalize and contain the experience versus entering into an acute emotional crisis.

It is important that patients are able to articulate to caregivers what they are experiencing in a way that facilitates being heard and understood as opposed to rejected, minimized, or disbelieved. When patients tell someone that they are not feeling "safe," it tends to elicit a different response from saying that "I can't take it anymore, I'm going to kill myself." Patients need to take responsibility for learning how to communicate to others that they are at risk and in distress in a way that elicits a response that meets their needs. Care providers, professional and personal, need to understand that the word *suicide* may simply be a way of communicating the intensity of the affect in that moment and that patients often have limited ability to express the intense affect directly. Patients often comment that threats of suicide are sometimes the only language that others will "listen to" and that such threats are needed to ensure that the intensity of their distress is taken seriously. Patients who are unable to identify or describe emotions can learn the language of emotions when it is modeled and directly taught. This would include the therapist asking or commenting, "Can you tell me what you understand the tears to mean?" If the patient is unable to identify the feelings, the therapist could offer, "for some people tears mean frustration, or anger, or being overwhelmed, and for some they mean happiness, like at a wedding. Do any of those resonate for you right now?" It is also important to ask patients what they want when they talk about suicide. "When you say suicide, can you tell me what it is you want to end? Some people use the word to indicate a strong wish to see the end of a given situation or the feelings they're experiencing." This information will provide the clinician with the purpose or desired outcome for the behavior. Working backward, the clinician can then help the patient to identify the varying emotions contributing to the desired outcome, normalizing and validating how the feelings are in fact providing important information.

Early Warning Signs

Early warning signs (EWS) are the feelings, behaviors, and cognitive "signs" that inform an individual that his or her sense of safety is changing. Patients have identified shortness of breath, gastric upset, sweating, thoughts of worthlessness or feeling "stupid," pacing, or locking themselves out of their homes as indicators that they are not as safe as when they are at baseline. Becoming aware of the EWS is the first step in allowing the individual to recognize that she or he may be at risk for suicide or self-harming. Using EWS, she or he can make a decision based on her or his own sense of control as to how to deal with the emerging risk situation.

Scale of Intensity

The scale of intensity, a modified brief solution-focused therapy scaling technique (Fiske, 1998), gives the patient the opportunity to identify his or her feelings, EWS, and choices to keep him- or herself safer. The scale also indicates the network of individuals to contact along the continuum of safe to unsafe. Some patients will use a stoplight image—green-yellow-red—to identify feeling safe, at risk, and unsafe. As their emotional literacy and self-awareness increases, we have found that the images then become more refined and specific; for example, flashing yellow or flashing red may come to be used to denote a higher intensity at each level.

Case Example

One patient used the example of a 13-floor elevator ride to identify his scale of intensity. At the first floor he felt "grounded," "safe," "calm." He reported no EWS, noting that his body felt relaxed, that he found himself humming or whistling a favorite tune, and that he could pretty much tolerate doing anything. In order to keep himself at this level, he identified strategies and skills to keep himself safe; for example, he learned that being active and doing something that gave him pleasure allowed him to maintain this "grounded" level sometimes for hours, even days, on end. At this level he did not need to be in contact with his psychiatrist and the treatment team. At the fifth floor on his scale of intensity, he reported feeling "not good" and "scared." His EWS included feeling agitated, beginning to stutter, and bursting into tears from time to time. He noted that the strategies to use at level 5 were to "keep mindlessly busy" and "not be alone." His network contacts included "calling my mom to come over to be with me. She can't do emotion because it upsets her to see me upset but she's really good at distraction. She will have me cleaning all my cupboards, the fridge, and washing the floor until the intensity passes." It is important for the person to recognize who to call and who *not* to call at varying levels of distress. At floor 12, he needed to go to the emergency department to keep him safe.

By being familiar with and using the scale of intensity, patients are then able to tell care providers and family how they feel and whether they are at risk for suicidal behavior, what they have done to keep themselves safe, and what might be needed to protect themselves from being more at risk. As a person's capacity to identify emotions increases over time, the scale of intensity usually becomes more specific and refined.

Connecting Behaviors to Events/Feelings/Thoughts

Many patients believe that once suicidal ideation is present, there is no choice but to act on the thoughts in order to obtain relief. Learning that "a feeling is a feeling, neither good nor bad, and that feelings are normal parts of the human experience" helps the patient to begin to differentiate thoughts and feelings from behavior and hence to recognize that she or he does not need to act on these thoughts or feelings. The idea that neither a feeling nor a thought can kill you, whereas an action can, is new and essential learning for many. Patients are taught that emotions are a primary signaling system that communicates intention and can be the "driver" to action (Greenberg & Pavio, 1997; Izard, 2002). When a person is emotionally flooded, problem-solving abilities can be compromised (Bergmans, Brown, & Carruthers, 2007). This is to say that when in crisis, a patient's ability to articulate her or his experience is hampered. The ability and skills are either "not available" in the moment, or the skills have never been learned. Often when in crisis, the patient with BPD is asked "What's wrong?" or "How can we help you?" Both questions require a vocabulary and problem-solving process that may not be present at the time. By teaching patients the language of emotion and to use their scale of intensity, they develop an awareness of their own risk and a script for communicating their needs when in crisis.

Fostering Curiosity or Interest

Fostering an interest or curiosity about "what's going on" creates a one-step-removed position and allows the patient to observe his or her emotions from the "outside." Initially the therapist can act as the "observer" and model through questions and observations, such as "I see your leg has made it halfway across town, what do you think might be happening there?" Oftentimes patients will say that they have no idea how it came to be that they hurt themselves, what they were feeling, or even "what happened." They become lost in the flood of emotions with no foothold to ground them. The image of Dorothy from *The Wizard of Oz* swirling around in the eye of the tornado comes to mind. In their distress, patients appear very "self-focused," but nevertheless, they are unable to observe themselves. Thus they are unable to identify the emotion to determine how they are going to be able to experience the emotion in the moment and yet keep themselves safe. Playfulness and humor enable the patient to take a "lighter" approach to self-observation. Taking a one-step-removed position might entail asking "What would Dorothy in the eye of the tornado be experiencing?" Another self-observation strategy might be to personify and name the feeling state as a participant in the situation; for example, in the earlier case of Ms. M, "I wonder what would happen if you decided not to take Anxiety with you on the next subway ride? What do you think you might feel? What might happen to Anxiety?"

Dealing with Crises and Collaborating with Emergency Departments

Working collaboratively with an emergency department (ED) is often necessary to deal with suicidal and other crises. A therapist's availability during crises varies across treatment services and settings. Often therapists cannot provide intersession telephone contact that includes after hours, and many therapists encourage patients to use the closest ED when in crisis. As a result, the therapist has an important role in assisting the ED staff to be more effective in managing patients with personality disorders and, equally important, in helping the patient to use emergency rooms effectively. During our studies we have found it useful to help emergency room staff understand suicidal crises in these patients and the specific strategies to employ in the emergency room. The ED staff was helped by having a model to explain suicidal behavior, and they were able to work with the concept that suicidal behaviors arose from the patients' inability to regulate their intense emotions. We drew the analogy to the patient who presents with a bleeding wound; the first task with patients in a suicidal crisis was to stop the "emotional bleeding." The ED staff can learn to recognize that these patients cannot participate in constructive problem solving until their emotional intensity was deescalated. In addition, the staff is able to comprehend that patients need to have their emotional experience validated and to feel that someone understood their emotional pain before they were able to begin problem solving. In working with the ED staff, we recognized that they seldom received feedback about their encounters with patients in a suicidal crisis. They had no idea whether their interventions were helpful or not. We assured them that interactions with these patients can be intense and that ED staff should allow themselves time for debriefing or seeking a consultation concerning their interventions with these patients.

During rounds for ED staff, two former patients spoke about specific strategies that they found helpful when presenting to the ED during a suicide crisis. The former patients spoke about the importance of being approached in a respectful manner, being called by name, and having their choice of coming for help reinforced as a positive step. From their experience, the former patients found that having a private space and some simple reminders to monitor their breathing were helpful to lessen their level of distress. They made concrete suggestions to staff about what the next step might be given the patients' difficulties with problem solving during the peak of the crisis.

Some other specific strategies that are typically useful to patients in crisis were taught to the ED staff. Simple strategies such as monitoring the patient's breathing, distraction techniques such as naming items in the room, or soothing strategies such as listening to an iPod were reviewed with staff. We encouraged the staff to point out examples of how the patient had made positive choices to be safer. For example, the staff could acknowledge the patient's progress in coming to the ED before making a suicide attempt. The importance of reducing access to means of suicide was stressed to the ED staff—for example, having someone remove large quantities of painkillers from the patient's home. Lastly, the ED staff could be instrumental in activating the patient's support network, particularly the supports that the patient identified as helpful during crises.

In a parallel fashion, we educated patients to be better consumers of the ED. As discussed earlier, patients prepared for the next crisis by developing their scale of intensity and recognizing their personal EWS. They were encouraged to prepare a crisis kit that they could bring to the ED. This kit would include a card with their medications, physicians' contact information, and important personal supports. The kit would include some distraction and soothing strategies that could be utilized in the ED. We rehearsed with the patients how the ED staff experience their presentations to the ED. The patients readily understood the multiple demands faced by the ED staff and recognized that clear, repeated attempts at communication were likely the best way to have their needs heard in such a chaotic setting.

CONCLUDING COMMENTS

In summary, working with patients with personality disorders at risk for suicide crises requires a team of people across a continuum of care. This team has to be able to discuss, support, and include the patient as a core member of the care team. With the appropriate preparation and collaboration, work with these patients can be both effective and rewarding.

REFERENCES

Allen, A., & Links, P. S. (2012). Aggression in borderline personality disorder: Evidence for increased risk and clinical predictors. *Current Psychiatry Reports, 14*, 62–69.

American Psychiatric Association. (2001). Practice guideline for the treatment of patients with borderline personality disorder. *American Journal of Psychiatry, 158*(10, Suppl.), 1–52.

Bateman, A., & Fonagy, P. (2007). The use of transference in dynamic psychotherapy. *American Journal of Psychiatry, 164*, 680.

Bergmans, Y., Brown, A. L., & Carruthers, A. S. H. (2007). Advances in crisis management of the suicidal patient: Perspectives from patients. *Current Psychiatry Reports*, *9*, 74–80.

Bergmans, Y., & Links, P. S. (2009). Reducing potential risk factors for suicide-related behavior with a group intervention for clients with recurrent suicide-related behavior. *Annals of Clinical Psychiatry*, *21*, 17–25.

Fiske, H. (1998). Applications of solution-focused brief therapy in suicide prevention. In D. DeLeo, A. Schmidtke, & R. F. W. Diekstra (Eds.), *Suicide prevention* (pp. 185–197). Dordrecht, The Netherlands: Kluwer Academic.

Greenberg, L. (2002). *Emotion-focused therapy. Coaching clients to work through their feelings.* Washington, DC: American Psychological Association.

Greenberg, L. S., & Paivio, S. C. (1997). *Working with emotions in psychotherapy.* New York: Guilford Press.

Gunderson, J. G., & Links, P. S. (2008). *Borderline personality disorder: A clinical guide* (2nd ed.). Washington, DC: American Psychiatric Publishing.

Izard, C. E. (2002). Translating emotion theory and research into preventive interventions. *Psychological Bulletin, 12,* 796–824.

Knox, J. (2011). *Self-agency in psychotherapy.* New York: Norton.

Lester, D. (1997). The role of shame in suicide. *Suicide and Life-Threatening Behavior, 4,* 352–361.

Linehan, M. M. (1993). *Cognitive-behavioral treatment of borderline personality disorder.* New York: Guilford Press.

Links, P. S. (1996). Introduction. In P. S. Links (Ed.), *Clinical assessment and management of severe personality disorders* (pp. xv–xix). Washington, DC: American Psychiatric Press.

Links, P. S., Heslegrave, R. J., Mitton, J. E., van Reekum, R., & Patrick, J. (1995). Borderline personality disorder and substance abuse: Consequences of comorbidity. *Canadian Journal of Psychiatry, 40,* 9–14.

Links, P. S., & Kolla, N. (2005). Assessing and managing suicide risk. In J. Oldham, A. Skodol, & D. Bender (Eds.), *Textbook of personality disorders* (pp. 449–462). Washington, DC: American Psychiatric Press.

Luminet, O., Vermeulen, N., Demaret, C., Taylor, G. J., & Bagby, R. M. (2006). Alexithymia and levels of processing: Evidence for an overall deficit in remembering emotion words. *Journal of Research in Personality, 40,* 713–733.

McMain, S. F., Links, P. S., Gnam, W. H., Guimond, T., Cardish, R. J., Korman, L., et al. (2009). A randomized controlled trial of dialectical behavior therapy versus general psychiatry management for borderline personality disorder. *American Journal of Psychiatry, 166,* 1365–1374.

Oldham, J. M. (2005). *Guideline watch: Practice guideline for the treatment of patients with borderline personality disorder.* Arlington, VA: American Psychiatric Association. Retrieved August 2, 2011, from *http://focus.psychiatryonline.org/cgi/content/full/3/3/396.*

Paris, J. (2004). Half in love with easeful death: The meaning of chronic suicidality in borderline personality disorder. *Harvard Review of Psychiatry, 12,* 42–48.

Perry, C. J., Fowler, J. C., Bailey, A., Clemence, A. J., Plakun, E. M., Zheutlin, B., et al. (2009). Improvement and recovery from suicidal and self-destructive phenomena in treatment-refractory disorders. *Journal of Nervous and Mental Disease, 197,* 28–34.

Ronningstam, E. (2009). Narcissistic personality disorder: Facing DSM-V. *Psychiatric Annals, 39,* 111–121.

Warwar, S. H., Links, P. S., Greenberg, L., & Bergmans, Y. (2008). Emotion-focused principles for working with borderline personality disorder. *Journal of Psychiatric Practice, 14,* 94–104.

Weare, K., & Gray, G. (2003). *What works in developing children's emotional and social competence and well-being?* (Research Report No. 456). London: Department for Education and Skills. Retrieved August 2, 2011, from *www.education.gov.uk/publications/eOrderingDownload/RR456.doc.*

Wilson, J. P., Drozdek, B., & Turkovic, S. (2006). Posttraumatic shame and guilt. *Trauma, Violence, and Abuse, 7,* 122–141.

Yoshida, K., Tonai, E., & Nagai, H. (2006). Long-term follow-up study of borderline patients in Japan: A preliminary study. *Comprehensive Psychiatry, 47,* 426–432.

Zaheer, J., Links, P. S., & Liu, E. (2008). Assessment and emergency management of suicidality in personality disorders. *Psychiatric Clinics of North America, 31,* 527–543.

Zanarini, M. C., Frankenburg, F. R., Hennen, J., Reich, D. B., & Silk, K. R. (2006). Prediction of the 10-year course of borderline personality disorder. *American Journal of Psychiatry, 16,* 827–832.

chapter 10

Psychopharmacological Considerations in Integrated Modular Treatment

Kenneth R. Silk and Robert O. Friedel

Pharmacological treatment of personality disorder is at an early state of development. The only disorder for which there is some empirical evidence of efficacy is borderline personality disorder (BPD) (Ripoll, Triebwasser, & Siever, 2011; Stoffers, Völlm, Rücker, Timmer, & Lieb, 2010). However, there is substantial evidence of dysfunction in neural circuits related to several core symptoms of BPD (e.g., Mauchnik & Schmahl, 2010; New, Goodman, Triebwasser, & Siever, 2008) that justify the use of medications and modest evidence that a combination of medication and psychotherapy is the most effective way to treat BPD (American Psychiatric Association, 2001; Gunderson, 2011; Simpson et al., 2004; Soler et al., 2005). This chapter briefly reviews evidence of the efficacy of medication in treating personality disorder and proposes general guidelines for combining pharmacotherapy and psychotherapy. Because most studies involve BPD, we focus primarily on this disorder and extrapolate findings to other personality disorders.

RESPONSE TO PHARMACOLOGICAL TREATMENT

Despite uncertainties and controversies, medications are used frequently in treating personality disorders, and many medications are regularly prescribed off label. In the Collaborative Longitudinal Personality Disorders Study (CLPS), Bender and colleagues (2001) reported that 81% of their cohort of patients with BPD, schizotypal personality disorder (STPD), avoidant personality disorder (AvPD), or obsessive–compulsive personality disorder (OCPD) had been prescribed psychotropic medication. Zanarini, Frankenberg, Hennen, and Silk (2004) found that 78% of patients with BPD took medications for 75% of the time over a 6-year period compared with 68% of patients with other personality disorders. Moreover, 37% of patients with BPD were on three or more medications at 6-year follow-up compared with only 8% of other participants with personality disorder; over half were taking one medication, and about a quarter were taking two. However, systematic randomized controlled trials (RCTs) of medication effects exist only for borderline, antisocial, and schizotypal personality disorders. In some disorders, such as AvPD, treatment recommendations are extrapolated from studies of social phobia or generalized social anxiety because of the presumed overlap between these diagnoses (Cox, Pagura, Stein, & Sareen, 2009; Reich, 2009; Reichborn-Kjennerud et al., 2007). Most studies report no statistically significant difference in medication response between participants with social phobia with and without AvPD, though there is a tendency for participants with comorbid disorders to demonstrate a greater drug–placebo difference. The comorbidity of social phobia and AvPD does not appear to hinder the pharmacological response that people with "pure" social phobia without AvPD attain (Herpertz et al., 2007). Similarly, recommendations for treating obsessive–compulsive personality disorder (OCPD) have been extrapolated from studies of OCD. Unlike the results for AvPD, OCD-based pharmacological treatment for OCPD is not effective unless OCD is also present; medications seem to affect OCD symptoms with little effect on OCPD cognitions and behaviors (Ansseau, Troisfontainesart, Papart, & von Frenckell, 1991).

Turning to the remaining current DSM-5 personality disorders, there are meager data supporting pharmacological treatment of STPD and antisocial personality disorder (ASPD). With STPD, one RCT (Koenigsberg et al., 2003) found that risperidone decreased positive and negative symptoms compared with placebo as measured by the Positive and Negative Syndrome Scale (PANSS). Although other open-label studies of antipsychotic medications have looked at psychopharmacological response in patients with STPD, these studies primarily involved patients with BPD, some of whom also met criteria for STPD (Goldberg et al., 1986). One might assume that the antipsychotic medications shown to be effective in treating schizophrenia would also be effective in STPD because of the genetic overlap between the two diagnoses (Kendler, Gruenberg, & Strauss, 1981; Siever et al., 1995). As with studies of BPD, in which some antipsychotic medications (aripiprazole and perhaps olanzapine) but not others (e.g., ziprasidone) have been shown to be effective, the same is probably true for STPD, although only risperidone has been shown to be effective in an RCT (Koenigsberg et al., 2003).

The studies of psychopharmacological agents in ASPD are inconclusive and not generalizable because they did not examine the effects of pharmacological agents on core ASPD symptoms that were not studied without confounding comorbidity or bias in participant selection. For example, some studies involved patients with comorbid substance or alcohol misuse, and outcome measures primarily examined the impact of medication on future substance use (Leal, Ziedonis, & Kosten, 1994; Powell et al., 1995). Other studies using prisoners with ASPD are confounded by issues of incentives, expectations tied to privileges, and complications surrounding the participants' ability to give truly informed consent; these confounds lead to findings that are at best marginally difficult to generalize to nonincarcerated individuals.

PHARMACOLOGICAL TREATMENT OF BPD

Until the late 1970s, conventional wisdom held that medication treatment of patients with BPD was not only ineffective but also contraindicated, a position that was challenged at the time in a review of the literature and the presentation of case studies by Brinkley, Beitman, and Friedel (1979). The ensuing RCTs and open-label trials primarily evaluated first-generation antipsychotic agents (FGAs) and the antidepressants amitriptyline, phenelzine, and fluoxetine. The initial, positive results encouraged subsequent studies of broader classes of medications, especially second-generation antipsychotics (SGAs) and antiepileptic agents (mood stabilizers). Research was also stimulated by the resistance of the disorder to traditional forms of psychotherapy (Stern, 1938). The results of these studies led to the American Psychiatric Association (2001) Practice Guideline for the Treatment of Patients with Borderline Personality Disorder, which concluded that "pharmacotherapy often has an important adjunctive role [to psychotherapy], especially for diminution of symptoms such as affective instability, impulsivity, psychotic-like symptoms, and self-destructive behavior" and that "pharmacotherapy is used to treat state symptoms during periods of acute decompensation as well as trait vulnerabilities. Symptoms exhibited by patients with BPD often fall within three behavioral dimensions—affective dysregulation, impulsive–behavioral dyscontrol, and cognitive–perceptual difficulties—for which specific pharmacological treatment strategies can be used" (American Psychiatric Association, 2001, p. 4; Siever & Davis, 1991; Soloff, 1998). Specifically, the guideline proposed using selective serotonin reuptake inhibitors (SSRIs) to treat affective dysregulation and impulse dyscontrol, with the addition of an SGA for patients with cognitive–perceptual disturbances.

Growing enthusiasm for the potential benefit of psychotropic agents in BPD resulted in further studies, including additional placebo-controlled RCTs. The accumulation of empirical data made it possible to conduct meta-analyses to increase analytic power. Seven such studies have been performed, generating varying results as new RCTs were reported. The most recent studies, though they did not analyze the same RCTs or use identical methodology, yielded reasonably consistent findings (Duggan, Huband, Smailagic, Ferriter, & Adams, 2008; Ingenhoven, Lafay, Rinne, Passchier, & Duivenvoorden, 2010; Stoffers et al., 2010). In addition, reanalysis of RCTs using a semiquantitative method developed by Saunders and Silk (2009) produced similar results. First, no individual or class of drugs improves BPD pathology in general or to the degree that the patient no longer meets criteria for BPD. However, medication may lessen a symptom or a diagnostic criterion, such as the affective dysregulation that is often considered the core feature of BPD (Linehan, 1993). Second, there is evidence that mood stabilizers, especially topiramate, valproate, and lamotrigine, are effective in reducing some of the symptoms of affective dysregulation, especially anger and impulse dyscontrol. Third, some SGAs, specifically aripiprazole and possibly olanzapine, as well as quetiapine (Black et al., 2014) and the FGA haloperidol, appear to reduce cognitive–perceptual impairment, particularly excessive suspiciousness and paranoid ideation. They also have significant effects on affective and impulse dysregulation. Finally, despite the American Psychiatric Association (2001) guideline recommendations, there is little evidential support that SSRIs have a therapeutic effect on the core symptoms of the disorder, such as emotion dysregulation (Healy, 1997, 2004; Kramer, 1993; Silk & Jibson, 2012), despite evidence of serotonin dysfunction in BPD (New et al., 2008). It may be that the few clinical trials of SSRIs were too underpowered to demonstrate efficacy, resulting in a Type II error. Current evidence suggests that SSRIs are primarily useful in treating active comorbid major depressive episodes. The American Psychiatric Association guidelines may reflect psychiatry's initial enthusiasm with the broad success and mild side-effect profile of SSRIs compared with other antidepressants. Thus research since the American Psychiatric Association guidelines were published supports a shift from the SSRIs to mood stabilizers and antipsychotic medications, particularly the SGAs.

No class of drugs has consistently demonstrated an effect on disturbed interpersonal relationships, although this outcome was not systematically measured in most RCTs. Further, studies have not evaluated medication effects on other core symptoms, including suicidal and self-injurious behaviors, dissociation, fear of abandonment, chronic feelings of emptiness, identity disturbances, and dichotomous thinking.

Open-label trials, consensus conferences of experts, and clinical experience provide additional evidence consistent with the conclusions of meta-analyses of RCTs. For example, open-label trials suggest that risperidone (Friedel et al., 2008; Rocca, Marchiaro, Cocuzza, & Bogetto, 2002) and quetiapine (Adityanjee et al., 2008; Van den Eynde et al., 2008; Villeneuve & Lemelin, 2005) appear to be effective. There is also reasonable agreement between our conclusions and those of the task force of the World Federation of Societies of Biological Psychiatry (WFSBP; Herpertz et al., 2007). Therefore, given the evidence, a reasonable therapeutic strategy in BPD is to use antipsychotic agents, especially aripiprazole, and mood stabilizers such as topiramate as first-line medications to treat appropriate symptoms (Abraham & Calabrese, 2008).

Our conclusions do not coincide with those of all reviews, particularly the American Psychiatric Association guidelines. Some differences reflect the existing literature when the reviews were performed. For example, the American Psychiatric Association guidelines and the initial Cochrane Report (Binks et al., 2006) preceded the publication of many influential studies. However, some reviewers have drawn different conclusions, even after examining the same studies that we have. Most notable is the guideline of the National Institute for Health and Care Excellence (NICE) in the United Kingdom (National Collaborating Centre for Mental Health, 2009, p. 297), which stated that "drug treatment should not be used specifically for borderline personality disorder or for the individual symptoms or behavior associated with the disorder (for example, repeated self-harm, marked emotional instability, risk-taking behaviour and transient psychotic symptoms)." In a review (Lieb, Völlm, Rücker, Timmer, & Stoffers, 2010) of the most recent Cochrane Report (Stoffers et al., 2010), the authors disagree with the NICE conclusions: "We suggest considering a reassessment of these recommendations, as there actually is encouraging evidence of the effectiveness of drug treatment for individual symptoms of borderline personality disorder" (Lieb et al., 2010, p. 10). The most recent Cochrane Report (Stoffers et al, 2010, p. 64), noted that "the scope of NICE and this Cochrane Collaboration review differ in asking different questions and using different means and methods to answer them." In the first case, the Cochrane analyses are intended to review all of the valid RCTs in the area, whereas "NICE has always focused on the most effective way to use NHS [National Health Service] resources" and that it "considers somewhat different sources of evidence." Although we agree with the intent of NICE to develop treatment guidelines by using a broad spectrum of evidence, and although we have done the same, our conclusions are dissimilar to those of NICE and consistent with those of the recent Cochrane Report and other recent quantitative reviews.

Greater agreement exists on the use of medications in crises. Both the American Psychiatric Association (2001) and NICE (National Collaborating Centre for Mental Health, 2009) guidelines state that medications may be used in crises, but both suggest discontinuation after the crisis has passed. The one RCT examining medium-term use (up to 16 weeks) of medications in BPD (Cornelius, Soloff, George, Ulrich, & Perel, 1993) demonstrated that there was little if any efficacy of maintenance treatment with haloperidol and phenelzine. There are more recent, but open, placebo-controlled studies of continued use of aripiprazole (Nickel, Loew, & Pedrosa Gil, 2007), topiramate (Loew & Nickel, 2008; Nickel & Loew, 2008), and lamotrigine (Leibenrich, Nickel, Tritt, & Pedrosa Gil, 2008) for 18 months that found significant efficacy for the medication versus the control group. Finally, the studies and reviews noted here and clinical experience suggest that there is benefit in treating patients with BPD with medications. The value of the maintenance use of medication treatment in patients with BPD is still debatable (Tyrer & Silk, 2011), but open trials and clinical experience suggest there is benefit in doing so with care and with the intention of reducing and discontinuing, if possible, the doses and medications as patients improve (see the case example later in the chapter).

Substantial improvements in the pharmacological treatment of BPD and other personality disorders await more RCTs and consistent use of disorder-specific methodological standards and outcome measures (Zanarini et al., 2010). Results of these studies are also likely to depend on designing future trials around fundamental psychological and neurobiological mechanisms as opposed to global diagnoses. Such efforts have been minimal, although some modest progress has been made for BPD (see New et al., 2008; Skodol et al., 2002). Nevertheless, given progress in the psychopharmacological treatment of BPD, it is likely that novel new classes of medications now under development may prove more effective and tolerable than those currently available (Stanley & Siever, 2010).

GUIDELINES FOR THE INTEGRATED USE OF MEDICATIONS AND PSYCHOTHERAPY

Collaboration between Providers in an Integrated Treatment Model

Patients with personality disorders, especially BPD, sometimes present in crises of great emotional pain, with poorly controlled behaviors and flawed thinking, pleading for something to help them rapidly. At other times, they desire help for chronic emotional, behavioral, cognitive, and interpersonal problems of varying levels of severity. Some research and much clinical experience support the proposal that the most reasonable and effective approach for many of these patients is the combined use of the right medications with the right form of therapy for each patient. That is, the most effective treatment strategy appears to be an integrated treatment approach, administered by a skilled and experienced treatment team working in a highly collaborative manner.

Principles of Collaboration

In some instances, medication management and psychotherapy may be administered by a single psychiatrist. However, the current trend in some jurisdictions is to assign the role of prescribing medications to a psychiatrist or other physician and the role of psychotherapy to another mental health professional. The latter approach requires a high level of collaboration if the work of treatment is to proceed optimally. This occurs only when there is a clear, mutual understanding (and perhaps even a formal agreement) between the treating professionals on how the patient's illness can be most effectively managed. *Management* appears to be the proper word here, as there are few clear indications as to which medications and forms of psychotherapy should be utilized at any particular phase in the treatment process (Silk, 2011).

To make the task even more difficult, attitudes held by psychopharmacologists and psychotherapists can seriously interfere with a collaborative approach.

- The psychopharmacologist believes that BPD is really an atypical presentation of an Axis I condition such as bipolar disorder that should be treated primarily with medications.
- The psychopharmacologist is disdainful of nonmedical mental health providers and has little understanding of the application of psychotherapy in the treatment of BPD.
- The psychopharmacologist believes that it is merely a matter of time before the right combination of medicines can be found to eliminate the patient's symptoms without the need for psychotherapy.
- The psychopharmacologist wishes to take over treatment during BPD crises in order to make unilateral changes in the medication regimen.
- The psychopharmacologist does not check on patient compliance with psychotherapy appointments, does not inquire about how therapy is progressing, and in other subtle ways undermines the process of psychotherapy.
- The psychotherapist is disdainful of psychiatry and psychiatrists and has little if any understanding of the biology of personality disorders and pharmacological treatment.
- The psychotherapist believes that medications have no role in the treatment of patients with personality disorder and is referring the patient to the psychopharmacologist only because the patient is demanding it.
- The psychotherapist does not inquire about patient medication compliance or ask about efficacy and side effects and in other subtle ways undermines pharmacotherapeutic interventions.
- The psychotherapist, by claiming confidentiality and exclusivity of the psychotherapy relationship, rationalizes an unwillingness to discuss essential issues of the therapy with the psychopharmacologist.

In contrast, several principles can be helpful in the development and maintenance of a solid collaboration between the two providers. These have been discussed in a number of places (Schlesinger & Silk, 2009) and can be summarized as follows:

- Understand and clarify the relationship between the therapist and the psychiatrist.
- Understand what the medications mean to the therapist and the psychiatrist.
- Understand and clarify what the medications mean to the patient.
- Understand the limits of effectiveness of medications and psychotherapy.

- Understand how medications and psychotherapy fit into the overall treatment plan for the patient.
- Understand the potential for medication side effects and, if used improperly, for lethality as well.
- Understand that interpersonal crises and affective storms cannot be relieved simply through initiation or modification of medications.
- Understand the proper roles of the therapist and the psychiatrist in the management of the patient in periods of acute crises.

Strategies for Integrating Treatment-Specific Psychotherapeutic and Psychopharmacological Interventions

A number of specific psychotherapeutic interventions that currently show promise are discussed at length in other chapters of this book. These, and the two-phase model of psychotherapy suggested herein, present a number of questions on the overall integration of pharmacotherapy and psychotherapy in the treatment plan of each patient. If we are to follow the preceding principle "Understand how medications and psychotherapy fit into the overall treatment plan for the patient," then we need to consider the role of the psychiatrist and how that role might differ from a generic form of therapy to one that is more specific. Although there are no data that support a specific collaborative posture for either type of psychotherapy, we need to consider carefully how the roles of the therapist and the psychiatrist may differ under these therapeutic conditions.

It would seem likely that the integration of pharmacotherapy and psychotherapy should not present substantial problems. However, when considering strategies for integrating psychopharmacology into a specific therapy, a number of questions arise. Three such questions might be: (1) How does the theory of therapy coincide with the concept of psychopharmacology? (2) What are possible challenges to integrating pharmacotherapy and psychotherapy? (3) What approaches should the psychopharmacologist and the therapist take? For example, with a specific treatment for BPD such as dialectical behavior therapy (DBT), when the patient has permission to contact the individual therapist for between-session consultations, should the patient always contact the individual therapist even when, at least in the patient's eyes, the issue or problem seems directly related to the medication? In transference-focused psychotherapy, when there is a collaborative relationship between the psychotherapist and the psychopharmacologist, should the patient call the psychopharmacologist when he or she experiences a sudden upsurge of anxiety or depressive symptoms? Or should one almost always make the assumption that the increase in these affects have underlying transferential drivers and that this should always be discussed with the psychotherapist prior to any contact or decision making about initiation or changing of medications? What do therapists who utilize mentalization-based therapy and schema therapy think about the specific usefulness of medications during psychotherapy?

Presently there are no clear answers to these questions as they apply to specific forms of therapy, but it would seem incumbent upon us to begin to explore potential alternatives. Designing and conducting RCTs to examine various options for prescribing psychotherapy within the context of each of the effective therapies for BPD remains many years away. In the meantime, we might begin by exploring, with the developers of each of the BPD-specific therapies, the most important treatment goals governing the selection and use of medications in their form of treatment. For example, two studies have examined the use of psychotropic medications in DBT with contradictory conclusions. When up to 40 mg of fluoxetine (Simpson et al., 2004) was added to DBT, there was less improvement in the active treatment group when compared with a placebo group. However, when olanzapine (at doses slightly above 8 mg) was added to DBT (Soler et al., 2005), olanzapine was associated with significant improvement in ratings of depression, anxiety, and impulsive, aggressive behavior when compared with a placebo control. Confounding variables may be that these studies do not describe how the medications were prescribed and how the medication fit into the overall treatment model of DBT. Another explanation of these results is that olanzapine appears to be an effective agent in the treatment of certain core symptoms of BPD, whereas fluoxetine is not.

There are other issues that need consideration at this point. Even if the prescribing psychiatrist sees him- or herself merely as a prescriber, this does not mean that the relationship between the prescriber and the patient is insignificant. A therapeutic relationship and a sense of trust need to be built into this relationship, just as they need to be built into a relationship in which psychotherapy is taking place. This entails the psychopharmacologist presenting him- or herself as a real person and means that validation of the patient's experience must be an essential facet of the psychiatrist's response to the patient and that that this validation must take place in a listening environment that would involve the psychiatrist setting aside enough time for the patient to speak and express feelings and ask questions and enough time for the psychiatrist to respond and for a dialogue to take place. Fifteen-minute "med checks" will not do here. At the same time the psychopharmacologist needs to make sure that the psychopharmacology visits do not turn into another session of therapy. Thus an understanding as to the range of the discussions with the psychopharmacologist may need to be clarified between the treaters and closely monitored because this is a situation that is ripe for splitting. Everything we have said here is even more important with a patient who is constantly expressing suicidal ideation. Trust, as best as it can be achieved, is essential here.

Splitting may be avoided to some degree if the psychopharmacology and the psychotherapy are performed by the same person. But there can also be problems with this situation. When the patient comes to the therapy in crisis, displaying substantial amounts of emotion dysregulation, it may be hard to decipher whether the dysregulation is being triggered by discussions that have taken place in the psychotherapy treatment that have been inflamed further as transference intensifies or whether this an instance in which the medications clearly are not working. It is hard to decipher which may be more prominent even when there are two people managing the treatment, the psychopharmacologist and the psychotherapist, and even when they have the opportunity to talk between themselves in an atmosphere (one hopes) of mutual respect. When both aspects of the therapy are being managed by the same person, this opportunity is not available, and although one might consider talking to oneself (not an unusual event when treating patients with BPD), the dialogue within oneself is not always positive and is contaminated by how the treater thinks about him- or herself at that particular moment.

It is important that the patient not only comply with the medication (or at least feel comfortable enough with the psychopharmacologist to say when she is not complying) but also use the medications as prescribed. Patients with BPD have high rates of suicidal ideation, acting-out behavior, and successful suicides. Fortunately, the lethality of some medications used to treat BPD, such as SSRIs and atypical antipsychotics, is low, although the mood stabilizers and benzodiazepines have significant lethality. However, even safe medications can become unsafe when combined with alcohol, benzodiazepines, or other drugs, either licit or illicit, or when the patient is in an extremely dyscontrolled or intense negative transferential state. Patients need to appreciate that medications carry a degree of risk and that therefore they must be taken as prescribed and not combined with other substances. A trusting and mutually respectful treatment relationship is important in promoting compliance and safety. Problems in the relationship can lead to the patient using the medication to act out feelings about life and about the psychopharmacologist, a situation that becomes more complicated if the patient has suicidal thoughts or plans. Transference and countertransference are not reserved solely for the psychotherapy, and the psychopharmacologist needs to be aware of these phenomena. Unrealistic expectations about the effectiveness of medication can foster negative feelings about the treatment in both the patient and the psychopharmacologist.

The multiple problems of patients with BPD and the variation in symptoms across appointments easily lead to polypharmacy, especially when symptoms are disruptive. Thus it is easy for patients to receive separate medications for depression, anxiety, mood changes, dissociative reactions, and perhaps intermittent panic and insomnia. Although there is no evidence that polypharmacy is useful, this approach almost ensures drug interactions and weight gain. Polypharmacy is best avoided by discussing your approach with the patient and pointing out that the effects of medication may be quite modest. It also helps to acknowledge the patient's pain and distress and the wish for an effective medication while noting that unfortunately such medications do not currently exist. The psychopharmacologist should also explain that there is little evidence that two medications work better than one and that the most reasonable approach is to: (1) agree upon a target symptom for medication; (2) use the medication for the length of time and dose needed to produce a response; and (3) stop the medication if there is no response and try a different medication. Patients also need to understand that medications do not prevent crises, that progress will largely result from psychotherapy, and that medication is being proposed to allow them to make the most use of therapy. Currently, the pharmacotherapy of personality disorder is at an early stage, and the therapeutic effects of medications vary from insignificant to moderate depending on the symptom in question (Stoffers et al., 2010). Ultimately, fully integrated treatment of personality disorders requires more systematic information on when to prescribe medications and what the most effective medications are for the specific symptoms of personality disorder.

CASE EXAMPLE

The following case example illustrates the application of the approach described in this chapter in the treatment of a young woman diagnosed with BPD and referred by her psychotherapist for evaluation and recommendations regarding medication.

Ms. S, a 25-year-old single woman, was prepared for a medication consultation by her psychotherapist, who explained that she thought that medications might facilitate their work together. The therapist explained that she had worked with the psychiatrist for many years and that he was knowledgeable about the biological, pharmacological, and psychotherapeutic aspects of BPD and left therapy to the therapist and patient. She emphasized that the final decision to use medications was the patient's. The therapist also noted that the suggestion to consider medication did not mean that she (the therapist) had given up or that the patient was sicker than when they first met. Rather, she felt that mood fluctuations and some behaviors and thought patterns that were hindering therapy might improve with medication, especially the patient's intense emotions that caused her to react quickly and prevented her from recognizing that other people might have thoughts, feelings, or motivations different from those she at times attributed to them (Fonagy & Bateman, 2006). The therapist also noted that because she saw the patient frequently, she would also monitor the patient's compliance with medications and their efficacy and side effects and that if the patient wished to stop or change medications, she should first discuss it with the therapist. The patient, therapist, and prescribing psychiatrist would then confer to arrive at a decision. The therapist emphasized the expectation that medications would be taken as prescribed, that the patient would refrain from using illicit drugs, and that alcohol, if used, should be limited to the occasional drink. The patient agreed that her judgment was affected by her moods but noted that she was worried about medication masking her individuality. The therapist acknowledged these concerns and suggested discussing them with the psychiatrist.

At the evaluation, Ms. S described a chronic low-grade level of depression, episodes of more severe depression, mood swings, intermittent cutting behavior, periods of feeling "unreal," and bouts of anger that disrupted relationships with parents and friends. The most troublesome symptoms were the "bad" (angry) and unpredictable mood swings that occurred when she felt that others were not treating her "right." Afterward she recognized that she had overreacted, but at the time she felt justified. She also reported feeling anxiety and depression that were often triggered when she felt her boyfriend, parents, or friends were angry with her or might leave her. On these occasions, she sometimes cut herself. She denied substance abuse but admitted to verbal and physical aggression and unprotected casual sex. She was chronically suspicious; she felt that people talked badly about her behind her back and that her boyfriend cheated on her. At these times she occasionally became more paranoid and believed that people were scheming against her. When very upset, she felt that she and the things around her were unreal. She agreed that she consistently thought in absolute, all-or-nothing terms. Sustaining relationships had always been difficult; when attracted to someone, she would seek their company almost exclusively but soon found they were inattentive to her needs, leading to the relationship ending.

Ms. S described two kinds of depressed states. The most common occurred when her security or self-worth was threatened. On these occasions, she became despondent, angry, and anxious and thought of harming herself. These episodes lasted for a few hours to several days. The second involved sustained low mood; increased sleep, appetite, and weight; low energy; anhedonia; decreased cognitive functioning; and impaired motivation resulting in a decline in activities of daily living, such as bathing. These episodes occurred most often during the fall and winter and lasted from several weeks to 2 months before resolving slowly.

Ms. S denied anxiety or panic attacks, disordered eating, decreased concentration, distractibility, and difficulty in completing tasks and organizing thoughts and possessions. She said she had been an anxious and emotionally hyperreactive child prone to temper tantrums and aggressive outbursts that could result in her destroying toys or striking siblings or parents. She denied emotional, physical, or sexual abuse. She felt she was "the black sheep of the family" because of her emotional and physical outbursts, her failure to perform academically as well as her siblings, and her choice of friends.

There was a history of depression in the father's family and of anxiety, depression, and alcoholism in the mother's family. Ms. S had an older sister who was married and employed, whom she reported (with some disdain) as "perfect," and a "moody" younger brother, age 19, who was attending college. When assessed, Ms. S was unemployed and living with her parents, on whom she was financially dependent. Relationships with parents were strained. Her social life was limited to a few "very close friends," but these seemed to change frequently. Boyfriends rarely lasted long because she said they "cheated" on her or ignored her needs or requests for attention. She had achieved mainly B's and C's in high school and found school "boring." Nevertheless, her parents insisted that she attend community college; she dropped out in the first semester. Subsequently, she had held multiple unskilled jobs, but none lasted long because she said her bosses were unreasonable and her coworkers hostile.

Mental status examination revealed a pleasant, attractive, mildly disheveled, cooperative young lady in a mild state of discomfort with above-average intelligence. Speech was spontaneous, relevant, and coherent. Her mood was "OK now." Affect was mildly guarded, restricted in range and reactivity. There was no evidence of psychotic symptoms. On occasion she would make a statement that she contradicted later in the session. When this was brought to her attention, she became perplexed and was unable to reconcile these remarks. Insight was adequate. She denied current suicidal or homicidal ideation.

The working diagnoses at this time were major depressive episodes, recurrent, with atypical and seasonal features, by history, and BPD, moderate severity. She wanted to know the psychiatrist's diagnostic impression. She agreed that she had depression and that she had discussed the diagnosis of BPD with her therapist. She thought she probably wasn't trying hard enough in therapy despite having an understanding therapist who wanted to help her. She then noted that the therapist had raised the idea that medication might help her to progress more easily and rapidly.

The nature of BPD was explained in biopsychosocial terms. The family history of psychiatric disorders was noted, and it was suggested that it raised the possibility of a genetic contribution to her symptoms. It was also noted that many people with BPD have experienced environmental adversities that, combined with genetic loadings, contributed to the development of BPD. The elaboration of this formulation and discussion of personal, severe traumas led to the following discussion.

MS. S: But that didn't happen to me.

THERAPIST: Yes, that's true, which suggests that genetic risk factors are especially important in your case. Your difficult behaviors began early, and you seemed to have difficulty interacting easily with your parents and family. These difficulties got worse as your symptoms increased in your early teens, as they often do in BPD. Though you did the best that you could under the circumstances, your biology probably held you back, and you were not able to develop the skills needed to function smoothly in a complicated world. I think you may benefit from medications, and both you and your parents might benefit from more information on the nature of your symptoms.

MS. S: So this means I can't do any better than I am now because my genes won't let me?

THERAPIST: I understand how you might think that, but there is a different perspective. Just as there are medications, dietary restrictions, and exercise for the treatment of diabetes and combined medicinal and behavioral treatments for other medical illnesses that have strong genetic risk factors, there are combined treatments for BPD involving medications and therapy. Both treatments appear to improve the function of specific brain pathways that are not operating as well as they should, and I hope that you might be willing to try medications to help normalize their activity. If effective, they may reduce the degree of your hyperemotional responses and other distressful feelings and allow you to think things through better, enable you to exert better control over your behaviors, and even reduce the frequency and severity of some of your depressions. However, medications alone don't lead you to find out who you really are, what behaviors you need to change, or give you the skills to change them. For this to happen, you need to remain in therapy.

MS. S: But therapy hasn't helped me very much with how bad I feel at times or helped me consistently change my reactions. Though I now know better in my mind, I still often feel and behave the same way as I did before I started therapy.

THERAPIST: Perhaps that is because your chemistry is still getting in your way and not because you aren't trying hard enough. I think that the medications might make things a bit easier for you. But I also want you to understand that the medications are far from a cure-all. They don't always work as well or as effectively as we would like, and that is another reason why you need to continue to work in therapy while taking the medications.

MS. S: But I really don't want to take medications because they'll change who I am, and I'm afraid of the side effects.

THERAPIST: I can certainly understand those worries, and I appreciate your bringing them up. You know, I'm not certain that you or any of us truly knows who you are. There has been so much commotion in your life that your true capabilities have not had the opportunity to be explored and used. It should be exciting to discover them in therapy. Also, you, your therapist, and I will spend time and attention weighing the positive effects versus the negative effects of the medication. I certainly do not want you to take medications that will make you feel worse. We will monitor side effects closely. In addition, I hope that the medications will not only allow you to feel better and to make better use of your therapy but also help you react more slowly and thoughtfully so you can avoid getting yourself into risky situations and make more sound decisions.

MS. S: Well, I just don't know what to do.

THERAPIST: I understand. If it's OK with you, I will call your therapist to brief her on my findings, and you and she can discuss them and my recommendations and your feelings about them. There is no need to rush into something about which you are uncertain.

Shortly afterward, Ms. S agreed to a trial on a medication. Because symptoms included suspiciousness, paranoid ideation, and dissociation, a morning dose of 2.5 mg of aripiprazole (Abilify) was started. After 1 week, with little therapeutic effect and no adverse drug reactions, the dose was increased to 5 mg. Over the next 6 weeks Ms. S experienced a moderate decrease in suspiciousness and no paranoid episodes. However, emotional dysregulation, thoughts of self-injury, and dissociative experiences were only moderately improved. An increase to 10 mg of aripiprazole resulted in rare dissociative episodes. Other symptoms remained moderately disruptive, and she reported an increase in her appetite and a modest weight gain.

Ms. S was then presented with the alternative of either increasing the aripiprazole further or adding topiramate (Topamax). After discussing the rationale for the latter (a complementary mechanism of action with aripiprazole to produce less emotional instability and impulsive behavior and possibly a stabilization of appetite), she agreed to start on 25 mg of topiramate initially at bedtime for 1 week, followed by a gradual increase in dosage to 200 mg per day. This led to a gradual and significant further decline in anger, emotional dysregulation, and impulsivity—changes confirmed by her therapist, who also noted that Ms. S was working more effectively in therapy. Occasional episodes of emotional dysregulation were handled successfully in therapy. Occasional, brief (as-needed) increases of aripiprazole by 2.5 mg once or twice a day were found to be beneficial when her acute episodes were not manageable otherwise.

In midautumn, Ms. S developed a major depressive episode with atypical features that interfered with her work and life in and out of therapy. A discussion of treatment options, such as light therapy and a course of bupropion (Wellbutrin), led to the patient choosing light therapy. This resulted in only modest improvement, so it was discontinued, and she agreed to take extended-release bupropion (morning dose of 150 mg). Over the course of the next month, she experienced a full remission of her depressive episode that lasted through the remainder of the winter.

About 6 months after initiating pharmacotherapy, the patient began complaining of daytime drowsiness. Aripiprazole was reduced to 5 mg per day, and this side effect resolved. She and her therapist agreed that they might further reduce the aripiprazole and topiramate as her work in therapy progressed. In addition, the patient subsequently needed bupropion only during the fall and winter.

CONCLUDING COMMENTS

The evidence supports the use of mood stabilizers and/or antipsychotic medications to treat BPD and of antipsychotic medication to treat STPD but provides little evidence that supports the use of medication to treat other personality disorders. The responsiveness of BPD to both medication and psychotherapy compared with other personality disorders has led to the suggestion that BPD may respond more like other mental disorders than like a personality disorder (Tyrer, 2009). The evidence especially supports the use of mood stabilizers such as topiramate, valproate, and lamotrigine to treat emotional dysregulation and impulsivity associated with BPD. Antipsychotic agents, especially aripiprazole, appear to be the only agents that significantly reduce cognitive–perceptual impairment, especially suspiciousness and paranoia. They also appear to reduce emotional and impulsive dysregulation. Open-label studies and RCTs, as well as clinical experience, suggest that the effectiveness of both mood stabilizers and antipsychotic agents differs across patients. It may be that genetic factors influence efficacy and side effects in specific patients (Houston, Kohler, Ostbye, Heinloth, & Perlis, 2011; Risselada, Mulder, Heerdink, & Egberts, 2011), suggesting that several medications may need to be tried before the most effective medication and dosage is determined for each patient.

The evidence leads us to recommend a conservative approach to using medications. A single medication should be prescribed for a length of time and at a dose sufficient to reveal some therapeutic benefit. If the medication does not then show any benefit for the targeted symptom(s), it should be discontinued before another medication for that symptom is tried. If the medication shows some (even modest) effect, the dose should be increased before adding another augmenting medication or before adding a medication to address a different target symptom. It should be noted that there is a reasonable biological rationale for the use of a second medication from another class for the same symptom if it cannot be controlled adequately by a single medication (Friedel et al., 2008). However, before doing so, the benefits and risks should be weighed carefully—that is, clinical improvement or more control over behavior versus the cost of adding another medication, such as weight gain, drug–drug interactions, and other adverse drug reactions. Extensive clinical experience suggests that the behavioral changes resulting from pharmacotherapy and psychotherapy are probably interactive, which is not surprising, as it seems likely that they each ultimately affect the same brain mechanisms (Saxena et al., 2009). We believe that both approaches are essential if patients with BPD with moderate to severe levels of psychopathology are to achieve optimal benefits from treatment.

Although the principles and guidelines for using medications as part of an integrated treatment model, as we have described and illustrated in the case example, seem easy to apply with a patient who is as cooperative as the patient described, they are also helpful when working with a more difficult patient or one in a crisis. They bring order to a situation that can rapidly become chaotic. Regular contact between therapist and psychiatrist, even if only at times of crisis, helps them work through difficult situations with the patient. Mutual respect and regular and straightforward communication reduce opportunities for misunderstandings and mutual recrimination and build a shared sense of responsibility and patience when the patient fails to improve.

Following these principles and expanding them with modification to others involved in the treatment can provide guidance and structure to the nature of collaboration in an integrated treatment approach involving more than two clinicians. They provide structure for the patient, minimize differences that can occur between treating clinicians, and offer an opportunity to resolve differences while leading to an agreed-upon strategy to move forward. Because the personality disorders involve both heritable and environmental factors, and because these factors affect interpersonal relationships, how we prescribe may at times be as important as what we prescribe (Silk, 2011). The "how" becomes more important when psychotherapist and prescriber are different people. This process requires mutual respect and collaboration and regular communication between the therapist and the prescriber, a collaboration that needs to be well understood not only by both therapist and prescriber but hopefully by the patient as well. This process also helps to avoid, or at least hopefully minimize, the potential for splitting so that it does not turn destructive to both the patient and the overall therapy.

Integrated therapy is more than just a collaboration between a therapist and a psychopharmacologist. Integrated therapy involves carefully considering all the models and theories existing within our field that strive to explain the underlying psychopathology and pathophysiology of personality disorders and choosing and blending those that are most appropriate for the patient and the clinical situation. In the treatment of a patient with BPD, the therapist and the psychopharmacologist need to base their clinical decisions on the specific psychopathology demonstrated by the patient, on current knowledge about the efficacy and limitations of pharmacotherapy and psychotherapy in the treatment of this psychopathology, and on our best understanding of the pathophysiological processes that are most likely involved. Over time, this iterative process should result in increasingly more rapid advances in each of these areas and eventually in more sophisticated and effective integrated uses of this knowledge in the clinical setting.

REFERENCES

Abraham, P. F., & Calabrese, J. R. (2008). Evidence-based pharmacologic treatment of borderline personality disorder: A shift from SSRIs to anticonvulsants and atypical antipsychotics? *Journal of Affective Disorders, 111,* 21–30.

Adityanjee, Romine, A., Brown, E., Thuras, P., Lee, S., & Schulz, S. C. (2008). Quetiapine in patients with borderline personality disorder: An open-label trial. *Annals of Clinical Psychiatry, 20,* 219-226.

American Psychiatric Association. (2001). Practice guideline for the treatment of patients with borderline personality disorder. *American Journal of Psychiatry, 158*(10, Suppl.), 1–52

Ansseau, M., Troisfontaines, B., Papart, P., & von Frenckell, R. (1991). Compulsive personality as predictor of response to serotoninergic antidepressants. *British Medical Journal, 303,* 760–761.

Bender, D. S., Dolan, R. T., Skodol, A. E., Sanislow, C. A., Dyck, I. R., McGlashan, T. H., et al. (2001). Treatment utilization by patients with personality disorders. *American Journal of Psychiatry, 158,* 295–302.

Binks, C. A., Fenton, M., McCarthy, L., Lee, T., Adams, C. E., & Duggan, C. (2006). Pharmacological interventions for people with borderline personality disorder. *Cochrane Database of Systematic Reviews, 1,* CD005653.

Black, D. W., Zanarini, M. C., Romine, A., Shaw, M., Allen, J., & Schulz, S. C. (2014). Comparison of low and moderate dosages of extended-release quetiapine in borderline personality disorder: A randomized, double-blind, placebo-controlled trial. *American Journal of Psychiatry, 171,* 1174–1182.

Brinkley, J. R., Beitman, B. S., & Friedel, R. O. (1979). Low-dose neuroleptic regimens in the treatment of borderline patients. *Archives of General Psychiatry, 36,* 319–326.

Cornelius, J. R., Soloff, P. H., George, A., Ulrich, R. F., & Perel, J. M. (1993). Haloperidol vs. phenelzine in continuation therapy of borderline disorder. *Psychopharmacology Bulletin. 29,* 333–337.

Cox, B. J., Pagura, J., Stein, M. B., & Sareen, J. (2009). The relationship between generalized social phobia and avoidant personality disorder in a national mental health survey. *Depression and Anxiety, 26,* 354–362.

Duggan, C., Huband, N., Smailagic, N., Ferriter, M., & Adams, C. (2008). The use of pharmacological treatments for people with personality disorder: A systematic review of randomized controlled trials. *Personality and Mental Health, 2,* 119–170.

Fonagy, P., & Bateman, A. (2006). Progress in the treatment of borderline personality disorder. *British Journal of Psychiatry, 188,* 1–3.

Friedel, R. O., Jackson, W. T., Huston, C. S., May, R. S., Kirby, N. L., & Stoves, A. (2008). Risperidone treatment of borderline personality disorder assessed by a borderline personality disorder-specific outcome measure: A pilot study [Letter to the editor]. *Journal of Clinical Psychopharmacology, 28*(3), 345–347.

Goldberg, S. C., Schulz, S. C., Schulz, P. M., Resnick, R. J., Hamer, R. M., & Friedel, R. O. (1986). Borderline personality disorders treated with low-dose thiothixene vs. placebo. *Archives of General Psychiatry, 43,* 680-686.

Gunderson, J. G. (2011). Clinical practice: Borderline personality disorder. *New England Journal of Medicine, 364,* 2037–2042.

Healy, D. (1997). *The antidepressant era.* Cambridge, MA: Harvard University Press.

Healy, D. (2004). *Let them eat Prozac: The unhealthy relationship between the pharmaceutical industry and depression.* New York: New York University Press.

Herpertz, S. C., Zanarini, M., Schulz, C. S., Siever, L., Lieb, K., Möller, H. J., et al. (2007). World Federation of Societies of Biological Psychiatry (WFSBP) guidelines for biological treatment of personality disorders. *World Journal of Biological Psychiatry, 8,* 212–244.

Houston, J. P., Kohler, J., Ostbye, K. M., Heinloth, A., & Perlis, R. H. (2011). Association of catechol-O-methyltransferase variants with duloxetine response in major depressive disorder. *Psychiatry Research, 189,* 475–477.

Ingenhoven, T., Lafay, P., Rinne, T., Passchier, J., & Duivenvoorden, H. (2010). Effectiveness of pharmacotherapy for severe personality disorders: Meta-analyses of randomized controlled trials. *Journal of Clinical Psychiatry, 71,* 14–25.

Kendler, K. S., Gruenberg, A. M., & Strauss, J. S. (1981). An independent analysis of the Copenhagen sample of the Danish adoption study of schizophrenia: II. The relationship between schizotypal personality disorder and schizophrenia. *Archives of General Psychiatry, 38,* 982–984.

Koenigsberg, H. W., Reynolds, D., Goodman, M., New, A. S., Mitropoulou, V., Trestman, R. L., et al. (2003). Risperidone in the treatment of schizotypal personality disorder. *Journal of Clinical Psychiatry, 64,* 628–634.

Kramer, P. (1993). *Listening to Prozac.* New York: Viking.

Leal, J., Ziedonis, D., & Kosten, T. (1994). Antisocial personality disorder as a prognostic factor for pharmacotherapy of cocaine dependence. *Drug and Alcohol Dependence, 35,* 31–35.

Leiberich, P., Nickel, M. K., Tritt, K., & Pedrosa Gil, F. (2008). Lamotrigine treatment of aggression in female borderline patients: Part II. An 18-month follow-up. *Journal of Psychopharmacology, 22,* 805-808.

Lieb, K., Völlm, B., Rücker, G., Timmer, A., & Stoffers, J. M. (2010). Pharmacotherapy for borderline personality disorder: Cochrane systematic review of randomised trials. *British Journal of Psychiatry, 196,* 4–12.

Linehan, M. M. (1993). *Cognitive-behavioral treatment of borderline personality disorder.* New York: Guilford Press.

Loew, T. H., & Nickel, M. K. (2008). Topiramate treatment of women with borderline personality disorder: Part II. An open 18-month follow-up. *Journal of Clinical Psychopharmacology, 28,* 355–857.

Mauchnik, J., & Schmahl. C. (2010). The latest neuroimaging findings in borderline personality disorder. *Current Psychiatry Reports, 12,* 46–55.

National Collaborating Centre for Mental Health. (2009). *Borderline personality disorder: Treatment and management.* Leicester, UK: British Psychological Society.

New, A. S., Goodman, M., Triebwasser, J., & Siever, L. J. (2008). Recent advances in the biological study of personality disorders. *Psychiatric Clinics of North America, 31,* 441–461.

Nickel, M. K., & Loew, T. H. (2008). Treatment of aggression with topiramate in male borderline patients. Part II. 18-month follow-up. *European Psychiatry: The Journal of the Association of European Psychiatrists, 23,* 115–117.

Nickel, M. K., Loew, T. H., & Pedrosa Gil, F. (2007). Aripiprazole in treatment of borderline patients: Part II. An 18-month follow-up. *Psychopharmacology, 191,* 1023–1026.

Powell, B. J., Campbell, J. L., Landon, J. F., Thomas, H. M., Nickel, E. J., Dale, T. M., et al. (1995). A double-blind, placebo-controlled study of nortriptyline and bromocriptine in male alcoholics subtyped by comorbid psychiatric disorders. *Alcoholism: Clinical and Experimental Research, 19,* 462–468.

Reich, J. (2009). Avoidant personality disorder and its relationship to social phobia. *Current Psychiatry Reports, 11,* 89–93.

Reichborn-Kjennerud, T., Czajkowski, N., Torgersen, S., Neale, M. C., Ørstavik, R. E., Tambs, K., et al. (2007). The relationship between avoidant personality disorder and social phobia: A population-based twin study. *American Journal of Psychiatry, 164,* 1722–1728.

Ripoll, L. H., Triebwasser, J., & Siever, L. J. (2011). Evidence-based pharmacotherapy for personality disorders. *International Journal of Neuropsychopharmacology, 14,* 1257–1288.

Risselada, A. J., Mulder, H., Heerdink, E. R., & Egberts, T. C. (2011). Pharmacogenetic testing to predict antipsychotic-induced weight gain: A systematic review. *Pharmacogenomics, 12,* 1213–1227.

Rocca, P., Marchiaro, L., Cocuzza, E., & Bogetto, F. (2002). Treatment of borderline personality disorder with risperidone. *Journal of Clinical Psychiatry, 63,* 241–244.

Saunders, E. F., & Silk, K. R. (2009). Personality trait dimensions and the pharmacological treatment of borderline personality disorder. *Journal of Clinical Psychopharmacology, 29,* 461–467.

Saxena, S., Gorbis, E., O'Neill, J., Baker, S. K., Mandelkern, M. A., Maidment, K. M., et al. (2009). Rapid effects of brief intensive cognitive-behavioral therapy on brain glucose metabolism in obsessive-compulsive disorder. *Molecular Psychiatry, 14,* 197–205.

Schlesinger, A. B., & Silk, K. R. (2009). Collaborative treatment. In J. M. Oldham, A. E. Skodol, & D. S. Bender (Eds.), *Essentials of personality disorders* (pp. 321–341). Washington DC: American Psychiatric Publishing.

Siever, L. J., & Davis, K. L. (1991). A psychobiological perspective on the personality disorders. *American Journal of Psychiatry, 148,* 1647–1658.

Siever, L. J., Rotter, M., Losonczy, M., Guo, S. L., Mitropoulou, V., Trestman, R., et al. (1995). Lateral ventricular enlargement in schizotypal personality disorder. *Psychiatry Research, 57,* 109–118.

Silk, K. R. (2011). The process of managing medications in patients with borderline personality disorder. *Journal of Psychiatric Practice, 17,* 311–319.

Silk, K. R., & Jibson, M. D. (2012). Personality disorders. In A. Rothchild (Ed.), *The evidence-based guide to antidepressant medication* (pp. 139–169). Washington, DC: American Psychiatric Publishing.

Simpson, E. B., Yen, S., Costello, E., Rosen, K., Begin, A., Pistorello, J., et al. (2004). Combined dialectical behavior therapy and fluoxetine in the treatment of borderline personality disorder. *Journal of Clinical Psychiatry, 65,* 379–385.

Skodol, A. E., Siever, L. J., Livesley, W. J., Gunderson, J. G., Pfohl, B., & Widiger, T. A. (2002). The borderline diagnosis: II. Biology, genetics, and clinical course. *Biological Psychiatry, 51,* 951–963.

Soler, J., Pascual, J. C., Campins, F., Barrachina, J., Puigdemont, D., Alvarez, E., et al. (2005). Double-blind, placebo-controlled study of dialectical behavior therapy plus olanzapine for borderline personality disorder. *American Journal of Psychiatry, 162,* 1221–1224.

Soloff, P. H. (1998). Algorithms for pharmacological treatment of personality dimensions: Symptom-specific treatments for cognitive–perceptual, affective, and impulsive–behavioral dysregulation. *Bulletin of the Menninger Clinic, 62,* 195–214.

Stanley, B., & Siever, L. J. (2010). The interpersonal dimension of borderline personality disorder: Toward a neuropeptide model. *American Journal of Psychiatry, 167,* 24–39.

Stern, A. (1938). Psychoanalytic investigation of and therapy in the borderline group of neuroses. *Psychoanalytic Quarterly, 7,* 467–489.

Stoffers, J., Völlm, B. A., Rücker, G., Timmer, A., & Lieb, K. (2010). Pharmacological interventions for borderline personality disorder. *Cochrane Database of Systematic Reviews, 16*(6), CD005653.

Tyrer, P. (2009). Why borderline personality disorder is neither borderline nor a personality disorder. *Personality and Mental Health, 3,* 86–95.

Tyrer, P., & Silk, K. R. (2011). A comparison of UK and US guidelines for drug treatment in borderline personality disorder. *International Review of Psychiatry, 23,* 388–394.

Van den Eynde, F., Senturk, V., Naudts, K., Vogels, C., Bernagie, K., Thas, O., et al. (2008). Efficacy of quetiapine for impulsivity and affective symptoms in borderline personality disorder. *Journal of Clinical Psychopharmacology, 28,* 147–155.

Villeneuve, E., & Lemelin, S. (2005). Open-label study of atypical neuroleptic quetiapine for treatment of borderline personality disorder: Impulsivity as main target. *Journal of Clinical Psychiatry, 66,* 1298–1303.

Zanarini, M. C., Frankenburg, F. R., Hennen, J., & Silk, K. R. (2004). Mental health service utilization by borderline personality disorder patients and Axis II comparison subjects followed prospectively for 6 years. *Journal of Clinical Psychiatry, 65,* 28–36.

Zanarini, M. C., Stanley, B., Black, D. W., Markowitz, J. C., Goodman, M., Lynch, T. R., et al. (2010). Methodological considerations for treatment trials for persons with borderline personality disorder. *Annals of Clinical Psychiatry, 22,* 75–83.

chapter 11

A Modular Strategy for Treating Emotional Dysregulation

W. John Livesley

Impairments in the regulation of emotions that are ubiquitous to personality disorders take two main forms: dysregulated and constricted. The dysregulated pattern involves reactive and unstable emotions that are associated with unstable relationships, arising from a need for closeness that conflicts with fear of rejection and abandonment. In contrast, the constricted pattern involves restricted expression of feelings associated with socially avoidant traits. This chapter discusses the treatment of emotional dysregulation, a central feature of DSM-IV/DSM-5 borderline personality disorder (BPD) and an important component of other forms of personality disorder.

Emotion regulation is a broad construct that refers to the processes influencing the occurrence, intensity, experience, and expression of emotions (Gross & Thompson, 2007). These processes include cognitive–emotional skills used to monitor, appraise, and modify emotional responses to internal and external events (Nolen-Hoeksema, 2012) and higher-order meaning systems and personal narratives. Impairments to these capacities and structures have widespread effects on personality functioning. When treating these impairments, the intention is to help patients to recognize the nuances of their emotional experiences, to regulate and modulate emotional expression, and to increase the capacity to process emotional experiences.

Although outcome research suggests that all specialized personality disorder treatments improve emotional dysregulation, the change mechanisms responsible are unclear. This is problematic because treatment methods differ across therapies. Some therapies, especially the cognitive-behavioral therapies and most notably dialectical behavior therapy (DBT; Linehan, 1993), target dysregulated emotions directly by enhancing emotion-regulating skills, improving the capacity to solve emotional problems, and restructuring cognitions associated with emotional arousal. In contrast, transference-focused psychotherapy (TFP; Clarkin, Yeomans, & Kernberg, 2006) adopts a more indirect approach, assuming that enhanced emotional control results from the resolution of structural impairments to personality that involve fragmented object relationships that are addressed in the context of the patient–therapist interaction. Mentalizing-based therapy (MBT; Bateman & Fonagy, 2006) similarly adopts a relatively indirect strategy, assuming that emotional control increases with improved mentalizing capacity. The contrast here is between the more skill-building approach of DBT and the greater emphasis that TFP and MBT place on developing an understanding of the interpersonal context of emotion and the capacity to process emotional experiences. As outcome studies show that these treatments are equally effective and that emotion dysregulation includes both deficiencies in emotion-regulating skills *and* in processing emotions, it is probably best to adopt a unified strategy that combines interventions from all therapeutic models until more definitive findings are available. This is the approach adopted in this chapter. Consistent with the theme of the volume, emotional dysregulation is decomposed into components and interventions are selected to treat each component based on evidence of efficacy and a rational analysis of potentially useful methods. This allows dysregulated emotions to be targeted synergistically from different perspectives. The first section of the chapter provides a context for identifying treatment goals and methods by examining the role of emotions in adaptive personality functioning, the structure of emotional traits, and the subjective experience of patients with intense, unstable emotions. The second section sets out a general framework for treatment, and the third section describes specific intervention modules.

NATURE AND STRUCTURE OF EMOTION DYSREGULATION

Dysregulated emotions are complex in structure and consequences. To identify effective treatment methods, we need to deconstruct this complexity. This requires an understanding of the role that emotions play in adaptive and maladaptive personality functions and the structure of emotional traits that underlie dysregulated emotional expression. However, this understanding is not sufficient to manage patients. To establish an effective working relationship, we also need to be able to relate empathically to patients' emotional experiences and align with their emotional distress. This requires an understanding of the subjective experience of dysregulated emotions and what it feels like to experience an emotional crisis.

The Role of Emotion in Personality Functioning

Dysregulated emotions lead to some obvious consequences, such as emotional crises, deliberate self-harm, and suicidality, and to some not-so-obvious consequences due to the impact of disorganized emotions on personality functioning. The most obvious manifestation of these impacts occurs in crises, when increasing emotional arousal progressively impairs cognitive functions involving information processing, problem solving, and impulse regulation, creating a positive feedback loop in which increasing cognitive impairment decreases control over emotions, leading to increased emotional arousal. More fundamentally, modulated emotions are necessary for adaptive personality functioning: Emotions are integral to coherent interchange with the environment, they contribute to stable relationships with others, and they guide the construction of meaning systems and personal narratives that have diverse influences on personality functioning, including emotional expression and interpersonal behavior. Emotions are also inherently motivational: They contribute to the establishment of long-term goals that give direction and purpose to action over time. Dysregulated emotions interfere with these processes, with widespread consequences for personal and interpersonal behavior. Consequently, comprehensive treatment of emotional dysregulation involves interventions to build emotional control, to correct the effects of unstable emotions on personality functioning, and to integrate emotions with other personality processes.

Adaptive interaction with the world requires a wide range of emotions expressed in regulated and nuanced ways. Emotions give meaning to experience: They shape our perception of the environment and our responses to it (Stanghellini & Rosfort, 2013). They tell us what is threatening and dangerous and what is rewarding and pleasurable, as well as the things that are important and the people who matter. And, in doing so, they help to anchor us to the world we occupy, thereby contributing to our sense of self and those aspects of identity that involve having a connection to the world and the sense of place that makes the world "our world." Without emotions, everything in the environment would seem equally important; nothing would stand out as significant and worthy of attention. But emotions do not only help to organize our perception of the environment; they also serve a motivational function by helping to link inner need states to external events that can satisfy these needs and by helping to identify goals that are worth attaining. The combined effects of these factors is that emotions play a large role in generating and organizing self-knowledge and self-understanding.

When emotions are unstable and disorganized, information inputs about the world are less consistent. The world, especially the interpersonal world, looks inconsistent and unpredictable. Because predictability contributes to feelings of safety and security, these feelings, coupled with the high levels of anxiousness associated with unstable emotions, leads to a perception of the world as threatening and malevolent. Labile emotions help to create an ever-changing social landscape that fails to provide the stable environmental input needed to construct stable representations of self and others.

As the hermeneutic tradition shows, humans are meaning-seeking and interpretative beings who seek to understand their experiences, moods, and personal qualities by constructing and reconstructing interpretative personal narratives (Ricoeur, 1981; Stanghellini & Rosfort, 2013). We do not passively receive informational input from our internal and external worlds but rather seek to impose meaning on our experiences, including the emotions that guide them. We do so not merely by representing emotions with schema we have acquired to organize and manage experience but also by elaborating meaning systems and constructing narratives around these experiences and the significance we believe them to have for understanding and organizing our lives. As they are elaborated, these narratives become important parts of our sense of self and identity, whereupon they assume a powerful organizing effect on behavior and help to regulate the emotions they are designed to understand (Leary, 2003). They can also generate emotions in themselves, and hence self-narratives can either contribute to emotional dysregulation or modulate emotional expression. The regulatory function of self-narratives is important. Hence, the treatment of emotional dysregulation needs to pay attention to the narratives patients construct around their emotional experiences and seek to restructure narratives that exacerbate and instigate emotional instability and strengthen those that modulate distress.

These phenomena are illustrated by the cases of two relatively typical patients. Both are young women forced to discontinue their studies due to similar levels of emotional instability, intense anxiety, and deliberate self-injury. Both responded to treatment with similar levels of symptomatic improvement. As a result, they completed their studies and went on to build productive careers. However, there are important differences in outcome. One has an active life and a positive outlook and is looking forward to a successful career. The other, although also doing well symptomatically and working successfully, remains fearful about becoming ill again and apprehensive about the future. This fear limits her life and career opportunities. These differences do not appear to reflect biological or psychological differences in emotion regulation. The difference seems to lie in the meaning and interpretation each patient attributed to her symptoms and emotional traits and the way this understanding became incorporated into her sense of self and identity. Consequently, we can only fully understood and treat these patients by taking into account the unique ways in which they react to their problems and their subjective experience of their emotions.

Both patients initially interpreted their dysregulated emotions as overwhelming and intolerable—what we could call *lower-level meaning*. These lower levels of meaning are subject to further self-reflection to create higher-order structures or narratives that become part of the self. This is an important process. A recurrent theme across several chapters of this book is the importance of working with narrative episodes (see Dimaggio et al., Chapter 8, this volume). It is at this level that differences emerge. One woman, a fearsome competitor in her chosen sport, accepted that her emotions were more intense than those of other people but interpreted this as a problem to overcome. She approached emotional dysregulation as she would a competitor—something she needed to vanquish. She was prepared to do whatever it took to win, and she expected to win. As a result, she was keen to learn skills to help her manage her feelings better, and this was sufficient for her to improve enough to get on with her life. As a result, her life became filled with positive goals that gave her a sense of purpose that facilitated emotion regulation. The other patient saw the same problems differently. She constructed a self-narrative of being a vulnerable person with inherent flaws who needed to be prudent and cautious. Each minor problem of everyday living was interpreted as proof of this vulnerability and hence as a reason for caution. Thus her life was filled with avoidance goals—situations and events she wanted to avoid. Unlike positive goals, negative goals are less rewarding and do not provide either a sense of integration or direction (Livesley, 2003). Unlike the first patient, the narrative she constructed amplified and often instigated emotional distress. Research on healthy participants suggests that when a problem behavior is linked to self or identity problems, a skill-building approach may help, but it is not sufficient (Walton, Paunesku, & Dweck, 2012). It is also important to address the associated belief system. This proved to be the case with the second patient. The skill-building and emotion-regulation strategies used with the first patient were helpful but not sufficient. It was also necessary to work with the self-narrative that helped to maintain and even instigate dysregulation.

Traits Associated with Unstable Emotions

Factor analyses of personality disorder traits are a useful starting point for understanding the structure of dysregulated emotions. Four factors are consistently identified that are variously labeled *asthenia/emotional dysregulation*, *antisocial/dissocial*, *asocial/social avoidance*, and *anankastic/compulsivity* (Livesley, Jang, & Vernon, 1998; Widiger & Simonsen, 2005). The large asthenia/emotional dysregulation factor consists of emotional, interpersonal, and cognitive traits. The emotional traits that underlie the clinical manifestations of emotional dysregulation are anxiousness and emotional lability (Livesley, 2008). The distinction between anxiousness and emotional lability is useful in helping patients to identify their feelings accurately and in selecting interventions. Anxiousness involves a lifelong tendency to worry and ruminate. Patients with high levels of anxiousness believe that they live in a threatening and hostile world. At times of crisis, they experience intense panic-like anxiety that creates a desperate urgency to end the feelings, which often leads to deliberate self-harm. Emotional lability is characterized by unstable, rapidly changing, and highly reactive emotions, variable moods, and intense anger. Anxiousness and emotional lability are associated with insecure attachment, submissive–dependency, social fearfulness, and cognitive dysregulation—the tendency for thinking to become confused and disorganized when stressed.

Like all personality traits (Plomin, Chipeur, & Loehlin, 1990), anxiousness and emotional lability are heritable (Livesley et al., 1998). Structural analyses suggest that anxiousness consists of a single genetic dimension, whereas emotional lability has two genetic components: (1) emotional reactivity that leads to rapid emotional arousal and irritability and (2) emotional intensity involving strong emotional reactions even to minor events. This structure is similar to Linehan's (1993) suggestion that the emotional responses of patients with BPD involve rapid arousal and slow return to baseline.

Anxiousness and emotional lability are often associated with generalized hypersensitivity, the tendency to experience things intensely; emotions, indeed any stimuli, feel intrusive and overwhelming, which amplifies distress. Many patients also show a fourth trait, a combination of anhedonia and pervasive pessimism, that is difficult to label succinctly. Such patients experience little pleasure or satisfaction, which impairs motivation and increases feelings of passivity and hopelessness because nothing is pleasurable, and experience a pervasive sense of pessimism that intensifies feelings of hopelessness and may increase suicidality. Emotional crises arise from the interaction of the four emotional traits, especially emotional lability and anxiousness, creating a perplexing mixture of feelings that patients find difficult to disentangle.

Phenotypic and genetic analyses have other clinical implications. First, the contribution of genetic factors needs to be understood by patients because this often helps to mute self-criticism. However, it is also important to ensure that the patient understands that this does not mean that emotional reactions cannot be changed with treatment. Second, these analyses show the value of decomposing emotional states into components that may respond to different interventions. They also draw attention to anxiousness—a feature that tends to be overlooked in favor of the more salient emotional lability—and thus the value of incorporating anxiety management strategies.

Subjective Experience

Although analyses of personality structure help to identify treatment targets, the management of emotional dysregulation also requires an understanding of the phenomenology of emotional instability and the patient's subjective experience of emotions. This understanding allows the therapist to align more empathically with the patient's distress. It also clarifies treatment goals.

Probably the most obvious feature of emotional dysregulation is the *undifferentiated nature* of intense emotional states. Patients experience a chaotic mixture of distress, intense panic-like anxiety, sadness, depression, anger, and frustration. Because these states are difficult to describe, patients often fall back on describing themselves as depressed, although depression is usually only part of the picture. The subjective complexity of these states suggests that a first step in treatment is to "unpack" emotional experiences by helping the patient to recognize the different feelings involved.

Another important feature of dysregulated emotions is how the individual *relates to his or her subjective experience of emotion.* As the acceptance-based behavioral therapies (Roemer & Orsillo, 2009) note, patients with emotional dysregulation have difficulty separating themselves from their feelings. This is especially true of patients with severe personality disorders; feelings are not treated as states that come and go but rather as enduring and all-encompassing states that define the self. In contrast, healthy individuals who feel sad or distressed recognize that these feelings are transient. They can also separate themselves from their feelings. This distinction is lost in patients with severe disorder who tend to "fuse" with their emotions (Hayes, Strosahl, & Wilson, 1999). Thus intense feelings permeate their whole being—rather than feeling angry or ashamed, the person sees him- or herself as an angry or shameful person. This fusion intensifies distress because it leads the patient to assume that he or she always has and always will feel this way. For example, a patient in a severely distressed state characterized by agitation, anxiety, and a painful sense of inner emptiness insisted that the feelings would never go away because he had always felt that way, even though in the preceding weeks he had talked about never having felt so well. The tendency to fuse with intense feelings suggests that an important therapeutic focus is to help patients to *decenter* from their experiences by reflecting on their experiences as opposed to simply reacting to them.

Despite experiencing intense painful emotions, patients with emotionally dysregulated personality disorder usually have limited awareness of the actual emotions involved. This almost paradoxical phenomenon is explained by the distinction between *self-focus* and *self-awareness.* These patients usually have an intense self-focus: They are acutely aware of, and hypersensitive to, inner experience, including the physiological sensations associated with emotional arousal, but have limited awareness of the nuances of these experiences. They experience acute distress without knowing the origins of this distress and pay little attention to the collage of feelings involved. Tendencies to fuse with feeling and difficulties with *self-reflection* and decentering leave these patients trapped in a distressed state that they cannot process or understand. Hence an important treatment strategy is to change a persistent self-focus first into self-awareness and self-understanding and subsequently into self-reflection by promoting the capacity to reflect on the nature and origins of emotional experiences.

Difficulty processing emotions leads to rapid and intense reactions. Treatment seeks to slow reactivity by creating a delay between events and action by enhancing the self-observation and self-reflection patients need to understand the meaning and significance of their feelings. As noted previously, these meaning systems help to regulate emotional arousal by creating an explanatory narrative that allows the patient to place emotional experiences within a broader interpersonal context, a process that enhances self-regulation and permits great flexibility in how emotions are managed.

Awareness is also limited by *emotional avoidance*. Intense distress often leads patients to conclude that emotions are harmful states to be avoided at all costs. Thus they suppress feelings and use cognitive and behavioral strategies to avoid exposure to situations and thoughts that evoke painful feelings. Emotional avoidance produces short-term reduction in distress, but in the long term, the urge to suppress or get rid of feelings intensifies distress and hinders the development of self-knowledge. As stressed by the acceptance-based behavioral therapies, emotional avoidance leads to *behavioral restriction* (Roemer & Orsillo, 2009). Patients become so preoccupied with avoiding feelings and situations that trigger them that their lives become increasingly constricted to the point that they even avoid activities that give pleasure and satisfaction. This is seen in individuals with severe disorders who become so preoccupied with avoiding unpleasant feelings that they even neglect the tasks of everyday living. When this happens, distress becomes almost self-perpetuating because patients create both a way of living that perpetuates distress and avoid situations that could potentially correct the maladaptive cognitions that generate distress.

Dysregulated emotions are usually accompanied by maladaptive ways of thinking about emotions (see Leahy, Chapter 12, this volume) that escalate distress. Patients tell themselves that their feelings are intolerable, that they cannot stand them, and that they will kill themselves if the feelings continue. This kind of self-talk perpetuates emotional distress. It also tends to be accompanied by intense self-criticism and self-invalidation—patients tell themselves that they should not have these feelings and that there is no reason for them, statements that often echo things heard from caregivers during childhood. One of the challenges in treating these patients is to help them to become more compassionate toward themselves and to show greater acceptance of negative feelings.

A GENERAL FRAMEWORK FOR TREATING EMOTIONAL DYSREGULATION

The overall goal in treating emotional dysregulation is to reduce the intensity and frequency of maladaptive emotional states and promote more adaptive use of emotions. The preceding discussion of emotional dysregulation helps to delineate four goals:

1. Increase knowledge about normal and dysregulated emotions.
2. Increase emotional awareness and understanding.
3. Increase emotional self-regulation skills.
4. Increase the capacity to process emotional experiences.

A multifaceted approach is needed to attain these goals and address the complex biological and psychosocial impairments affecting emotional expression. Reliance on a one-dimensional approach such as either medication or a skill-building approach—two strategies commonly used by mental health systems—is unlikely to be sufficient, although each may contribute to a unified approach. Medication may help to settle emotional reactivity and facilitate psychotherapeutic interventions (see Silk & Friedel, Chapter 10, this volume, for medication strategies), and skill building is helpful in enhancing self-regulation. However, other treatment strategies are needed to enhance the emotional processing capacity and restructure the meaning systems and narratives implicated in emotional expression.

Livesley and colleagues, in earlier chapters (Chapters 1–3) in this volume, noted the value of conceptualizing interventions in terms of general strategies based on common change mechanisms and specific interventions that are more directly tied to specific impairments. The general intervention strategies create the treatment process needed to contain emotional reactivity and incorporate interventions to enhance the motivation, self-reflection, and metacognitive functioning that underpin the use of more specific interventions. The specific treatment of emotional dysregulation begins with case formulation. As noted by Clarkin and Livesley (Chapter 4, this volume), the formulation used to plan treatment requires revision throughout therapy as new information becomes available. The first opportunity to do this occurs when the patient is sufficiently engaged to work on improving emotion regulation.

Formulation

The formulation is most conveniently organized using the framework for understanding emotional crises adopted by most therapies for personality disorder (Swenson, 1989). This assumes that crises consist of an escalating emotional state triggered by a specific event that evokes feelings of rejection, abandonment, or intrusion. These schemas activate intense emotions that lead to various cognitive, emotional, and behavioral reactions, including deliberate self-harm. Cognitive responses involve maladaptive thoughts and modes of thinking, such as rumination, catastrophic thinking, and self-criticism (see Leahy, Chapter 12, this volume) that serve to escalate distress until it feels intolerable. At this point, the patient often engages in some form of deliberate self-harm that terminates the distress. This model of crisis postulates the occurrence of deficits in the mechanisms that regulate emotions and impulses arising from a combination of biological or environmental factors. This implies a modular approach in which components in the sequence—event, dysphoric emotions, and consequential behaviors—are potential targets for intervention. This sequence organizes information about crises in a way that is readily understood by patients, as illustrated in the following clinical vignette.

Case Example

Jennifer, a young woman in her early 20s, was forced to discontinue her studies due to intense, unstable emotions and rapid, unpredictable mood changes associated with self-harming behaviors, including cutting, overdoses, and binge eating. When referred for therapy, she was in an almost constant state of distress, lurching from one crisis to another. Therapy was initially dominated by the most recent crisis and was largely concerned with providing support and containing reactivity. Gradually, within-session distress began to settle, although between sessions the crises continued unabated. With this minor improvement, the alliance improved, and Jennifer began discussing problems in more detail. She revealed that she was horrified about the risks she had been taking in recent months and that she was especially concerned about what she had done during her most recent crisis. This provided an opportunity to formulate a more detailed understanding of crisis behavior prior to more systematic work on improving emotion control and reducing self-harm.

The event was explored using the behavioral sequence described previously. Jennifer revealed that a few days earlier, she had had a sexual relationship with a stranger she had met in a bar. Now she was concerned about what she had done. After dealing with the practicalities of her concern, the therapist asked about what had happened. During the evening in question, she was distressed and desperately needed company. She went to a bar, started talking to a man she had just met, and spent the night in his apartment. The next morning, she was suddenly confronted with the risks she had taken. Although considerable time was spent dealing with the seriousness of this event, our concern here is with formulation. It transpired that during the late afternoon and early evening, she had felt increasingly distressed, and then panicky, about being alone. The loneliness and distress became intolerable, so she went looking for company. On entering a bar, she almost immediately started talking to a stranger. He was interested in her, and she almost instantly felt better. However, as she talked to him, she began to feel obliged to please him to ensure that he liked her and wanted to be with her.

When the therapist asked her when she first felt upset, Jennifer initially said she could not remember. With gentle but persistent inquiry, she recalled that she had felt this way earlier in the day but insisted that nothing had happened to upset her. In fact, she thought that she woke up feeling that way. The therapist commented that things do not happen without a reason. Jennifer said that she understood that but nevertheless insisted that nothing had happened. When asked what she did from the moment she woke up, she recalled an early-morning telephone conversation with her mother during which her mother refused to help her with a relatively minor matter. The therapist asked how she felt about this. She said she was angry. It was so unfair because her mother did not treat her brother in this way. She did everything he asked. The injustice of it infuriated her, and she ruminated about it all morning. She felt unloved, hurt, and rejected. She also felt alone and needed to feel that someone cared. The rumination continued throughout the day and she became increasingly distressed until the feelings became intolerable.

At this point, the therapist noted that they had a good picture of what happened and used the behavioral sequence of event–escalating emotional state–response to discuss the episode. The therapist recalled how, during their first meeting, Jennifer had said that she wanted to overcome episodes of intense distress that seemed to occur for no reason. However, it was clear that with the latest episode there was a cause—she felt hurt and rejected by her mother. Jennifer said she recognized this now and noted that these feelings always occurred when she felt rejected and unloved. The therapist asked about other events and then noted that these events activated thoughts about being out of control, worthless, and unloved. It was also noted that she brooded over what happened, which caused the feelings to escalate until they became intolerable. At that point, she felt she had to do something to change them. On this occasion, she had engaged in risky sexual behavior because she needed to feel wanted, but on other occasions she had harmed herself in other ways, such as cutting. All these actions made her feel better for a while, but later, when she realized what she had done, she felt much worse.

During the discussion, the therapist constructed a diagram of the sequence of events that was then given to Jennifer. Together the therapist and Jennifer worked over the event again, and Jennifer added new details to the diagram. This helped her to connect emotional states to specific events and to recognize that these feelings did not occur spontaneously. She was also able to see the connection between feelings and different forms of self-harm, which she had not recognized as connected. Now she realized that cutting, bingeing, and risky sexual behavior were different ways to make herself feel better. As she provided more details about triggering events, Jennifer also recalled other episodes that fit the pattern. She commented: "This makes absolute sense. I did not realize these things were connected—it was all confusing." Subsequently, the alliance deepened, and Jennifer became more motivated to change. For example, she began to wonder whether she could deal with distress differently and what she could do to stop harming herself.

These developments were a turning point in therapy. The formulation helped to contain emotional instability by helping Jennifer to understand why she was so upset, which reduced the feeling that everything was out of control. Of course, crises continued, but they were less frequent and intense. This seems to be a common occurrence. Davidson (2008), writing about formulation in cognitive therapy, noted how a successful formulation has a settling effect that reduces distress and demoralization and facilitates engagement.

Role of the Common Factors

The modular approach to treating emotional dysregulation assumes that specific modules will be delivered using an integrated model that combines a common-factors approach with technical eclecticism (see Livesley, Dimaggio, & Clarkin, Chapter 1, this volume). The general treatment modules used to operationalize common change mechanisms serve two functions (see Livesley & Clarkin, Chapter 2, this volume). First, they establish the within-therapy conditions necessary for change, namely, a structured approach and a collaborative alliance. Second, they establish within-patient conditions fundamental to change, namely, motivation and self-reflection.

The motivation module seeks to build and reinforce a commitment to change, an important condition because, although many patients express a strong desire to change, this desire is often compromised by the overwhelming nature of unstable emotions and feelings of passivity and helplessness that often accompany emotional dysregulation and that can make patients fearful and reluctant to try new ways to master their distress and practice key skills. Consequently, an important part of treating emotional dysregulation is to maintain a commitment to change, address obstacles, and reinforce any step the patient takes to change. This means that most sessions involve an interweaving of general and specific interventions to create the conditions needed for patients to try new ways of thinking and acting and then using even modest changes to build the alliance and motivation.

Change also requires the capacity for self-reflection—a consistent preparedness to reflect on the nature, origins, and consequences of emotional arousal, a process that is fundamental to improving both the self-regulation and the processing of emotions. As noted earlier, intense emotions impede self-reflection, so that a major part of therapy is to help the patient to reflect on all aspects of emotional experiences. Especially important is the development of an understanding of the interpersonal context of emotional experiences. This depends on improving the metacognitive processes involved in understanding the mental states of self and others (Dimaggio et al., 2012). A possible reason for the effectiveness of mentalizing-based therapy is the careful and systematic use of the mentalizing component of self-reflection that enables the patient to begin processing emotions rather than merely reacting to them.

SPECIFIC TREATMENT MODULES

The specific interventions may be conveniently organized into four modules: (1) a psychoeducation module that provides information about the nature of emotional dysregulation and emotions, the adaptive origins of emotions, the way emotions affect thoughts and actions, and the role emotions play in everyday behavior and normal personality functioning; (2) an awareness module designed to increase awareness and recognition of different emotions, develop the ability to track emotional experiences, and reduce emotional avoidance; (3) a self-regulation module that consists of treatment methods to increase the self-management of emotions to permit more flexible and nuanced expression of emotions; and (4) an emotion-processing module to enhance emotion processing and increase the capacity to reflect on emotions and their consequences.

Each module consists of interventions selected on the basis of outcome studies and a rational analysis of the interventions that are likely to be useful in treating specific impairments. An important practical issue is whether modules should be delivered as discrete packages using a predetermined number of sessions or whether the interventions should be incorporated into the therapeutic process as the opportunity presents. Both methods are used in treating personality disorder. The more structured shorter-term therapies such as systems training for emotional predictability and problem solving (STEPPS; Blum et al., 2008) adopt the former structure, whereas other therapies adopt a more flexible approach, introducing interventions when problems emerge in session. The latter approach is adopted here not only to ensure coverage of emotion-regulation impairments but also to improve emotion-processing capacity.

Psychoeducation Module

Although psychoeducation is used extensively in treating conditions such as schizophrenia and eating disorders, it has been used less systematically in treating personality disorder. Nevertheless, it is important (Ruiz-Sancho, Smith, & Gunderson, 2001) because most patients are poorly informed about personality disorder and emotions. Besides the general information provided when discussing the treatment contract, more specific information is required about emotional dysregulation because many patients have little understanding of why they are so distressed and their lives so chaotic. Many also believe that emotions are bad or dangerous and do not understand the role emotions play in adaptive behavior. As a result, they berate themselves for having feelings and seek to avoid or suppress them. Many also seek therapy hoping that the therapist will "stop or take away" negative feelings. These ideas may be partly corrected with information about how emotions are an inherent part of human nature that are essential for social interaction and how emotions such as anxiety, fear, and anger evolved because they alert us to important events that need to be dealt with. The idea that feelings serve a useful purpose is often new for many patients. Information on the genetic origins of emotions also helps to build tolerance and acceptance. Besides information on the adaptive significance of emotions, it is also helpful to provide information on emotion avoidance and its effects and on how suppression and behavioral avoidance can actually increase distress in the longer term.

A recent crisis is often an opportunity to discuss the collage of feelings involved and to help the patient distinguish between anxiety and fearfulness and more general intense emotional reactions. This distinction is useful because many patients (and clinicians) focus on emotional lability and neglect the panicky fearfulness that adds to dysphoric states. It is also useful to explain how intense emotions reduce the ability to think, which in turn reduces cognitive control over feelings, causing them to spiral out of control. The behavioral sequence (triggering event–emotion–responses to emotion) can subsequently be used to organize a discussion of the origins and consequences of emotional arousal, especially how emotional distress escalates until it becomes intolerable, at which point acts such as deliberate self-harm reduce distress. This explanation is validating because it explains the adaptive aspect of these acts.

The module is not intended to be delivered within a fixed time period or through a designated number of sessions. Rather, information is imparted gradually, as different aspects of the patient's emotional life become the focus of treatment, to avoid overwhelming patients who are vulnerable to information overload. As with all other modules, the assumption is that specific interventions are integrated into the flow of therapy and become part of the therapeutic narrative.

Awareness Modules

The awareness module has three components aimed at developing the ability to recognize and identify feelings, promote greater present-focused awareness of emotions, and develop an understanding of emotional, cognitive, and behavioral responses to emotional states.

Identifying and Labeling Emotions

Emotional control begins by learning to recognize, identify, and label emotions; it is difficult to control behaviors that are poorly recognized. Although most patients think that they are acutely aware of their feelings, they often have little actual awareness of the origins and complexities of emotional reactions or of how feelings of anger and rage can mask more vulnerable feelings of fearfulness and sadness. Increased awareness requires that the patient learn to decompose emotional states into specific components and to label each component. The goal here is to help the patient to progress from an intense self-focus to self-awareness and later to self-reflection. Although emotion recognition is often taught as a separate exercise aided with handouts, it often easier, at least initially, to clarify and label feelings as they emerge in therapy because accurate identification of feelings requires a degree of self-observation and this skill is often poorly developed. Patients often label the most obvious or least painful feelings present in any emotional state and often need the therapist's help to observe and label the nuances of their experiences. In-session work also allows the therapist to deal with emotion avoidance, to provide support when feelings threaten to be overwhelming, and to validate feelings as they are recognized, thereby strengthening patients' confidence in the authenticity of their experience.

It is also helpful for patients to recognize the different components of each emotion, physiological sensations as well as the more cognitive aspects of emotions, including the meanings and narratives associated with expressed emotions. In the philosophical literature, the physiological component is sometimes referred to as *feelings*, in contrast to the cognitive component, which is labeled *emotion*. However, these terms are used interchangeably in the mental health literature. Nevertheless, it is helpful to differentiate the two components because patients do not always recognize that the physical sensations are related to emotions, and this misunderstanding may result in physiological sensations that are linked to emotion being misinterpreted, leading to health anxieties.

Tracking Emotions and Emotional Responses

Besides learning to identify emotions accurately, it is also important that patients learn to track emotional experiences by recognizing their origins, the flow of emotional responses and their subsequent escalation, and the impact of emotional states on subsequent action. This can be accomplished by applying the event–emotion–response–consequences model discussed earlier to a recent crisis as illustrated in the description of the case formulation. Because patients are often unable to recognize triggers, therapists need to be patient but persistent in searching for triggers to ensure that the patient becomes skilled at recognizing them. The important point for patients to learn is that feelings do not simply occur spontaneously but rather that they are activated by specific events. Hence an important part of this process is to focus on the details of triggering events and to help the patients to recognize distress early so that they can use emotion-regulation skills before the feelings become uncontrollable. This process is important for another reason: Because most triggers are interpersonal events, such as a perceived rejection or humiliation, this process begins to situate emotional responses in an interpersonal context—an important step toward improving emotion-processing ability (see also Dimaggio et al., Chapter 17, this volume; Leahy, Chapter 12, this volume).

Once triggering events have been explored, attention can be given to examining the consequences of emotions, especially how distress escalates into a crisis state, by exploring the thoughts, additional feelings, and behaviors evoked by the initial emotional experience. Because patients often have difficulty identifying reactions across all three areas, an understanding of these reactions begins to link events that were often considered unrelated and hence promotes integration. Especially significant is recognition of maladaptive ways of thinking, such as rumination and catastrophizing, that increase distress. Many of these processes and the self-talk involved are so automatic that the patient is often unaware of the pervasiveness of these modes of thought and the contribution they play in increasing and maintaining distressed states (see Leahy, Chapter 12, this volume). Linked to maladaptive emotional schemas are secondary emotions initiated by the first emotional response. Distress activated by the initial trigger often evokes other emotional responses, such as intense fearfulness and anxiety, not only about the initial event but also about the emotions activated.

The various responses to intense emotional states have short-term and long-term consequences. Most patients are familiar with short-term consequences of responses to reduce distress that reinforce these responses and increase the likelihood that they will occur in the future. This is most apparent with acts of deliberate self-harm, such as cutting, that serve to punctuate the distress. Less apparent to most patients are the long-term consequences of responses to intense emotions in terms of the impact on their lives and how others react to them. The distinction is important in building a commitment to learn more adaptive ways to self-regulate distress. Hence it is useful to spend time discussing the short-term and long-term benefits and costs of the various responses. Throughout this process, within-session work is helpful. By carefully monitoring the patient's emotional state, the therapist models both attention to detail and empathy in the way the patient's emotions are tracked.

Developing Moment-by-Moment Awareness of Emotions

Increased emotion awareness and control depend on the development of present-focused or moment-to-moment nonjudgmental awareness of emotions (Barlow et al., 2011; Kabat-Zinn, 2005). As Barlow and colleagues (2011) note, a key skill is the capacity to objectively observe experiences as they occur. Patients with personality disorders with severe levels of emotional dysregulation lack this ability; they tend to "fuse" with their experience and have difficulty decentering from the experience sufficiently to view it objectively.

As Barlow and colleagues (2011) noted, the initial emotional response to an event is often adaptive and directly relevant to the event—for example, fear in response to a perceived threat. However, this is often quickly followed by additional reactions that tend to be more judgmental. The case example of Jennifer, discussed earlier, illustrates this point: Jennifer's initial irritation at her mother's refusal to help was understandable, but this was quickly followed by more evaluative reactions, such as feeling rejected and unloved, that increased distress by establishing a ruminative process. Patients need to learn to attend to the flow of reactions that accompany emotional arousal if they are to modify their responses. Judgmental and self-critical reactions to initial emotional responses are common in patients with personality disorders; patients blame themselves for being upset and tell themselves that they "should not feel this way," that there is something fundamentally wrong with them, or that their intense emotions are indications of weakness and vulnerability.

Awareness of the various reactions to emotional arousal is increased by working through examples of specific episodes. Doing this allows the therapist to "invite" the patient to observe what happened in a more detached way rather than simply reliving the event in therapy. A focus on specific details of the event and consistent use of comments such as "How did you see it?" "Could we look at this another way?" "What do you think the other person was thinking?" and "Why were you so critical of yourself?" help to draw the patient into a more objective, observational stance. Mindfulness exercises also have an important role to play in building the ability to experience in the moment and to observe experience getting caught up in evaluative ruminations. Mindfulness is not discussed further here as it is explored in detail by Ottavi and colleagues (Chapter 13, this volume).

Promoting Emotion Acceptance and Tolerance

Awareness, tolerance, and acceptance are closely intertwined; the open, nonjudgmental momentary focus on experience needed for emotion regulation can be fully realized only with increased emotion tolerance and acceptance. This means that although the different aspects of awareness are being discussed as if they are distinct, most interventions incorporate all components. As indicated previously, for most patients emotional experiences activate evaluative and self-critical responses that add to inner confusion and turmoil, creating an intolerance of emotions that limits awareness. Increased tolerance begins by encouraging patients to examine feelings as they occur in session by drawing patients' attention to small changes in emotional state and asking them describe and "hold" these feelings. This uses the treatment relationship to provide what Winnicot (1960) called a "holding environment" that helps to contain and regulate emotional arousal. An increase in the patient's capacity to tolerate distress is then used to build the alliance and promote self-efficacy. This process illustrates the reciprocal use of general and specific interventions in integrated modular treatment to enhance the other.

Intolerance of distress is often increased by cognitive reactions to negative emotions. Ruminative and critical self-talk increases distress, although many patients are aware that these thoughts are occurring. Change requires increased awareness of these modes of thought and how they increase distress. Consequently, increased tolerance depends on challenging and restructuring these thoughts and associated emotional schemas (see Leahy, Chapter 12, this volume). An important part of this process is also to build self-compassion and reduce self-derogation and criticism. Again, patients often fail to recognize how self-punitive they are and how they are more critical of themselves than they are of others.

Countering Emotional Avoidance

Emotional awareness is also reduced by cognitive and behavioral strategies used to suppress feelings and avoid situations that activate distress. As with self-talk, patients are often unaware of these behaviors. The problem can be managed using a two-step process. First, after noting several examples of avoidance, the therapist uses an event to draw the patient's attention to avoidance as a general response to distress. Patients vary in their awareness-avoidant behavior. Some clearly recognize that they act in this way, although they may not always recognize all instances, but others are almost totally oblivious. Identification of the broad pattern helps the patient to see links among behaviors that may have seemed to be unrelated. Recognition may be facilitated by discussing how emotions are suppressed or avoided, so that a psychoeducational component is woven into therapy. This introduces the second step in the process: recognition of specific avoidance behaviors, first in therapy and later in everyday situations. This process is aided by helping the patient to construct a list of avoidance behaviors, such as rapidly changing a topic when emotions begin to emerge, using distracting behaviors, or avoiding eye contact, and of specific cognitive avoidance strategies, such as deliberate suppression of feelings, self-reassurance, or focusing on positive things (see also Dimaggio et al., Chapter 17, this volume). In most instances, it is sufficient simply to draw the patient's attention to his or her avoidant response. At other times, however, it is also necessary to address fears and concerns that motivate avoidance, a process akin to the defense interpretation format of psychodynamic therapy in which attention is drawn to an avoidant response and anxieties that motivated the avoidant act, such as fear of losing control or guilt.

An important part of this process is to ensure that the patient fully recognizes short-term and long-term consequences of avoidance, especially how suppression of important aspects of self-experience limits awareness and self-understanding, with attendant effects on personality functioning. It also prevents the person from learning how to manage feelings and hence dooms him or her to having to continue grappling with distress. Moreover, suppression does not work in the longer term: Suppressed and avoided feelings do not go away permanently and often emerge more powerful than before.

Emotional Regulation Module

This module is intended to build on the increased cognitive control of emotions achieved through increased awareness by developing specific skills to compensate for regulatory deficits. As with other specific interventions, skills may be developed using specific training sessions or integrated into therapy. Either way, it is important to ensure that these skills are fully integrated with other components of treatment. Skill acquisition can be introduced using relatively simple interventions, such as distraction and self-soothing, early in treatment to reduce distress and subsequently supplemented with more complex interventions that require more training.

Distraction

Although distraction is a simple way to self-regulate emotions as the first step in building greater control, the idea seems inconsistent with the earlier discussion of distraction as an avoidance strategy. The distinction is that with emotional avoidance, distraction is usually used chronically with limited awareness, but, as a self-regulating behavior, it is used intentionally to control distress until other methods are acquired. The intentional use of distraction is an important step in challenging the idea that emotions are uncontrollable. Even modest success in delaying or reducing distress helps to promote beliefs of self-efficacy. To be effective, distracting activities, such as the self-soothing behaviors discussed in the next section, need to be used early in the sequence of emotional arousal. This is the reason that awareness and self-monitoring of emotions is so important. If they are not deployed early, the patient becomes so preoccupied with the distress that he or she forgets to use them. For this reason it may be helpful for patients to compile a list of suitable activities that they can refer to when they first notice something is amiss.

Promoting Self-Soothing

Like distraction, self-soothing is widely used by healthy individuals to self-regulate distress. People with emotionally dysregulated personality disorders have difficulty self-soothing presumably because early attachment problems hindered the learning of simple self-regulatory behaviors. Many patients also feel guilty or undeserving of pleasure, which makes self-soothing a source of guilt rather than relief. As with other interventions, self-soothing is more effective if it is used before feelings get too strong. Hence, it is useful for patients to construct a list of activities that are potentially soothing that they can refer to when distressed.

Grounding Techniques

Patients who experience intense, panic-like anxiety and dissociative reactions, such as loss of contact with immediate reality, depersonalization, or derealization, may learn to thwart these responses using grounding techniques. In these states, the panic creates a positive feedback loop in which intense anxiety leads to loss of contact with surroundings and a preoccupation with inner experience, leading to further panic. Simple acts such as placing one's feet firmly on the ground; feeling a solid object, such as the arms of the chair, and concentrating on the texture and solidity of the object; looking around and focusing on specific objects in the environment; and increasing abdominal breathing by placing one's arms around the back of the chair help to settle the panic and the tendency to dissociate because they force the patient to attend to external stimuli rather than painful inner experiences.

Grounding is best introduced early in therapy, when the patient begins to dissociate in a session or describes a recent dissociative experience, by taking the patient through the different steps. Success depends on a satisfactory alliance, so it is not productive to introduce the exercise when rapport is poor. The exercise is a useful way to initiate active collaborative work, and any success can be used to enhance the alliance and the commitment to change. It is often useful to teach the exercise to significant others or friends who can remind the patient of what to do when he or she feels overwhelmed. Often significant others feel helpless and do not know what to do when dissociative crises occur, which contributes to the panic and distress. The exercise involves significant others in treatment and helps to ensure that the exercise is used in everyday situations.

Relaxation

Relaxation training is useful in managing the anxious component of emotional dysregulation. It also forms the foundation for other interventions.

Although a variety of techniques are available that differ in complexity, it is best to use a simple method, such as breath training involving slow abdominal breathing, because patients with severe pathology often lack the patience and motivation to use more complex methods, especially early in treatment. When breathing out, patients are instructed to say simple word, such as *calm* or *relax*, and to let themselves go loose. Over time, the word becomes a conditioned stimulus that, when said, initiates relaxation. This method is easy to learn and produces almost immediate benefits. It also tends not to evoke fear of losing control, which often occurs when patients try to relax. When teaching the exercise in session, relaxation can be introduced as a way to counter anxiety and fearfulness. It also helps to explain that relaxation is a skill and that, as with all skills, practice leads to improvement.

As with other methods, relaxation is best introduced when the patient is not too stressed and the alliance is satisfactory to ensure that the first experience is positive. Patients should also be encouraged to practice relaxation regularly when they are feeling relatively calm until proficiency is achieved, when it can then be used to self-manage negative feelings. The value of teaching a simple form of relaxation is that it is easy to use in everyday situations to manage various feelings such as fear, stress, assumed slights, anger, and jealousy.

Attention Control

Affect regulation requires the ability to switch attention from unpleasant thoughts rather than ruminating about them. Attention control can be improved by learning to switch attention between a painful, triggering stimulus and a more pleasant, relaxing one. The exercise is a version of systematic desensitization (Wolpe, 1958), which uses the relaxation exercise described previously. Systematic desensitization seeks to extinguish the fear evoked by a specific stimulus by presenting a low level of intensity of the stimulus while encouraging relaxation. Here, it is used to demonstrate that emotions can be controlled, to build emotion tolerance and control, and to desensitize fear reactions to traumatic stimuli.

The first step is to identify the stimulus that triggers emotional distress and dissociation—for example, painful or traumatic memories, words or phrases used by an abuser, interpersonal events that activate maladaptive schemata, and painful events such as bereavement. When memories evoke uncontrollable emotions, it is helpful to identify components of the stimulus that evoke less intense reactions, rather like the hierarchy used to desensitize phobias. Next, the patient is asked to identify an easily visualized pleasant scene, which is then used to help the patient to relax. When relaxed, the patient is asked to switch attention from the pleasant scene to the triggering stimulus. When anxiety increases, the patient is asked to switch attention back to the pleasant stimuli and helped to focus on it and relax until the anxiety settles. Initially, attention is diverted to the pleasant stimulus as soon as distressing emotions are aroused, which may be only a matter of seconds. This helps to ensure that the patient succeeds in switching attention and relaxing. When relaxation occurs, the cycle is repeated. On the first occasion, it is useful to complete three or four switches, which may take only about 10 minutes. The length of time that the patient is asked to focus on the traumatic stimulus is gradually increased as his or her ability to tolerate and control distress increases. Over time, more traumatic stimuli are introduced.

This intervention is best introduced in session so that the therapeutic relationship can be used to contain and regulate anxiety. Once the patient understands the process and is able to regulate distress, he or she can begin to practice between sessions. As with the grounding exercise, some patients also benefit from involving significant others. The exercise is interactive and involves the patient working collaboratively with the therapist. Reviewing the experience immediately afterward provides an opportunity to use a successful outcome to strengthen the alliance and motivation for change.

Emotion-Processing Module

The treatment methods discussed so far seek to improve emotion control by increasing awareness and building requisite skills. These changes are a necessary part of treatment, but they are not sufficient: It is also important to increase the capacity to process emotional experiences. This means increasing the patients' understanding of the nuances of their experiences, recognizing the interpersonal factors that influence the flow of emotions, developing greater flexibility in the ways events are interpreted, appreciating the reciprocal relationship between emotional reactions and other mental processes, and helping patients to recognize and restructure the ways emotions are incorporated into higher-order meaning systems and personal narratives. This final component of treating emotional dysregulation seeks to integrate emotions with other aspects of personality function and the relationship between the individual and his or her unique environment. With these developments treatment becomes less structured; consequently, the following discussion is more concerned with principles than techniques. Treatment also changes in the sense that the focus becomes more interpersonal. Hence these developments pave the way for the next phase of therapy, which is primarily concerned with exploring and changing maladaptive interpersonal patterns.

Developing Flexibility in Emotion Processing

Emotional dysregulation is usually accompanied by considerable rigidity in the way emotional events are interpreted that extends to all aspects of emotional experience. Patients tend to assume that their view of events is accurate and the only conceivable way to interpret them. They do not fully recognize that perceptions are merely interpretations and that alternative interpretations are possible. This rigidity extends to other reactions to emotion arousal and increases with emotional intensity.

Steps taken to increase flexibility in emotion processing begin to change therapy in subtle but important ways. To this point, the focus has been on promoting change largely by increasing skills related to self-awareness, self-reflection, and emotion control. Now change focuses more on restructuring well-established cognitions and emotional responses that are important components of the patient's beliefs and habitual modes of functioning. Patients often experience these developments as more challenging, which places a greater strain on the alliance. Hence therapists need to be increasingly attentive to the alliance and to be prepared to stop work on emotion processing and focus on repairing and building the alliance as needed.

Earlier discussions of the events that trigger emotional reactions can now be extended to develop a greater understanding of the kinds of events that activate intense emotions and the reasons for the patient's sensitivity to these events and to open up the possibility of restructuring how some events are perceived. Because most events are interpersonal in nature—the patient feels rejected or mistreated—this means that emotions need to be understood in terms of their interpersonal context. Exploration of this context connects emotions to underlying interpersonal schemas, such as fears and expectations of abandonment and rejection. A focus not only on the event but also on how the event was perceived opens up the possibility that the event could be interpreted differently. For example, in the earlier case formulation, Jennifer felt rejected and unloved by her mother. At this phase of therapy, Jennifer could be encouraged to consider other interpretations and to suggest alternative ways of understanding her mother's behavior—that her mother refused to help not because she did not care but because of a prior commitment—and to consider that her sensitivity to rejection may lead her to misinterpret some events. Realization of this possibility is promoted by inquiring about what her mother may have been thinking and feeling at the time. Encouragement to "take the role of the other" and see things from the other's perspective is important to more effective processing of emotional reactions, and it can be supplemented with standard cognitive therapy intervention that helps the patient to challenge and restructure interpretations based on misperceptions and misconceptions and by metacognitive strategies (see Bateman & Fonagy, Chapter 7, this volume; Dimaggio et al., Chapter 8, this volume).

The next step on the pathway to more adaptive emotion processing is further exploration of the cognitions that accompany emotional arousal. Beliefs and self-talk that escalate distress can be worked through again and the patient taught to challenge them using standard cognitive therapy strategies. For example, whenever one patient was distressed, she did not describe herself as sad or stressed but rather as "falling apart." This evoked even more panic. It was only after she developed greater flexibility in the way she thought about her emotions and began to describe feelings in more specific and less catastrophic terms that self-regulation improved. Besides specific maladaptive beliefs, distress is also increased by maladaptive modes of thought such as rumination and catastrophizing. The problems with these reactions to intense emotions are that they increase the self-focus and the preoccupation with the actual feelings at the price of trying to understand and solve the problems that caused them. This work was begun earlier in treatment; however, improved affect regulation provides an opportunity to work over this material at greater depth with a view to consolidating changes and increasing cognitive and behavioral flexibility.

Reformulating Narratives

Thus far the treatment of impairments in emotion regulation has focused on remedying relatively low-level impairments in regulatory mechanisms by improving emotion awareness, by learning skills to compensate for deficiencies in self-regulation, and by restructuring low-level schemas and personal constructs. However, previous discussion of the role of emotions in personality functioning noted how emotions shape higher-order meaning systems that subsequently play an important role in emotion regulation. Throughout treatment it is important that therapists keep these higher-order structures in mind and avoid an exclusive focus on lower-order regulatory skills. Earlier discussion of higher-order structures made reference to two patients with similar problems with emotion regulation who had somewhat different outcomes due to differences in the way emotional dysregulation shaped their personal narratives. These cases illustrate the important point that the effects of unstable emotions are not confined to relatively circumscribed impacts on symptoms and general functioning. They also influence the development of self-structures and self-narratives, with widespread effects on personality across all functional domains. With one patient, emotional dysregulation was construed as a problem to be overcome. This construction was motivating and allowed the patient to marshal multiple resources that aided improvement. She drew upon experiences in learning the skills needed to excel in her favorite sport to acquire emotion-regulation skills. As the more intense emotions settled, she began to realize that she could actually use her intense feelings in adaptive ways. This was an important realization. Although patients often embark on therapy with the hope that treatment will rid them of these feelings, this is an unrealistic expectation. Genetic influences on emotion control, the biological impacts of severe adversity, and the impact of learning mean that most patients will remain to some degree vulnerable to emotional lability. Eventually patients have to moderate their expectations and accept that they may always be more emotional than the average person and hence learn how to continue using the skills and strategies learned in therapy after treatment ends. This process is facilitated with recognition that not all feelings are negative and that feelings can be used constructively. This happened with this patient. She came to realize that she could manage anxiety and mood, that she could draw on these feelings to motivate her when competing in her sport, and that modest levels of anxiety could also facilitate her studies. The previous fearfulness about having intense feelings gave way to acceptance that these feelings were part of her and that she could use them. As this higher-order narrative evolved, the emotions that were previously considered a liability were incorporated into a self-narrative that helped to define her identity. This had a stabilizing effect that helped to modulate emotional reactivity.

The second patient described earlier was different. For her, intense emotion was not a problem to be overcome but rather an indication of vulnerability. Early in development, she began to think of herself as flawed and as having substantial limitations. She did not push herself to learn self-regulatory skills but rather approached them cautiously and without much hope of success. A sense of vulnerability and impairment defined who she was. Although she improved symptomatically to the point of completing studies and finding good employment, her sense of self remained unchanged. Rather than helping to regulate her emotions, her self-narrative exacerbated emotional distress and on some occasions actually initiated crises. More substantial progress occurred only when she learned to be more flexible in the way she construed situations and began to construct a new self-narrative that was less predicated on a sense of vulnerability and impairment.

I have introduced these cases to draw attention to the importance of viewing emotional control and dyscontrol within the broad context of the overall personality system. Current therapies understandably stress skill building. This aspect of treatment is readily measurable and lends itself well to treatment using specific, clearly defined protocols. However, personality is an organized system with rich interactions among components. The pathology of personality disorder is never confined to one part of the system but inevitably affects functioning across all domains. To treat emotion dysregulation effectively, we need to attend to the ramifications of emotions on other personality processes and to both lower- and higher-order regulatory mechanisms.

CONCLUDING COMMENTS

This chapter has attempted to offer a transtheoretical, unified approach to treating emotional dysregulation associated with severe personality disorder. Following an examination of the structure of emotional traits and the subjective experience of unstable emotions, a modular framework was proposed consisting of general modules designed to establish the conditions needed for effective treatment and specific modules designed to increase awareness and control of emotions and to promote more effective processing of emotional experiences. A modular approach was adopted for several reasons. It provides a convenient framework for organizing an eclectic array of treatment methods that relates interventions to specific impairments. It also emphasizes the heterogeneity of personality pathology and the importance of tailoring treatment to the individual: Not all modules will be needed to the same degree with all patients. However, the modularity structure is not intended to imply that treatment follows a predictable sequence. In practice, most sessions will require the use of interventions from multiple modules to match the flow of the therapeutic dialogue. Nevertheless, most treatments do show a consistent pattern—treatment methods become less structured with progress, and the scope of interventions progressively broadens.

With progress, therapy gradually moves from focusing on the patient's capacity to self-manage emotions to viewing emotions more broadly within the context of the overall personality. This means that an interpersonal focus is increasingly incorporated into treatment because emotions are essentially interpersonal phenomena. As this occurs, attention begins to move from emotion regulation to the treatment of interpersonal impairments. Emotions, however, are an intimate part of all personality functioning, and hence, even though the primary focus changes, it will be necessary to work on most aspects of emotion regulation, especially the processing of emotions, throughout therapy.

REFERENCES

Barlow, D. H., Farchione, T. J., Fairholme, C. P., Ellard, K. K., Boieseau, C. L., Allan, L. B., et al. (2011). *Unified protocol for transdiagnostic treatment of emotional disorders*. Oxford, UK: Oxford University Press.

Bateman, A., & Fonagy, P. (2006). *Mentalization-based treatment for borderline personality disorder*. Oxford, UK: Oxford University Press.

Blum, N., St. John, D., Pfohl, B., Stuart, S., McCormick, B., Allen, J., et al. (2008). Systems training for emotional predictability and problem solving (STEPPS) for outpatients with borderline personality disorder: A randomized controlled trial and 1-year follow-up. *American Journal of Psychiatry, 165*, 468–478.

Clarkin, J. F., Yeomans, F. E., & Kernberg, O. F. (2006). *Psychotherapy for borderline personality: Focusing on object relations*. Washington, DC: American Psychiatric Publishing.

Davidson, K. (2008). *Cognitive therapy for personality disorders*. London: Routledge.

Dimaggio, G., Salvatore, G., Fiore, D., Carcione, A., Nicolò, G., & Semerari, A. (2012). General principles for treating the overconstricted personality disorder: Toward operationalizing technique. *Journal of Personality Disorders, 26*, 63–83.

Gross, J. J., & Thompson, R. A. (2007). Emotional regulation: Conceptual foundations. In J. J. Gross (Ed.), *Handbook of emotion regulation* (pp. 3–24). New York: Guilford Press.

Hayes, S. C., Strosahl, K. D., & Wilson, K. G. (1999). *Acceptance and commitment therapy: An experiential approach to behavioral change*. New York: Guilford Press.

Kabat-Zinn, J. (2005). *Coming to our senses: Healing ourselves and the world through mindfulness*. New York: Hyperion.

Leary, M. R. (2003). The self and emotion. In R. J. Davidson, K. R. Scherer, & H. H. Goldsmith (Eds.), *Handbook of affective sciences* (pp. 773–786). New York: Guilford Press.

Linehan, M. M. (1993). *Cognitive-behavioral treatment of borderline personality disorder*. New York: Guilford Press.

Livesley W. J. (2003). *Practical management of personality disorder*. New York: Guilford Press.

Livesley, W. J. (2008). Toward a genetically informed model of borderline personality disorder. *Journal of Personality Disorders, 22,* 42–71.

Livesley, W. J., Jang, K. L., & Vernon, P. A. (1998). The phenotypic and genetic architecture of traits delineating personality disorder. *Archives of General Psychiatry, 55,* 941–948.

Livesley, W. J., Jang, K. L., & Vernon, P. A. (2003). Genetic basis of personality structure. In T. Millon & E. J. Lerner (Eds.), *Handbook of psychology* (Vol. 5, pp. 59–83). Hoboken, NJ: Wiley.

Nolen-Hoeksema, S. (2012). Emotion regulation and psychopathology: The role of gender. *Annual Review of Clinical Psychology, 6,* 161–187.

Plomin, R., Chipeur, H. M., & Loehlin, J. C. (1990). Behavior genetics and personality. In L. A. Pervin (Ed.), *Handbook of personality: Theory and research* (pp. 225–243). New York: Guilford Press.

Ricoeur, P. (1981). The narrative function. In P. Ricoeur, *Hermeneutics and the human sciences* (J. B. Thompson, Ed. & Trans.) (pp. 165–181). Cambridge, UK: Cambridge University Press.

Roemer, L., & Orsillo, S. M. (2009). *Mindfulness- and acceptance-based behavioral therapies in practice.* New York: Guilford Press.

Ruiz-Sancho, A. M., Smith, G. W., & Gunderson, J. E. (2001). Psychoeducational approaches. In W. J. Livesley (Ed.), *Handbook of personality disorders: Theory, research, and treatment* (pp. 460–474). New York: Guilford Press.

Stanghellini, G., & Rosfort, R. (2013). *Emotions and personhood.* Oxford, UK: Oxford University Press.

Swenson, C. (1989). Kernberg and Linehan: Two approaches to the borderline patient. *Journal of Personality Disorders, 3,* 26–35.

Walton, G. M., Paunesku, D., & Dweck, C. S. (2012). Expandable selves. In M. R. Leary & J. P. Tangney (Eds.), *Handbook of self and identity* (2nd ed., pp. 141–154). New York; Guilford Press.

Widiger, T., & Simonsen, E. (2005). Alternative dimensional models of personality disorder: Finding a common ground. *Journal of Personality Disorders, 19,* 110–130.

Winnicott, D. W. (1960). Ego distortion in terms of true and false self. In *The maturational process and the facilitating environment* (pp. 158–165). New York: International Universities Press.

Wolpe, J. (1958). *Psychotherapy by reciprocal inhibition.* Stanford, CA: Stanford University Press.

chapter 12

Treating Emotional Schemas

Robert L. Leahy

In this chapter I describe a social–cognitive–behavioral model of how individuals conceptualize emotion and implement strategies of emotion regulation based on these conceptualizations. In addition, I examine how beliefs about emotions—and strategies of emotion regulation—are related to personality disorders. This model—*emotional schema therapy*—draws on cognitive models of schematic processing, behavioral models of experiential avoidance, attribution models of explanatory style, the dialectical behavioral model of emotional myths, metacognitive models of conceptualizing thought processes, and other cognitive-behavioral models. It proposes that emotion entails a social construction of emotional experience, emotional display, and emotional regulation. I describe empirical support for the processes underlying emotional schemas and their relationship to individual differences in psychopathology. Furthermore, I outline various techniques and strategies that are employed in identifying and modifying these emotional schemas. Finally, I illustrate their relevance to the treatment of borderline personality disorder.

A META-EXPERIENTIAL MODEL OF EMOTION

The Metacognitive Model of Psychopathology

Wells has proposed that a variety of psychopathological problems arise because of problematic beliefs about thought that give rise to unhelpful coping strategies (Wells, 2008). Wells's model places little emphasis on the content of thoughts (which, in the Beckian model, would include automatic thought distortions, maladaptive assumptions, and core beliefs or schemas). Rather, the emphasis is on the *function and process* of thinking about thoughts. According to this model, individuals have both positive ("I need to worry to be prepared") and negative ("My worry is going to make me sick") beliefs about worry. Moreover, worry is characterized by five factors that underlie beliefs *about* worry: (1) positive views of worry ("It helps me solve problems"), (2) danger and control ("It's out of control"), (3) cognitive competence ("I can't trust my memory"), (4) cognitive self-consciousness ("I pay a lot of attention to my thoughts"), and (5) negative beliefs about worry ("If I think positively, something bad will happen").

Wells views worry and rumination as part of the cognitive attentional syndrome, which is characterized by excessive focus or attention on the content and meaning of cognition (Wells, 2002, 2004). Thus the individual who has the thought "I might freeze up in my talk" then activates a process of paying attention to the thought, taking the thought seriously, fearing the thought, suppressing the thought, answering the thought, and attempting to obtain reassurance that things will work out. All these strategies lock the individual in an endless struggle with the content of thinking and prevent more adaptive strategies—such as facing the fear, problem solving, or accepting the thought but acting anyway. Metacognitive therapy has been shown to be effective for a wide range of disorders, including generalized anxiety disorder, social anxiety, obsessive–compulsive disorder (OCD), panic disorder, posttraumatic stress disorder (PTSD), and depression (especially the ruminative component) (Wells, 2008). There is preliminary evidence for the efficacy of metacognitive therapy in the treatment of borderline personality disorder (BPD) (Nordahl, 2011).

Metacognitive therapy assists the patient in identifying her or his beliefs about the nature of thinking strategies (such as rumination, worry, threat detection, suppression, and reassurance seeking), examining the costs and benefits of these strategies, engaging in attentional redeployment, using metaphors to gain distance from thinking ("Imagine your thoughts in a cloud"), engaging in more direct exposure and problem solving, and utilizing detached mindfulness to examine the "need" to control and direct thinking. The goal of therapy is to modify the patient's concern about the content and "process" of thinking.

Social Construction of Emotion

The emotional schema model is based on a social-cognitive model of emotional intelligence and draws from the metacognitive model advanced by Wells (Leahy, 2002, 2003; Leahy, Tirch, & Napolitano, 2011). It is proposed that each of us has an implicit theory of emotion, emotion regulation, emotional display, and the emotions of others. Although it is acknowledged that there is a strong biological and evolutionary basis of emotion, there are also significant historical, cultural, and individual differences in the social construction of emotion. Briefly, the "history" of emotion indicates that rules for emotional expression have dramatically changed. Norbert Elias's classic work on this topic, *The Civilizing Process: Sociogenetic and Psychogenetic Investigations* (1939/2000), traces the development of rules for internalization of aggressive and sexual behavior and emotion with the rise of courtly manners and the increased urbanization and social control of behavior. Similarly, Max Weber (1992) described the rise of internalization, guilt, and conscientiousness as part of the spread of Protestant emphasis on these qualities and the corresponding spread of capitalism. Historian Peter Stearns, in *American Cool: Constructing a Twentieth-Century Emotional Style* (1994), describes the increased emphasis on self-control, reduced emotional display of intensity, and the emphasis on a "cool" and aloof demeanor, and he links these developments to changes in child rearing from the 19th to later 20th centuries (Stearns, 1994). There are considerable cultural differences in the "legitimacy" of emotion, including differences in the "appropriateness" of physical touching, expression of emotion, crying behavior, and other displays of emotion. For example, Lutz (2001), in *Crying: A Natural and Cultural History of Tears*, describes significant variations across culture and across historical periods in the "appropriateness" of crying.

Linehan's (1993a) dialectical behavior therapy (DBT) emphasizes the role of "emotional myths"—that is, beliefs about emotion that lead to fear of emotion and problematic strategies of emotional dysregulation. Similarly, Gottman (Gottman, Katz, & Hooven, 1997) has identified a variety of "emotional philosophies" that affect how partners think about, evaluate, and respond to their partner's emotional state. Thus some partners may view emotion as a burden and therefore employ a dismissive or even disparaging style. Others may view emotions as an opportunity to get closer, to get to know and get to help. Along related lines, Greenberg's (2002) emotion-focused therapy stresses the role of emotional "schemas" as the emotion experience that "contains" beliefs, sensations, behavioral dispositions, and interpersonal styles. Psychodynamic theory has addressed the importance of beliefs about the danger and uncontrollability of intense emotion, which leads to the use of defense mechanisms. The recent emphasis on "affect phobia" by McCullough and colleagues (2003) in their book *Treating Affect Phobia: A Manual for Short-Term Dynamic Psychotherapy* illustrates the importance of beliefs about emotion in the maintenance of pathology. Similar to these other models that suggest that concepts of emotion may lead to problematic emotion regulation, emotional schema therapy proposes that individual differences in the beliefs, strategies, and displays of emotion have significant implications for psychopathology. We turn to this model now.

Emotional Schemas

The classic cognitive-behavioral model of stress was advanced by Lazarus (1999; Lazarus & Folkman, 1984), who identified three components—a stressor (threatening or demanding event), evaluation of coping ("I can't handle this"), and stress ("I feel overwhelmed"). Thus stress is based on a *cognitive appraisal* model—focused on the event that elicits the appraisal. The cognitive model, however, has expanded beyond automatic thoughts about external events (e.g., loss, threat) to incorporate models of how sensations, intrusive thoughts, and other "symptoms" are evaluated. For example, recent cognitive models of OCD and other disorders have focused on appraisals of the nature of an intrusive thought, indicating that perseverative focus on these thoughts is enhanced by beliefs that an intrusive thought (e.g., "I am contaminated") is exacerbated by excessive attention to the thought that results from beliefs that the thought is personally relevant, says something negative about the person, needs to be suppressed, will escalate in intensity, cannot be tolerated, and will continue indefinitely (Purdon & Clark, 1994; Purdon, Rowa, & Antony, 2005; Salkovskis, 1996). Similarly, cognitive models of social anxiety, panic, and PTSD emphasize the negative appraisals of sensations and symptoms, such as the belief that anxious sensations are dangerous, that overt signs of anxiety are humiliating and are noticed by everyone, and that intrusive sensations and images are a sign that the initial trauma is happening again (Salkovskis & Clark, 1991, 1993; Steil & Ehlers, 2000; Wells & Papageorgiou, 2001). Thus the problem is not simply the appraisal of external threat but also the appraisal of the nature of the stress experience itself.

In an attempt to extend these formulations to a model of emotional processing, I have advanced a model of "emotional schemas" (Leahy, 2002, 2007). *Emotional schemas* are one's beliefs, explanations, evaluations, and strategies about the emotions of oneself and others (see Figure 12.1). For example, imagine the following: Ned hears from his girlfriend, Mary, via text message, that she is breaking up with him after 3 months of a rather troubled and complicated relationship. She indicates that she sees no reason for further communication and that he should "move on." He responds with feelings of confusion, anger, anxiety, loneliness, and some relief. However, he now has his own thoughts and responses to these emotions. He believes he should feel only *one way* ("Either happy or sad"), that he doesn't understand why he feels so upset, and wonders whether others would have this range of emotions—with the accompanying intensity. He feels ashamed about his feelings, thinking it is a sign that he is "not a real man," and he is reluctant to express them. He doesn't think anyone would understand him, and he fears that letting himself go with his feelings would lead to a complete breakdown. In attempts to control these feelings, he avoids places and people associated with the ex-girlfriend, he tries to suppress any thoughts of her, and he finds himself ruminating about what happened and worrying about the future. He has taken to eating more junk food and drinking more wine while he sits at home, alone, wondering, "What is wrong with me?"

In contrast, Michael has also experienced a similar breakup under exactly the same conditions. But his beliefs and strategies about emotion are quite different. He thinks, "It makes sense that I would have mixed feelings—there

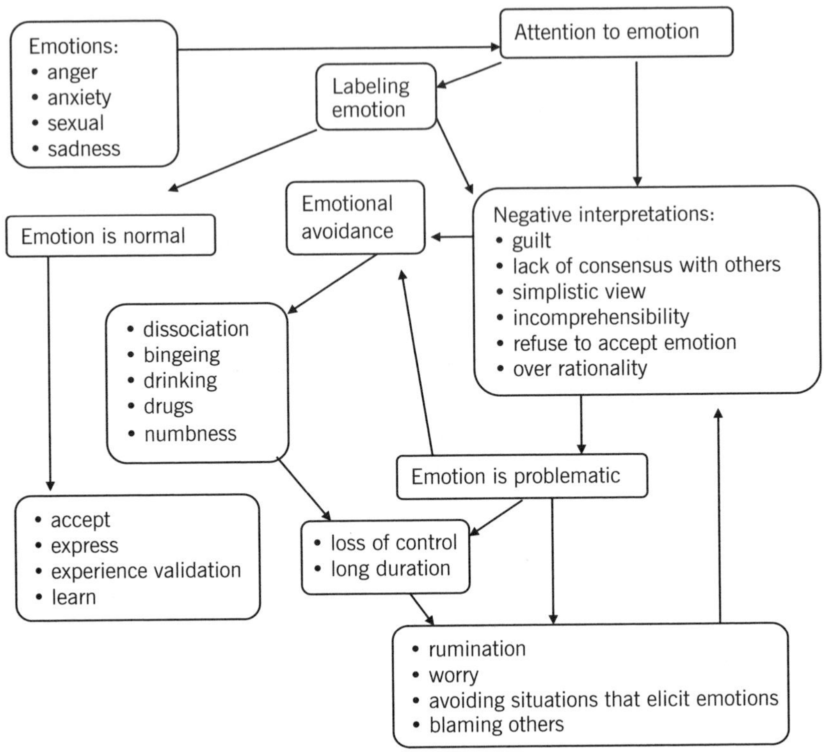

FIGURE 12.1. Emotional schemas.

were some good things, some problematic things, and she broke up in an insensitive way." He is able to tolerate ambivalence and recognize that painful feelings come from meaningful experiences. He thinks others might feel the same way. He views his emotional range as a sign of being a complete human being, expresses these feelings to his friend Ellen, and experiences validation and some clarification of his feelings. He knows that his emotions can get the best of him at times, but he also knows that he will survive the feelings because he knows to get past it means to go through it. He doesn't ruminate, worry, suppress, or overdrink, and he gradually, with some difficulty, moves forward, each step realizing that he has learned something, lost something, and can grow through even the most painful experiences.

As the foregoing examples indicate, individuals experiencing the same stressful event may respond with different evaluations *about* their emotions. Ned believes that painful emotions are dangerous, confusing, unique to him, and a sign of weakness and that they need to be suppressed or eliminated lest they go out of control and drive him completely insane. Similar to the cognitive attentional syndrome identified by Wells, the emotional schemas that are activated precipitate a series of unhelpful strategies, such as rumination, worry, avoidance, and substance abuse. In contrast, Michael, imperfect though he may be, employs more adaptive evaluations and strategies to his emotions and is thereby saved from the problematic strategies that characterize a more "neurotic" response to emotion. For Michael, painful emotions are not dangerous and do not need to be eliminated. Indeed, they can point to his higher values—attachment, intimacy, the fact that people matter—and he can experience the pain while recognizing its temporary and possibly illuminating nature.

The emotional schema model proposes that people have different theories about emotion. I have identified 14 dimensions of emotional schemas that include the following: comprehensibility, control and danger, duration, consensus with others, shame/guilt, expression, validation, relation to higher values, blame, rumination, simplistic view, numbness, overemphasis on rationality, and acceptance (Leahy, 2002). These dimensions are measured by a 50-item self-report form, the Leahy Emotional Schema Scale (LESS).

EMPIRICAL SUPPORT FOR THE EMOTIONAL SCHEMA MODEL

There is empirical support for the emotional schema model as related to anxiety, depression, and other forms of psychopathology. Emotional schemas are correlated with scores on the Beck Depression Inventory, the Beck Anxiety Inventory (Leahy, 2002; Leahy, Tirch, & Melwani, 2012), psychological flexibility, mindfulness, and metacognitive factors underlying worry (Leahy, 2011a, 2011b; Tirch, Leahy, Silberstein, & Melwani, 2012). In a study on satisfaction in intimate relationships, every one of the 14 LESS scores is significantly correlated with marital satisfaction (Dyadic Adjustment Scale; Leahy, 2012). The borderline personality dimension of the Millon Clinical Multiaxial Inventory (MCMI) revealed the following predictors: comprehensibility, rumination, validation, numbness, blame, simplistic view of emotion, control, higher values, and rationality (lower ratings; Leahy, 2015). These data strongly suggest the importance of emotional schemas in psychopathology. Individuals scoring higher on avoidant, dependent, and borderline personality had overly negative views of their emotions, whereas individuals scoring higher on narcissistic and histrionic personality had overly positive views of their emotions.. In a separate study of the emotional schemas endorsed by individuals scoring higher on borderline personality, multiple regression analysis of the specific dimensions of BPD indicated that the most predictive were comprehensibility, validation, rumination, blame, numbness, and control, reflecting the fact that individuals with BPD believe that their emotions do not make sense and that they are not validated, that they ruminate about their feelings, blame others, experience numbness, and feel out of control. Contrast this with the multiple regression for individuals scoring higher on narcissistic personality: They produce lower scores on guilt, expression, rumination, and higher values. These data suggest that individuals with narcissistic personality have less guilt about their emotions, believe that they can express their feelings, ruminate less about how they feel, and believe that their emotions are related to their higher values.

EMOTIONAL SCHEMA THERAPY: CONCEPTUALIZATION, STRATEGIES, AND TECHNIQUES

The goals of emotional schema therapy are to enhance emotional processing and tolerance for emotional experience and to decrease the utilization of problematic strategies—such as rumination, worry, avoidance, isolation, substance abuse, disordered eating, excessive reassurance seeking, emotional suppression, and dissociation. Although clearly related to the metacognitive model advanced by Wells, emotional schema therapy is a *meta-experiential* model that examines and modifies beliefs and strategies about *experience or emotion* rather than beliefs about *thoughts*. Thus therapy utilizes emotionally evocative strategies to enhance the recognition that powerful emotions need not be feared. The goal is not necessarily to "feel better" or "to think rationally." The goal is to be capable of a wider range of human feelings in a life of greater meaning and to decrease reliance on unhelpful strategies of regulation or avoidance. Moreover, emotional schema techniques and conceptualizations can be integrated into a variety of other therapies, including DBT, cognitive therapy, behavioral activation, mentalization approaches, and transference-based psychodynamic therapy. Whether one views emotional schema therapy as "stand-alone treatment" or as a set of principles, concepts, and strategies to weave within one's approach is a decision for the clinician.

Interventions

Assessing the Patient's Emotional Schemas

Using the LESS, the therapist can identify problematic beliefs and strategies and inquire as to the specific emotions and what these beliefs are. For example, the patient who responds, "I worry that if I have certain feelings I might go crazy," will be asked, "Which particular feelings will drive you crazy?" Some patients believe that anxiety or anger will lead to insanity, others believe that allowing feelings of sadness will risk suicidal despair. Further inquiry may lead to identifying problematic strategies such as "When I feel anxious, I binge" or "When I feel sad, I ask my friends to tell me it's going to be OK." One patient indicated that she felt ashamed of her feelings and that her emotions made no sense: "I don't know why I am depressed, I have so many good things in my life." On further inquiry, it was revealed that both her parents had suffered from depression and that depression was widespread through both sides of her family, suggesting a strong genetic link. She also viewed depression as a sign of weakness and thought others would disparage her if they knew she was depressed. Individuals with BPD often endorse a wide range of dysfunctional beliefs about their emotions. For example, a patient with BPD indicated that her emotions did not make sense, that they seemed to come out of nowhere, that others did not understand her feelings, that she had a hard time tolerating mixed feelings about herself and other people, that her emotions seemed to be out of control, and that she thought her feelings would last indefinitely. As the therapist reflected to her these responses, she commented, "This is the first time I have felt really understood in therapy."

As reflected in the study of personality disorders and emotional schemas, patients who have narcissistic or histrionic personality disorders may have overly positive beliefs about their emotions. For example, the initial assessment may indicate that the patient with narcissistic personality disorder believes that he or she is entitled to his or her anger and, thereby, entitled to ridicule and humiliate other people. These beliefs about emotion and the utility of emotional display can be helpful to the patient and therapist in developing treatment strategies aimed at more effective coping with emotion dysregulation and expression.

Emotionally Evocative Strategies

The therapist can use imagery and memories of experiences that are powerfully associated with emotion. In the earlier example of the jilted gentlemen, the therapists can ask the patients to recall in considerable detail the experience of receiving the rejecting messages, identifying the place, time, surroundings, sensations, and thoughts associated with that memory. Similar to the cognitive-behavioral therapy view that the fear schema must be activated in order to "habituate" and "learn new responses" (Foa & Kozak, 1986), the emotional schema model proposes that accessing the emotional experience associated with the memory can facilitate new learning. This new learning involves recognizing that the emotion can be tolerated, that it is not overwhelming, that the emotion can be shared and validated, and that one can make sense of the emotion. Rather than viewing emotional intensity as requiring a decrease or elimination of emotional intensity, the emotional schema model suggests that new ways of relating to, experiencing, tolerating, and using emotion can be facilitated. The goal is not a decrease in the emotion—although patients may view that as desirable—but rather the ability to "make room" for painful experiences as part of a complete emotional repertoire. Thus, recalling the details of the emotionally evocative events can facilitate this process. For example, Ned could recall the email message in which Mary announced the end of the relationship. He was sitting at home, alone, just back from a difficult day at work, hungry and tired, opening his email on his smartphone, feeling his heart beating rapidly as he read the message, feeling disoriented, "as if I was watching myself, as if I were not real," feeling a sad, heavy feeling coming over him, and thinking, "I am all alone."

Similarly, using imagery to develop "portrayals" of emotion can also facilitate access to intensity and meaning (Holmes & Hackmann, 2004). With Ned, the imagery of "your picture of the worst outcome" was "I see myself lying in bed, alone, with the sheets pulled up, in an empty room. I see myself crying, feeling depressed." Alternatively, Ned provided the following imagery of the best possible outcome: "I am lying in bed holding a woman I love who loves me. I feel content." Ned then began to cry in the session and commented, "I can't imagine that this could ever happen."

Patients with avoidant personality disorder also have difficulty identifying their emotional experience, often distancing themselves from their experiences. One patient commented that his emotions seemed vague, hard to identify, and that he often found himself fantasizing about being somewhere else. He acknowledged his fear that, if he allowed himself to accept his emotional experience, he would become more depressed and would cease to function. His intolerance of emotion led him to self-medicate with alcohol. He also feared that if he cried during sessions he would feel humiliated and that the therapist would think of him as a weak loser. His feared fantasy was that the therapist would laugh at him, disparage him for being childish, and not want to see him. This reminded him of his experience as a child when his mother was busy on the telephone, having no time to talk with him, and would tell him to stop acting like a "baby." The therapist suggested a role play in which he was asked to assert himself with his mother in the image and tell her how he deserved to be treated. This led to greater acceptance of his right to have negative feelings and his willingness to share them in therapy.

Identifying Problematic Coping Strategies

Further inquiry may help to identify problematic strategies such as "When I feel anxious, I binge" or "When I feel sad, I ask my friends to tell me it's going to be OK." Another patient with avoidant and dependent features indicated that when she was depressed she felt enervated and attempted to conserve her energy by lying in bed, which was also associated with greater rumination. She also said that when she socialized with friends she couldn't "help herself" and had to tell them everything bad that she was feeling. This led her to believe that she was a burden to her friends, which may have been partly true. She endorsed a belief about expression and total validation that had an inadvertent self-defeating component: "I have to be myself and tell people what I am feeling to get the support that I need." Although there may have been some grain of truth in this thought, its inflexibility meant that she either inundated her friends with depressive rumination or completely isolated herself.

Ned's unhelpful strategies were to isolate himself, spend excessive amount of time lying in bed, ruminate, worry, blame Mary, blame himself, complain to friends when he saw them, drink, and overeat. Some of these strategies provided him with avoidance or escape from the emotion, the feeling of self-righteous disdain, and momentary reassurance. However, they also maintained his feeling "stuck" in the rut of the experience of the breakup, prevented him from living his life more fully, and added to his sense of despair about future relationships.

Patients with personality disorder utilize a wide range of problematic strategies for coping with their emotional experience. The person with avoidant personality isolates, withdrawing into a private world of fantasy and rumination, looking for any signs of rejection. The person with dependent personality turns to others for comfort, often resulting in dependence on unreliable people. The person with BPD, seeking validation, may inundate others with complaints and tales of suffering, only to alienate the very people he or she would rely on. The person with narcissistic personality blames others for his or her negative emotions and attempts to punish them. Because everyone has negative emotions at times, the therapist can continue to explore these problematic strategies: "When you feel down or feel anxious, what do you do next?"

Examining Costs and Benefits of Coping Strategies

Coping strategies are used because the patient expects to gain from them. For example, Ned would binge eat when he felt distressed. The therapist asked him to list the advantages and disadvantages to this coping behavior. Initially, Ned denied any benefit—"I know it isn't useful"—but the therapist gently directed him to the possibility that almost every strategy can have some expected benefit. Ned acknowledged the following: "When I feel lonely, out of control, at least I can soothe myself with junk food. I can feel better immediately. I can get my mind off of things." The therapist commented that each of these is a powerful reason to continue bingeing, as they are immediate reinforcers that allow him to avoid painful experiences in the short term. The disadvantages were longer term—both immediately after the binge was completed (guilt, feeling physically uncomfortable) and longer after, in gaining weight and feeling out of control. Underlying the use of these problematic coping strategies were the following emotional schemas: "Painful feelings cannot be tolerated. They will escalate. They have to be suppressed. They will last indefinitely. I can't stand these feelings." If the therapist and Ned could show that these underlying emotional schemas are false, then there would be less need for bingeing.

Ned's avoidant tendencies maintained his belief that he was alone, that his emotions did not make sense, that no one could validate him, and that there was no way out. His reliance on bingeing further reinforced his belief that emotions needed to be controlled but could not be eliminated and therefore were problematic. His reliance on rumination as part of his avoidance kept him stuck in the emotional quagmire of self-absorption, not allowing him the opportunity to feel effective in pursuing productive behavior either on his own or with others. Helping the patient understand that these coping strategies may maintain the negative emotional experience can provide some motivational force toward more adaptive strategies.

Modifying Specific Schemas

GUILT AND SHAME

Therapy won't get very far if the patient feels so guilty or ashamed that he will not share his emotional experience. The therapist can anticipate this and comment, "Many of us feel confused, guilty, or ashamed about our feelings. But our emotions tell us about our needs and who we are. I wonder if there are certain feelings that you might feel reluctant to tell me about—perhaps feelings that you are ashamed of." With Ned, this led to his acknowledging that he felt ashamed of feeling so sad and lonely, as he equated these emotions with weakness and as a sign that he wasn't a "real man." In addition, he acknowledged fantasies of revenge against Mary, commenting that he thought of "blasting her out" on her Facebook page before she took the initiative to "unfriend" him. Guilt over emotions that are felt is based on a set of beliefs that one should always have the "right emotions," that one is responsible for one's emotions, and—sometimes—the belief that emotions will inevitably lead to behavior. It is helpful for patients to recognize that emotions and behavior are different and that true moral or ethical choices are possible only if there are forces (such as emotions) pulling oneself in the opposite direction. Feeling angry is not the same thing as acting in a hostile manner. Similarly, the belief that "real men" don't feel sad is countered by the recognition that great heroic or tragic figures experience sadness and even shed tears—figures in literature such as Achilles, Odysseus, Hamlet, and King Lear. Moreover, the therapist can inquire whether the patient believes that the therapist might have judgmental thoughts about the patient's emotional experience or emotional display.

GOOD AND BAD EMOTIONS

Some patients label certain emotions as "good"—happiness, hope, curiosity, excitement, love—and other emotions as "bad"—anger, sadness, anxiety, jealousy, and envy. The assumption is that one must never feel the "bad" emotions and that these emotions will damage you or that they are a sign of weakness, poor character, or pathological tendencies. Linehan refers to these beliefs as "emotion myths" (Linehan, 1993a). The current wave of "happiness" psychologies adds to this myth about the possibilities of human existence. Thus, when the patient is not feeling happy, he becomes concerned that there is "something wrong" with him. And, when he feels jealous or angry, he thinks that he is neurotic or even despicable. Ned reported feelings of anger, the desire for revenge, and jealousy about the possibility that Mary might be with other men. He labeled these as *bad emotions*—emotions that he had to get rid of.

The therapist can ask the patient to list the good and bad emotions separately, indicate what "makes an emotion good or bad," and examine the costs and benefits of viewing emotions in these evaluative terms. Some patients believe that an emotion is "bad" if it is associated with "negative" feelings or can lead to antisocial or problematic behavior. The therapist can inquire whether people attending a funeral should feel happy. "What would it mean to tell people who have lost someone that their sadness is a bad emotion and one that should be eliminated immediately?" Most patients recognize that this is not only invalidating and inappropriate but also dehumanizing. Then the question arises, What makes a painful emotion "appropriate"? Who decides?

Some patients believe that by labeling an emotion as "bad" they can avoid the emotion and thereby prevent themselves from acting out if they have the emotion. Ned said, "I don't want to feel jealous because it just makes me upset and I don't want to be the kind of guy who just harbors these feelings." Note that Ned's concern was acting on the jealousy and ruminating about it—which are different from simply acknowledging that one has these feelings. In contrast to this "myth" about good and bad emotions, the therapist can explore the possibility that emotions evolved because they have some adaptive value. For example, anger helps in the defense of self and family, anxiety may alert you to real dangers, regret may help you learn from your mistakes, jealousy may help you drive off competitors, and envy may help you recognize the value of imitating the behavior of people who are successful. One patient, who complained of "envy attacks" (the way some patients complain of panic attacks) found this evolutionary interpretation quite helpful. It assisted him in normalizing his envy and allowed him to examine how he could turn his envy into admiration and his admiration into imitation. We labeled this "constructive use of envy." He didn't have to fear or suppress the envy—he only had to acknowledge the envy, examine his possible action choices, and pursue behaviors that would be in his ultimate self-interest. Similarly, Ned was assisted in normalizing his jealousy: "Don't people feel jealous about their recent partner being intimate with others?"

INVALIDATION

Patients with BPD are especially sensitive to any sign of invalidation and often view attempts to change in therapy as invalidating the experience of suffering and victimization. Similarly, patients with avoidant personality disorder, such as Ned, have often been told that their emotions do not make sense, that their emotions are a burden to others, and that they should control their feelings. The therapist can ask how parents responded when the patient, as a child, expressed painful feelings. Ned recalled: "I never would go to my father because he would simply tell me to act more like a man and to stop crying like a baby. My mother had too many problems of her own. I often felt like I was interrupting her on the phone when she was talking to her friends. She would tell me to leave her alone, she was busy." Ned got the emotional messages that his emotions would be criticized, that he would be humiliated, that he wasn't strong, and that others did not have time for his feelings. As a result he thought that expressing emotion with friends would lead to further humiliation, so he refrained from sharing his feelings, further isolating himself and adding to his risk for depression.

SELF-INVALIDATION

Many patients have internalized these invalidating messages and invalidate themselves. Patients with BPD vacillate between what appear as excessive demands for validation with excessive self-invalidation. One patient commented, "My feelings just don't make sense. What's wrong with me? I should get a handle on things." Self-sacrificing and dependent patients may fear that their emotional needs are excessive and may alienate the people on whom they depend. A self-sacrificing, dependent married woman claimed that her desires for affection and sexuality in her marriage may be too excessive and unrealistic: "Maybe I am asking too much." Her strategy of self-invalidation contributed to the difficulty in asserting herself with her alcoholic husband.

With Ned, self-invalidation could be seen in his facial expression—an awkward smile as he recalled the humiliating breakup. The therapist commented, "I notice that you are smiling as you recall this painful message from Mary—almost as if you are trying to communicate to me and to yourself that this isn't a big deal. I wonder if you tend to minimize your emotions with other people—and with yourself." Ned acknowledged that he didn't want to "sound like a downer" and that he often minimized his feelings with friends—and with Mary. In fact, one of the reasons that Mary had difficulty with him, she said, was that "I never seem to know what you are feeling." Other typical self-invalidation thoughts are "My emotions are a drag. I need to stop feeling this way. I'm just a whiner. I should just get on with things and stop complaining and stop worrying. I should be stronger, less emotional."

INCOMPREHENSIBILITY

As indicated by our research findings, patients with BPD believe that their emotions do not make sense. With their earlier and current invalidating environments and their sense that their emotions are overwhelming, patients with BPD are wrapped in a dilemma of feeling a need to express their emotions and a fear that their emotions overwhelm them. A common belief that patients like Ned have is that their emotions don't make sense. Ned said, "I don't know why I feel so bad about this breakup. It was only a few months, and I had mixed feelings for a long time. Why do I feel so upset? Why can't I just move on and forget about it?" These beliefs are based on the assumption that the intensity of an emotion should match the length of a relationship. In addition, some patients believe that their emotions don't make sense if they have mixed feelings. A consequence of the belief that emotions don't make sense is the corollary belief that "If they don't make sense, I won't know how to cope with them, they can come out of nowhere, and I am helpless with my emotions." Making sense of emotion is part of therapy. For example, Ned's mix of emotions—"sadness, shame, confusion, anxiety, and relief"—can be linked to a set of automatic or spontaneous thoughts, each of which leads to a specific emotion. These include: "I have nothing in my life now" (sadness); "I must be weak if I feel so sad" (shame); "I should only feel one way—this doesn't make sense to have mixed feelings" (confusion); "Will I ever be happy again? Will anyone ever want to be with me?" (anxiety); and "I don't have to deal with her mood swings anymore" (relief). Emotions make sense when they are linked to reasons.

DURABILITY

Affective forecasting often involves the belief that emotions, once they occur, will last indefinitely. Ned endorsed several such beliefs—"I will feel anxious and sad and lonely for a long time." Sometimes the durability is expressed in dichotomous thinking: "I always feel sad now." The belief in the durability of emotion adds to a sense of helplessness and hopelessness about overcoming the present mood. This can be addressed by asking the patient, "What are the costs and benefits of believing that your mood will last indefinitely? What is the evidence for and against this belief?" Some patients believe that by lowering their expectations their negative mood will change and they can avoid further disappointment. "I don't want to get my hopes up," Ned said. "I've been hurt too many times." Of course, the disadvantage is hopelessness. Ned believed that the evidence that he would be unhappy indefinitely was that he felt so unhappy now—a form of overgeneralization and emotional reasoning. The therapist then asked him if he had had these beliefs about negative moods in the past. He said, "Yes, almost every time I feel down I think it's going to last indefinitely." The evidence from past experiences suggested that his moods inevitably changed. The idea that moods last indefinitely can be further challenged through the use of activity scheduling, pleasure predicting, and assigning activities that are pleasurable and involve some sense of mastery. Ned charted his moods every hour of the week, noted the activities, and—on a separate chart—listed his predictions for specific activities that he and the therapist agreed on as "experiments" in seeing whether moods changed. Collecting these data helped him realize that his mood improved substantially when he was concentrating on tasks at work, talking with friends, working out at the gym, or watching an interesting football game on television. His moods were negative when he lay in bed after waking up and when he ruminated, criticized himself, and sat at home doing nothing. Thus his moods were not as durable as he thought, as they could change within an hour. Patients with BPD hold strong beliefs about durability of emotions. One patient said, "I think that if I allow myself to feel sad it will never go away. I will feel bad forever." Learning how to improve the moment, ride the wave of the emotion, distract oneself, have daily behavioral goals, and identify longer-term life strategies can assist patients in recognizing that what feels like "forever" is another emotional myth that needs to be dispelled.

LOSS OF CONTROL

Many patients believe that if they begin to feel an emotion it will go out of control and overwhelm them. Thus they attempt to avoid situations that elicit emotions, use emotion suppression strategies, and become more anxious once they feel an emotion—which leads to further escalation of that emotion. Some patients attempt to suppress crying in a session. Ned said, "I feel I have to keep my crying in because—if I start—it will just go out of control. I think, 'I'll never stop crying.'" The therapist should be aware of any attempts that can be seen in the patient's facial expression that crying is being suppressed. The therapist can inquire, "What would it look like if your emotions went out of control? What do you see yourself doing?" One patient believed that if he allowed himself to tolerate any anxiety when he was in a subway car, he would lose all control, start running around, screaming, bang on the door to get out, and completely humiliate himself. The therapist can then inquire, "Has any of this ever happened? Why not?" Some patients attribute their "ability to control their emotions" to superstitious behavior. For example, Ned claimed that he was able to keep himself from losing all control by telling himself that he would be OK. This self-reassurance was then viewed as the reason that he didn't lose control. He still maintained the belief that he would "go crazy" if he didn't control himself by this kind of self-statement. One way of challenging this superstitious belief is to have the patient activate memories of the feared experience (in this case, Mary's breakup with Ned) and then repeat for 10 minutes, "I will go out of control and go crazy." This exposure to the feared feeling and the feared thought—without neutralization—can be helpful in dispelling the erroneous belief that one needs to reassure oneself or one will go insane.

Patients with BPD often claim that their emotions are out of control—a message that may reflect their earlier experiences of invalidation. Indeed, because they have been taught that their emotions do not make sense and are illegitimate and shameful, they have developed a fear of their feelings that may spiral out of control. This "Catch-22" leads to dysfunctional coping strategies, such as drug and alcohol abuse, binge eating, cutting, or—in many cases—isolation and avoidance. Learning how to tolerate some emotion, while being able to distract, improve the moment, and employ mindful awareness and acceptance, can help mitigate these extreme beliefs that one either has total control or no control.

RELATION TO HIGHER VALUES

The emotional schema model proposes that painful emotions and experiences may arise from the pursuit of higher values. If "things matter," then painful emotions may be a consequence of their loss or of the frustration in not achieving valued goals. For example, if a relationship matters, then its ending is likely to involve painful emotions of sadness, loss, loneliness, and even despair. Martha Nussbaum notes in her fascinating book, *Upheavals of Thought* (2001), that not to feel great sadness after her mother has died—but to claim that she loves her mother—would seem to contradict the statement that she really cared about her mother. Loss of what matters carries with it the painful emotions. What is valued can often point to what can bring us pain. For example, Ned's jealousy was linked to his values of commitment, fidelity, and exclusiveness in an intimate relationship: "It makes sense, Ned, for you to feel jealous because you have had such a strong, intimate attachment to Mary for some time and things matter to you. Your painful emotions come from your ability to experience strong feelings and have a meaningful relationship. You are obviously not a shallow person." One can accept that certain things "come with the territory"—such as painful feelings about what matters.

Rather than discount the importance of his relationship with Mary, Ned can become focused on the values that he believes have been affected. In this particular case, these values included intimacy, commitment, sharing life, doing things for another person, and being close to one another. These values can be affirmed—once again—as important values to aim for in life. Some of these values can be pursued in friendships, others through helping others (e.g., volunteer activities), and other values (such as intimacy and closeness) may have to wait for their realization. But values add hope, and they give meaning to tolerating the difficulties that one must tolerate during the more difficult times. The therapist noted, "It's one thing to lose the relationship with Mary, as problematic as it was. But it would be an even greater loss to lose the values that you were pursuing."

Kierkegaard once said, "If you marry you'll regret it, if you don't marry you'll regret it." This inevitability of regret and difficulty may be part of the nature of commitment. Ned's belief—"I'm afraid that if I get involved I'll get hurt again"—reflected a belief that "I wouldn't be able to take another disappointment" and "I have to avoid pain in the future." In contrast to this fear of disappointment and loss is an alternative view of the value of a mortal and imperfect life. As I said to Ned, "It may be true that if you fall in love again, you might suffer. In the end, all is lost because all of us are mortal and the people we love are mortal. The issue, though, is not to avoid suffering at all costs—because the cost may be a life that is empty and meaningless. The goal might be to live a life worth suffering for." This recognition that it was hopeless to avoid suffering—because the only alternatives were a life cut off from intimacy or a life with intimacy and the possibility of loss—helped Ned understand that, if he could go through his pain to get past it during the current loss, he might be able to pursue a life that had meaning, that brought both happiness and sadness, a life that was more complete—and possibly more challenging.

APPLICATION TO BPD

Linehan proposed that BPD is characterized by a wide range of areas of dysregulation, including self, emotion, behavior, interpersonal functioning, and identity (Crowell, Beauchaine, & Linehan, 2009; Gratz, Latzman, Tull, Reynolds, & Lejuez, 2011; Linehan, 1993a, 1993b). Linehan's model stresses the interaction between early invalidating environments, impulsivity, increased probability of abuse, and poor skills in emotional regulation. Even as it recognizes the importance of these putative etiological factors in BPD, the emotional schema model proposes that BPD is characterized by a wide range of dysfunctional beliefs about emotion. These dysfunctional emotional schemas include beliefs that one's emotions are incomprehensible, unlike the emotions of others, out of control; that they need to be suppressed, will continue indefinitely, cannot be expressed, will not be validated, and are shameful. Moreover, individuals with BPD utilize a range of dysfunctional strategies to suppress emotions, including self-injurious behavior, bingeing, substance abuse, blaming, rumination, worry, and avoidance. The LESS is helpful at intake in directing the clinician toward these problematic concepts of emotion. For example, the clinician can immediately inquire about beliefs about emotion: "You said that there are some emotions that you think don't make sense. Which emotions are these? What makes you think these emotions don't make sense? What does that make you feel? Think?" "You indicate that you believe that your emotions might last forever if you don't control them. Which emotions will last forever? What do you do when you think that? What would happen if you did not suppress these emotions?" "You indicate that you feel ashamed about your emotions. Which emotions? Why?" We have found that the LESS helps to enrich assessment by allowing the clinician to evaluate immediately one of the most central issues for individuals with BPD— their beliefs about their own emotions. One patient said, "This is the first time I felt someone really understood me." It certainly addresses the primary concern about invalidation.

The clinician can link current beliefs about emotion with emotion myths in the family: "Could you tell me how your mother or father responded to you when you were a kid when you were upset?" Patients who indicate that parents were dismissive or ridiculing can see a connection between these messages of invalidation and current beliefs about their emotions—such as beliefs about the futility of expression and validation, incomprehensibility, or the uniqueness of one's emotions. Moreover, the clinician can inquire about problematic strategies to seek validation, such as escalating, dramatic displays, pouting, attempts to elicit painful emotions in others, blaming, and parasuicidal acts.

The initial evaluation—which may take several sessions—allows both patient and clinician to develop a sophisticated model of the patient's theory of emotion, emotional display, emotional socialization, and emotional regulation. We have found it useful to provide patients with the schematic (Figure 12.1) that illustrates the emotional schema model. This allows them to understand how their problematic beliefs about the legitimacy, control, and danger of emotion lead to dysfunctional strategies of emotional suppression. By clearly identifying the content of these schemas, the patient and clinician can identify targets for change—that is, their beliefs and problematic strategies about emotion.

For example, the patient who believes that her or his emotions do not make sense will also believe that an experience that is incomprehensible is unpredictable, uncontrollable, and—possibly—evidence of basic defectiveness. Therapy utilizes several techniques to "make sense" of emotion: monitoring emotion (and intensity of emotion), identifying automatic thoughts and maladaptive assumptions associated with emotion, imagery induction (activating imagery that is associated with an emotion and then identifying the thoughts associated with the image), and identifying early experiences of the emotion (e.g., memories from childhood that help identify the source of problematic beliefs about the emotion). For example, Wanda had a history of BPD. She monitored her sadness and found that it was higher when she was alone. This was associated with thoughts that "I am alone because no one loves me," "I will always be alone," and "I am alone because I am damaged goods." Her maladaptive assumption was "If you have emotional problems no one will accept you. You have to hide your real self." She recalled an early experience when she was 16 of an attempted suicide by overdose after a breakup with her boyfriend when her mother told her, "There's nothing wrong with you. It must be jet lag from your trip back from Europe." She felt alone, invalidated, ashamed, and overwhelmed by her emotions. The therapist was able to link the emotions of sadness, shame, frustration, and anger with the sense that no one in her family appeared to have much time for her emotion. Further exploration of her beliefs about invalidation revealed family "myths" about emotion—that is, the family insisted on "loyalty" to the image that "nothing is wrong with you," that "having problems reflects poorly on the family," and the implicit assumption that she was there to serve their needs. Thus, having emotions like sadness, anxiety, and anger were signs of being unlovable, defective, and disloyal.

The patient also indicated that she needed to smoke marijuana or drink excessively to get rid of emotions. "If I don't stop feeling this way, then I won't be able to function, I won't be able to sleep." Her combination of beliefs that her emotions made no sense and were a sign of defectiveness led to increased self-invalidation and attempts to hide emotion from others. The therapist observed, "I notice that when you talk about your emotions you have a smile on your face as if you are saying to me, 'Don't take me seriously.' It's as if you are trying to tell me that your emotions don't count." She responded that she didn't want to sound pathetic and weak, didn't want the therapist to feel sorry for her, and didn't want anyone to know the "real me." These beliefs about expression, invalidation, defectiveness, incomprehensibility, and uniqueness of her emotion led to a discussion of how she had two selves, which the therapist labeled "back stage" and "front stage." The front-stage self was the image she wanted others to see, "the Party Girl." "I put on an act. I'm the one who dances at the party. I make everyone laugh." The back-stage self was one that was alone, misunderstood, afraid, feeling unlovable, and hiding from the world. "If they knew the back-stage me they would hate me." The patient's image of herself was merged with her dysfunctional emotional schemas—she equated herself with concepts of her own emotions: "bad emotions = bad me." The therapist indicated that the behavior that others might find problematic was not her emotions of sadness, anger, anxiety, and hopelessness; these were human emotions that everyone has experienced. Rather, the difficulty people might have was in her solutions to the problem—that is, her use of cocaine, bingeing, self-injury, sexual acting out, and alcohol abuse. The difficulty was less with her emotions and more with the solutions she utilized for these emotions.

In contrast to these dysfunctional solutions, the therapist suggested several, more helpful strategies. These included identifying and differentiating emotions, linking emotions to thoughts, modifying these thoughts with cognitive therapy techniques (examine the cognitive distortions, evaluate costs and benefits, look at the evidence, argue back against the thought, ask what advice you would give a friend). In addition, the therapist suggested that it might help for the patient to examine her beliefs about emotion, such as evaluating whether an emotion lasts indefinitely (e.g., using activity scheduling to chart variation in intensity and occurrence of emotions) and challenging her ideas that her emotions made no sense, that she should feel ashamed and guilty about her emotions, and that her emotions were a sign of weakness or defectiveness. Universalizing painful emotions, such as sadness, anger, shame, anxiety, and loneliness, not only assists in normalizing emotion but also provides examples of how "others" can cope with painful experience. The patient's self-critical thoughts about her emotions were examined using the following techniques: identifying her "should" statements about emotion ("I shouldn't feel sad"), developing a rationale for why her sad feelings made sense (given her automatic thoughts and her invalidating experiences growing up), using a double-standard technique ("What would you think of someone else who had these emotions?"), evaluating the evidence that her emotions come and go, and evaluating how others tolerate emotions.

The patient's beliefs that she could not accept her emotion were challenged by practicing radical acceptance ("What if you were to accept that this is how you feel at this moment rather than struggling against it?"), mindful detachment ("Stand back and observe, in a nonjudgmental way, without controlling your emotion, how you feel, where you feel it, what is going on"), describing the sensations and emotions with a detached mindful stance, accepting the emotion as part of a context of many other emotions and experiences—that is, "making space for the emotion"—and "riding the wave" of the emotion rather than sinking into it or struggling against it. Her beliefs that she should condemn herself for her feelings—"I am bad because I have bad feelings"—was addressed by examining the socialization experiences that led to these beliefs, evaluating whether there were better ways that her parents could have handled things, role plays with the imaginary figure of her mother while the patient challenged the mother's dismissive attitude toward the patient's emotions, and using an imaginary compassionate figure that could soothe her emotions with "loving kindness" and recognize her right to feel bad (Gilbert, 2010; Leahy, 2015; Leahy et al., 2011).

The patient's emotions of loneliness and her thoughts that she was unlovable were linked to her "higher values" of intimacy, commitment, and connectedness with others. The therapist observed, "You have these feelings of loneliness because being connected to others, being in an intimate relationship where you can love and be loved, are central to who you are. Your pain, right now, may come from something that is good about you, something that yearns for connection and commitment." By linking her pain to a "good enough reason to tolerate the pain," she could make sense of her feelings, while feeling better about accepting them as the cost of a meaningful life. The therapist observed, "You may try to present yourself as shallow so that others won't see your need, but you are not really a superficial person. Just like so many of us, you want to feel loved and you want to love. It would be sad to lose that desire, that need." This patient had viewed her "need" to feel cared for as a weakness, but the therapist reframed this need as linking her to a universal set of emotions, needs, and values: "You have been afraid to accept your needs because your parents were not good at meeting these needs and made you feel ashamed of having needs. But why shouldn't you be like all of us who are human—needing each other, needing to feel cared for?"

Therapy also involved the patient's recognition of how her beliefs about emotion affected the transference and countertransference. For example, she indicated that she believed that the therapist might think that she was weak and defective for having these emotional problems and for having needs, and she recalled a dream: "I dreamed that you dropped me as a patient." She indicated that she wanted the therapist to believe that she was strong, defiant, and did not have any needs for nurturance or validation: "I don't want to appear needy. It's pathetic." This led to a discussion and recognition that her interpersonal choices outside of therapy were directed toward self-defeating objects of attachment—men who she knew would not be nurturing or trustworthy. By managing her expectations downward, she would ensure that she would not be disappointed, not betrayed in any "meaningful" way, and not hurt like she had been by her former boyfriend or by her dismissive and minimizing parents.

Over the course of a 2-year period of treatment, the patient dramatically reduced drug misuse, although she had one relapse of cocaine abuse during that time. Her binge-and-purge cycles were significantly reduced—and eventually eliminated. Her drinking became less regular and less problematic. After several short-term relationships, she eventually developed a long-term relationship with a more appropriate partner, about whom she initially felt ambivalent. Her ambivalence was linked to her beliefs that she was unlovable and that he would eventually leave her, so that her best strategy was to sabotage the relationship. Recognizing her past pattern of self-defeating choices, however, she maintained the relationship. Two years after finishing treatment she married the man.

To summarize the course of treatment of this patient, we can identify the following goals and treatment interventions and strategies:

- Identify emotional schemas.
- Identify problematic emotion-regulation strategies.
- Identify self-invalidation and minimizing needs.
- Identify avoidance strategies.
- Use "compassionate confrontation."
- Label, mirror, validate, and expand emotions.
- Normalize emotions.
- Help the patient view emotions as temporary, connected to needs, and having validity.
- Eliminate emotional avoidance behaviors (bingeing/purging, drinking, marijuana).
- Identify fear of crying ("I was able to cry in front of my cat"), that is, crying = weakness, humiliation.
- Examine masochistic/self-defeating relationships.
- Challenge self-schema (unlovable/defective).
- Develop a "bill of rights" for relationships and feelings.
- Overcome a fear that "ending relationships is devastating."
- Develop an "affirming" model of a healthy, intimate relationship.

CONCLUDING COMMENTS

Cognitive-behavioral approaches are sometimes criticized for being overly rational and for not addressing emotional experience or the socialization effects on the patient. The approach described in this chapter focuses on the importance of emotional experience, individual differences in beliefs about emotion, problematic strategies of emotional regulation and avoidance, and different styles of communicating emotions and perceiving the emotions of others. Indeed, in the case of the woman with borderline personality who minimized her severe problems, the usual cognitive therapy model of "letting the patient set the agenda" did not guide the treatment because the patient's emotional avoidance led to trivializing the treatment. In fact, some patients may deliberately seek cognitive-behavioral therapy because they wish to avoid emotionally salient material. The emotional schema model allows the therapist to identify these transferential issues in a compassionate style of confrontation, while eliciting beliefs and fears of emotional "exposure" and concerns about loss of control and humiliation. Because of its specific focus on these emotional schemas and strategies, emotional schema therapy may be particularly helpful in treating patients with BPD.

REFERENCES

Crowell, S. E., Beauchaine, T. P., & Linehan, M. M. (2009). A biosocial developmental model of borderline personality: Elaborating and extending Linehan's theory. *Psychological Bulletin, 135*(3), 495–510.

Elias, N. (2000). *The civilizing process: Sociogenetic and psychogenetic investigations* (E. Jephcott, Trans.). Oxford, UK: Blackwell. (Original work published 1939)

Foa, E. B., & Kozak, M. J. (1986). Emotional processing of fear: Exposure to corrective information. *Psychological Bulletin, 99*, 20–35.

Gilbert, P. (2010). *Compassion-focused therapy: Distinctive features.* New York: Routledge.

Gottman, J. M., Katz, L. F., & Hooven, C. (1997). *Meta-emotion: How families communicate emotionally.* Mahwah, NJ: Erlbaum.

Gratz, K. L., Latzman, R. D., Tull, M. T., Reynolds, E. K., & Lejuez, C. W. (2011). Exploring the association between emotional abuse and childhood borderline personality features: The moderating role of personality traits. *Behavior Therapy, 42*(3), 493–508.

Greenberg, L. S. (2002). *Emotion-focused therapy: Coaching clients to work through their feelings.* Washington, DC: American Psychological Association.

Holmes, E. A., & Hackmann, A. (Eds.). (2004). *Mental imagery and memory in psychopathology.* Hove, UK: Psychology Press.

Lazarus, R. S. (1999). *Stress and emotion: A new synthesis.* New York: Springer.

Lazarus, R. S., & Folkman, S. (1984). *Stress, appraisal, and coping.* New York: Springer.

Leahy, R. L. (2002). A model of emotional schemas. *Cognitive and Behavioral Practice, 9*(3), 177–190.

Leahy, R. L. (2003). Emotional schemas and resistance. In R. L. Leahy (Ed.), *Roadblocks in cognitive-behavioral therapy: Transforming challenges into opportunities for change* (pp. 91–115). New York: Guilford Press.

Leahy, R. L. (2007). Emotional schemas and self-help: Homework compliance and obsessive–compulsive disorder. *Cognitive and Behavioral Practice, 14*(3), 297–302.

Leahy, R. L. (2011a, June). *Emotional intelligence and cognitive therapy: A bridge over troubled waters.* Paper presented at the International Congress of Cognitive Psychotherapy, Istanbul, Turkey.

Leahy, R. L. (2011b, April). *Emotional schemas and implicit theory of emotion:*

Overcoming fear of feeling. Paper presented at the International Conference of Metacognitive Therapy, Manchester, UK.

Leahy, R. L. (2012). *Emotional schemas as predictors of relationship dissatisfaction.* Unpublished manuscript, American Institute for Cognitive Therapy.

Leahy, R. L. (2015). *Emotional schema therapy.* New York: Guilford Press.

Leahy, R. L., & Tirch, D. (2011, June). *Emotional schemas, psychological flexibility and borderline personality.* Paper presented at the International Congress on Cognitive Psychotherapy, Istanbul, Turkey.

Leahy, R. L., Tirch, D., & Napolitano, L. A. (2011). *Emotion regulation in psychotherapy: A practitioner's guide.* New York: Guilford Press.

Leahy, R. L., Tirch, D. D., & Melwani, P. S. (2012). Processes underlying depression: Risk aversion, emotional schemas, and psychological flexibility. *International Journal of Cognitive Therapy, 5*(4), 362–379.

Linehan, M. M. (1993a). *Cognitive-behavioral treatment of borderline personality disorder.* New York: Guilford Press.

Linehan, M. M. (1993b). *Skills training manual for treating borderline personality disorder.* New York: Guilford Press.

Lutz, T. (2001). *Crying: A natural and cultural history of tears.* New York: Norton.

McCullough, L., Kuhn, N., Andrews, S., Kaplan, A., Wolf, J., & Hurley, C. L. (2003). *Treating affect phobia: A manual for short-term dynamic psychotherapy.* New York: Guilford Press.

Nordahl, H. M. (2011, May). *The ERIS Protocol: MCT for Borderline Personality.* Paper presented at the Metacognitive Therapy Conference, Manchester, UK.

Nussbaum, M. C. (2001). *Upheavals of thought: The intelligence of emotions.* Cambridge, UK: Cambridge University Press.

Purdon, C., & Clark, D. A. (1994). Obsessive intrusive thoughts in nonclinical subjects: II. Cognitive appraisal, emotional response and thought control strategies. *Behaviour Research and Therapy, 32*, 403–410.

Purdon, C., Rowa, K., & Antony, M. M. (2005). Thought suppression and its effects on thought frequency, appraisal and mood state in individuals with obsessive–compulsive disorder. *Behaviour Research and Therapy, 43*(1), 93–108.

Salkovskis, P. M. (1996). The cognitive approach to anxiety: Threat beliefs, safety-seeking behavior, and the special case of health anxiety and obsessions. In P. M. Salkovskis (Ed.), *Frontiers of cognitive therapy* (pp. 48–74). New York: Guilford Press.

Salkovskis, P. M., & Clark, D. M. (1991). Cognitive therapy for panic attacks. *Journal of Cognitive Psychotherapy, 5*, 215–226.

Salkovskis, P. M., & Clark, D. M. (1993). Panic disorder and hypochondriasis. *Advances in Behaviour Research and Therapy, 15*(1), 23–48.

Stearns, P. (1994). *American cool: Constructing a twentieth-century emotional style.* New York: New York University Press.

Steil, R., & Ehlers, A. (2000). Dysfunctional meaning of posttraumatic intrusions in chronic PTSD. *Behaviour Research and Therapy, 38*(6), 537–558.

Tirch, D. D., Leahy, R. L., Silberstein, L. R., & Melwani, P. S. (2012). Emotional schemas, psychological flexibility, and anxiety: The role of flexible response patterns to anxious arousal. *International Journal of Cognitive Therapy, 5*(4), 380–391.

Weber, M. (1992). *The Protestant ethic and the spirit of capitalism.* New York: Routledge.

Wells, A. (2002). Meta-cognitive beliefs in the maintenance of worry and generalized anxiety disorder. In R. G. Heimberg, C. L. Turk, & D. S. Mennin (Eds.), *Generalized anxiety disorder: Advances in research and practice.* New York: Guilford Press.

Wells, A. (2004). A cognitive model of GAD: Metacognitions and pathological worry. In R. G. Heimberg, C. L. Turk, & D. S. Mennin (Eds.), *Generalized anxiety disorder: Advances in research and practice* (pp. 164–186). New York: Guilford Press.

Wells, A. (2008). *Metacognitive therapy for anxiety and depression.* New York: Guilford Press.

Wells, A., & Papageorgiou, C. (2001). Social phobic interoception: Effects of bodily information on anxiety, beliefs and self-processing. *Behavior Research and Therapy, 39*(1), 1–11.

chapter 13

Adapting Mindfulness for Treating Personality Disorder

Paolo Ottavi, Tiziana Passarella, Manuela Pasinetti, Giampaolo Salvatore, and Giancarlo Dimaggio

Patients with personality disorders often worry about what occurs in interpersonal relationships. They ruminate over wrongs suffered and mistakes made and fears of being rejected, humiliated, or dominated that leave them trapped in emotions such as anxiety, anger, and guilt that are difficult to overcome. The results are often symptom disorders, such as depression, anxiety, and obsessive–compulsive disorder (Alnæs & Torgersen, 1988; Dimaggio, Semerari, Carcione, Nicolò, & Procacci, 2007). Such symptoms, frequently associated with personality disorders, respond to mindfulness-based interventions, such as mindfulness-based stress reduction (MBSR; Kabat-Zinn, 1982, 1990) or mindfulness-based cognitive therapy (MBCT; Segal, Williams, & Teasdale, 2002). A training course of eight sessions in mindfulness improved stress-correlated symptoms (Kearney, McDermott, Malte, Martinez, & Simpson, 2012; Shapiro, Oman, Thoresen, Plante, & Flinders, 2008), chronic distress (Schmidt et al., 2011), generalized anxiety (Evans et al., 2008), social phobia (Goldin & Gross, 2010), major depression (Chiesa & Serretti, 2011; Piet & Hougaard, 2011), eating disorders (Kristeller & Wolever, 2011; Wanden-Berghe, Sanz-Valero, & Wanden-Berghe, 2011), and substance abuse (Bowen, Chawla, & Marlatt, 2010; Zgierska et al., 2009). When such symptoms are associated with personality disorders, it could, therefore, be useful to include mindfulness interventions in treatment. However, patients suffering from personality disorders also present problems different from symptomatic disorders, such as difficulties in forming and maintaining a therapeutic alliance; interpersonal rumination; poor compliance with homework; a tendency to suffer from several comorbid symptoms, which renders the application of one single protocol problematic; and being overwhelmed by interpersonal problems in addition to the symptoms themselves. In this chapter we therefore propose how to adapt mindfulness interventions in order to make them applicable to personality disorders.

WHAT IS "MINDFULNESS"?

The term *mindfulness* is used in several ways. First, it is used to refer to a transitory and involuntary mental state involving high vigilance, average relaxedness, and attention directed at what is happening in the present, with a prevailing focus on sensory information and minimal cognitive processing. Second, it refers to mental exercises, derived from Buddhist tradition, designed to train a person to voluntarily achieve a state of noncritical observation of one's stream of consciousness at a given moment. Third, the term is also applied to a cognitive metaskill (Baer, 2003; Linehan, 1993) on which other skills, such as emotional and interpersonal regulation, are based. Mindfulness is a form of being in touch with one's mental states, in which one observes and describes one's inner experience without judging it and without attempting to modify or correct it. It is the ability to explore and comprehend one's ever-changing mental states. Research confirms that practicing mindfulness improves the ability to monitor one's mental states "online" and thus renders them more aware (Siegel, 2007, 2010).

MINDFULNESS SYMPTOM PROTOCOLS

The various mindfulness-based therapies consist of short manualized protocols, generally involving eight weekly sessions, with experiential and psychoeducational components that can be delivered in a group format (Fjorback, Arendt, Ornbøl, Fink, & Walach, 2011; Kabat-Zinn, 1990; Segal et al., 2002). However, the main therapeutic factor in mindfulness-based therapies is the experiential part, which consists of two components: meditation and group discussion/inquiry. Meditation is usually led by an instructor who assists participants in exploring their inner experience. The most common forms of meditation concentrate on (1) senses (especially hearing and cenesthesia); (2) breathing; (3) movement (walking meditation and mindful yoga); and (4) stream of consciousness. Inquiry consists of an investigation by the instructor aimed at shedding light on the most noteworthy elements experienced during meditation. Effective inquiry enables the participant to pinpoint the automatisms underlying his or her suffering and maximizes the therapeutic alliance and compliance by immediately tackling any difficulties the patient encountered during meditation.

PRACTICING MINDFULNESS AND PERSONALITY DISORDERS

Mindfulness is used in dialectical behavior therapy (DBT) to treat borderline personality disorder (BPD) and other disorders from the impulsive–dysregulated spectrum (Chapman, 2006; Linehan, 1993; Wupperman, Neumann, Whitman, & Axelrod, 2009). Given that mindfulness stimulates observation and description of inner experience without judgment, it provides the foundation for improving emotional and interpersonal self-regulation—which are both impaired in these patients—thereby reducing impulsiveness and the tendency to act out in self-harming and aggressive ways that are often used as dysfunctional emotion regulation strategies. Until now there has not been a mindfulness-based program explicitly designed for personality disorders other than BPD that feature dysregulation. In this chapter we try to bridge this gap, illustrating the major obstacles we encountered with these clients and how we adapted mindfulness protocol to work with these personality disorders.

INTERPERSONAL RUMINATION IN PERSONALITY DISORDERS

Just as do patients with pure symptom disorders, patients with personality disorders use maladaptive coping strategies to manage negative affects. Among these a central role is taken on by what we name *interpersonal rumination*, that is, a particular kind of thinking that is passive and nonresolutive and that has distressing relational contents as its subject. Some kind of repetitive negative thought can be found in many patients with symptom disorders, and therefore it seems to constitute a pathogenetic and transdiagnostic maintenance mechanism (Ehring & Watkins, 2008). The repeated negative thought involved is termed *rumination* (especially in mood disorders) or *worry* (especially in anxiety disorders). The difference between rumination and worry consists in the fact that with the former the negative thought is directed toward the past, whereas in worry the thought is directed toward anticipating negative consequences in the future. Here we shall always use the term *rumination* in a broader sense, defining it as a way of dysfunctional coping consisting in a form of repetitive negative thought, which can be directed toward the past, the future, and also the present and which takes on disorder-specific contents.

Rumination has been studied in mood disorders (Nolen-Hoeksema, 2000; Papageorgiou & Wells, 2009); anxiety disorders, such as generalized anxiety disorder (Borkovec, 1994; Borkovec, Alcaine, & Behar, 2004; Dugas et al., 1998); and obsessive–compulsive disorder (Wells & Papageorgiou, 1998) and eating disorders (Startup et al., 2013). Rumination takes on specific contents: Patients with major depression ruminate about the causes and significance of their negative mood ("Why do I feel so down? What's happening to me?"), those with generalized anxiety disorder about the negative consequences of uncertain situations ("And now what's going to happen? It will all go wrong. It will be a disaster"), and patients with obsessive–compulsive disorder about the possibilities of their having contaminated themselves or caused harm to others or themselves with their thoughts and actions ("I'm afraid I'm going to do something very bad and it disgusts me"). Patients with eating disorders dedicate much time to worrying and thinking about putting on weight, becoming fat, and so on. In eating disorders, rumination has a more markedly interpersonal connotation similar to personality disorders. Patients anticipate and fear a long chain of negative social consequences linked to the way in which their bodies appear to others' eyes. For example, they fear denigration by parents or peers.

In personality disorders, rumination mainly involves interpersonal relationships, with patients devoting their attention and memory to recalling, analyzing, or anticipating distressing relational situations in which they were offended, criticized, humiliated, neglected, misunderstood, or abandoned and in which they fear they have hurt or will hurt others, making them feel guilty. The patients recall memories of problematic relationships and focus on negative details. They also anticipate negative reactions from others. Patients with avoidant personality disorder spend much time trying to foresee others' potential responses to a certain behavior of theirs; they are constantly reviewing various potential interpersonal scenarios, in which, on each occasion and in each scene, they try to change their behavior and be more assertive, passive, or detached but then anticipate others' potential reactions (well disposed, indifferent, sarcastic, disdainful, or ridiculing). This mental exercise keeps them busy sometimes for hours on end, during which their feelings of social anxiety increase, leaving them paralyzed with regard to choices and making them avoid social contact.

At other times ruminative thought is of the counterfactual type, that is, it attempts to modify the consequences of an event already occurred by manipulating its antecedents: "Uh, why didn't I do . . . ?" "Why didn't I tell him . . . ?" "How would things have gone if only I'd . . . ?". This kind of thinking easily becomes an endless and inconclusive repetition of alternative scenarios and leads to unfavorable outcomes, such as the blocking of actions or amplifying of emotions such as shame, blame, regret, and guilt.

Interpersonal rumination can be broken down into three dimensions. First, it can be directed toward the present—a biased search for proof to confirm that there is an environmental risk, similar to threat monitoring in anxiety disorders (Wells, 2008). This is very frequent in patients with paranoid and avoidant disorders and leads them to be hypervigilant and to process every interpersonal signal in order to not neglect any indications of danger or threats. Second, rumination can be directed toward the past, a retrospective search for proof and reevaluation of others' behavior with counterfactual thought. Third, it can be directed toward the future, concentrating on anticipating the feared outcomes of an interaction, as with anxious worry, or on the interpersonal strategies to be adopted to forestall a problem or tackle it.

In paranoid personality disorder, in particular, patients worry when they think back over occasions on which they were provoked, threatened, humiliated, dominated, or cheated. Patients with narcissistic personality disorder ruminate when they think about situations in which some of their needs were not recognized, they did not feel gratified, or they sensed a challenge or an offense. Patients with avoidant personality disorder worry about situations in which they felt excluded, judged negatively, criticized, derided, or humiliated. Patients with dependent personality disorder ruminate about situations in which there is a potential or real loss of relationships. Finally, those with obsessive–compulsive personality disorder worry about actions of theirs that could have harmed others or could trigger negative consequences or else about the pros and cons of a decision by going over the horns of the dilemma hundreds of times.

ADAPTING MINDFULNESS TO PERSONALITY DISORDERS: RATIONALE

In our clinical practice, we evaluated whether it was possible to apply the mindfulness protocols developed to treat symptom disorders to personality disorders, especially disorders involving overmodulation and inhibition of emotional expression, such as avoidant, narcissistic, paranoid, dependent, and obsessive–compulsive disorders. Our experience suggested the need to modify the standard mindfulness protocols for several reasons.

Limited Awareness and Difficulty Describing the Nuances of Experience

First, patients have difficulty identifying and describing the nuances of their mental states (Dimaggio et al., 2007; Dimaggio & Lysaker, 2010), which makes it difficult to perceive qualitative differences in their mental states (e.g. irritation, frustration, anxiety) during meditation. Such difficulties can be frustrating, leading to decreased motivation and early dropout. Also, when patients are unaware of the antecedents of relational problems, it is difficult to treat the related symptoms. Hence, meditation has to be adapted to allow patients to become more aware of the emotions experienced during interpersonal encounters and the link between these emotions and dysfunctional beliefs about oneself and others (e.g., "I can't seem weak; otherwise they'll take advantage of me").

Rigid Constructions and Lack of Cognitive Decentering and Flexibility

Second, even when patients are aware of thoughts and feelings about interpersonal encounters, they treat these thoughts as fixed rather than as points of view that could change if events were observed from different viewpoints. This rigidity can make mindfulness challenging because mindfulness treats mental states as constructions, not as mirror images of reality. For example, an instructor's suggestion to consider mental states as simple products of the mind may be threatening to a patient with paranoia because relinquishing thoughts of being threatened can cause unbearable anxiety in that lowering one's guard is assumed to expose one to great risks from an ill-intentioned world. These points are illustrated by the following vignette:

> When Giulio, a therapy-naive patient with avoidant and obsessive–compulsive personality disorders started in an MBCT group, he was strongly motivated and had the goal of tackling the depression he had been living with for several months. However, when he experienced difficulties with meditation, he quickly became afraid of being judged negatively by the therapists because he was unable to keep up with the rest of the group. During inquiry, he feared he would show weaknesses that would expose him to criticism. He started to avoid sharing his experiences with the group or produced fictitious and problem-free reports. During the meditations, he felt isolated and a failure and criticized himself for being inferior to the other participants. After the fourth session, he left the group.

We adopted two strategies to deal with these problems: (1) mindfulness was used only when patients had developed an understanding of their dysfunctional interpersonal schemas and how it is often their construction of events, not the events themselves, that cause problems; and (2) specific meditation sessions were dedicated to interpersonal schemas. Here, patients are guided to explore painful interpersonal memories, varying their scene's observation point so as to learn to assume a decentered position.

The best time for a patient with personality disorder to benefit from mindfulness training is likely when he or she is capable of understanding his or her mental states, of giving them a name and linking them to the specific situations generating them, and aware that his or her suffering originates from his or her own ideas about him- or herself and others. At this point mindfulness is useful in dealing with dysfunctional coping strategies such as rumination, worry, threat monitoring, and avoidance in interpersonal situations.

Tendency to Externalize Responsibility

There are other problems associated with personality disorder that create difficulties using standard mindfulness interventions. One is the tendency, seen especially in patients with narcissistic, paranoid, or passive–aggressive features, to show conflicted relationships with authority that may lead to antagonism toward instructors, which undermines participation in the program and compliance with home exercises. Patients often feel anger, impotence, incapacity, defiance, frustration, and so on toward the therapist or therapy when prescribed homework, which increases the dropout risk. Patients with personality disorder also often ascribe their suffering to the external world and can thus see an approach centered exclusively on exploring their inner world to be ineffective or capricious. In other cases, they think that they themselves are the cause of their problems and self-ascribe faults that they consider facts and unchangeable; as a result, they have difficulty believing that a program based on a modification of their mental states can be of any use.

Impaired Sense of Agency

Linked to this problem are more pervasive problems with a sense of agency. These patients have difficulty seeing themselves as the authors of their own experiences and actions, which makes mediation difficult because they may initially see meditation and the idea of modifying the course of their thoughts as not within their reach. Usually during therapy the sense of agency improves. Nevertheless, we consider it important to foresee a work plan that proceeds more gradually compared with standard mindfulness protocols, with shorter meditation sessions and greater attention to inquiry, so as to help patients sense their ability to control their own mental states and make use of some simple exercises that we describe later.

SPECIFIC TECHNIQUES FOR ADAPTING MINDFULNESS TO PERSONALITY DISORDERS

Based on the problems that patients with personality disorder typically experience using mindfulness exercises, we made the following adaptations to the MBCT protocol.

Briefer Meditations and More Time Dedicated during Sessions to the Inquiry Process

To make up for patients' gaps in identifying mental contents and sense of agency, it is essential to use briefer meditations (around 15–20 minutes maximum) in the first five sessions and to spend more time on careful inquiries accompanied by accurate explanations of mental functioning.

Commutation Exercises

A technical expedient for tackling a deficit in sense of agency is commutation exercises aimed at making patients more aware of their ability to shift voluntarily between two modes of cognitive processing—what some authors (Segal et al., 2002) call the "doing mode" and the "being mode" and others (Wells, 2008) the "object mode" and the "metacognitive mode." The "doing/object" mode refers to an ordinary state of mind in which mental events are experienced as perceptual events in an undifferentiated manner; for instance, when we are concentrating on solving a problem or when we are absorbed in fantasies or reasoning. The "being/metacognitive" mode is related to a state in which our minds consider thoughts and emotions as inner events and identify and differentiate them from reality; for example, when we are aware of what is passing through our minds in a given moment, when we are present and careful about what is happening within ourselves and in the external world. These exercises last just a few seconds, or at most 1 minute, and are focused exclusively on simple experiences such as seeing or hearing. For example, patients can be asked to voluntarily let go of every thought they have at that moment and, for a few seconds, focus on a single part of their bodies, without actually meditating. Learning to shift between the two modes allows patients to grasp more deeply the representational nature of their thoughts and thus to assume a more decentered position toward their mental activity. Consequently, this promotes the abandonment of dysfunctional coping mechanisms based on interpersonal rumination, worry, and threat monitoring.

The brevity of the exercise often helps participants to appreciate the different properties of their current mental states and to discover differences between their usual streams of thought and the mindful state. Once they have recognized the difference, they can train themselves to switch from one mode to another. These simple exercises increase self-monitoring and a sense of agency that makes it easier to engage in more complex formal meditation.

Homework: More Emphasis on Practicing Informal Rather Than Formal Meditation

As we mentioned earlier, a goal in using mindfulness with personality disorders is to manage negative emotions directed at therapists (as holders of authority) and certain therapy aspects (e.g., prescribing homework). Consequently, it is important to establish a strong therapeutic alliance and adopt a flexible approach to homework. The instructor may find it more productive to suggest short and easy exercises as homework that emphasize the value of observing and carefully recording any difficulties experienced in meditating ("When you are at home, sit on a chair and observe your aversion to practicing/your difficulty in interrupting what you are doing for just 1 minute").

Use of the Rumination Questionnaire

The use of a structured questionnaire as part of standard mindfulness protocols is not aimed at an assessment; its purpose is rather to make patients aware of and to educate them about mental processes and contents that cause subjective suffering. With personality disorders, it is important to make patients aware of interpersonal rumination and its typical contents. For this reason, in the mindfulness training for personality disorders that we are describing, we created a 10-item self-report questionnaire that we called Scale of Interpersonal Worries. This scale addresses six components of interpersonal rumination: rumination, worry, threat monitoring, gap filling, counterfactual thinking, and wishful thinking. In session 4, patients are asked to fill in the scale and discuss their responses within the group. This aims at illustrating and clarifying the different ways in which dysfunctional thinking may increase the patients' suffering instead of solving it.

More Emphasis on Interpersonal Aspects of Emotional Distress

Given that relational topics predominate in the ruminations of individuals with personality disorders, such patients need to be helped to see that the problems to which they dedicate time and mental energy by ruminating are for the most part the result of their schema-dependent readings of interpersonal relationships. This should be done first of all in individual psychotherapy (see Dimaggio et al., 2015). However, adapted mindfulness can offer a preferential field of observation by promoting a detailed exploration of distressing memories of an interpersonal nature. This is carried out via specific forms of meditation in which patients are assisted in recalling a specific distressing interpersonal situation and pinpointing their emotions, thoughts, and sensations of self and other at that time. Later on there will be a detailed description of the structure of meditations about the interpersonal schema, one of the most significant innovations in our model vis-à-vis ST–mindfulness.

ADAPTED MINDFULNESS FOR PERSONALITY DISORDER: CHARACTERISTICS AND STRUCTURE OF TRAINING

The protocol of what we will call metacognitive interpersonal mindfulness-based training (MIMBT) for personality disorders consists of nine weekly sessions developed for use in the context of metacognitive interpersonal therapy for personality disorders (Dimaggio et al., 2007, 2012, 2015), although it can be used either independently or as part of another form of integrated treatment. Groups are made up of 5–10 participants who have already carried out or are currently carrying out individual psychotherapy. There is homework in the form of self-observation and formal and informal meditation tasks. Formal meditation at home is done under the guidance of the voice of one of the instructors, recorded on a compact disc. The nine sessions are structured so that participants can proceed gradually at their own pace to learn the required skills. These include learning to identify precisely one's mental states, being aware of one's momentary mental functioning, learning to shift attention from emotionally arousing images (avoiding every form of mental control), understanding others separately from one's own point of view, and increasing the ability to access self-soothing feelings.

The program's structure is summarized in Table 13.1. The first session provides an introduction to the program and the therapists and participants. An explanation is offered of the pathogenic mechanisms that will be dealt with—especially interpersonal rumination and other mental control mechanisms—and a few rapid commutation exercises are used to introduce the difference between a mind that thinks, controls, and evaluates and a mind that is aware as it observes its continuously changing inner landscape. Questions and concerns are dealt with, and the instructors explain what mindfulness *is* and what it is *not* (relaxation, control or suppression of thoughts, solving of existential problems, surrogate psychotherapy, etc.).

Sessions 2–4 introduce guided meditations that stimulate an attentional focus on the body (Kerr, Sacchet, Lazar, Moore, & Jones, 2013) (see Table 13.1).

Using specific guided meditations, in sessions 5 and 6 patients become more familiar with both pleasant and unpleasant mental contents (thoughts and emotions). In particular, they are led in session 5 to evoke positive thoughts and identify the effects on their mood and affective sphere and in session 6 to evoke negative thoughts and related states of mind. For example, patients are asked to recall a currently distressing issue and to try not to react or avoid it but rather to be aware of the effects on their bodies and affectivity.

In sessions 7–9, meditation is focused more on the interpersonal aspects of emotional experience. Patients are asked to explore a memory of an unpleasant interpersonal event and are helped to (1) identify the expectations and desires associated with the event ("What were you expecting?", "What would

TABLE 13.1. The Structure of Metacognitive Interpersonal Mindfulness-Based Training

Sessions	Focus	Contents
1	Introduction	Presentation of course topics; rapid commutation exercises.
2–4	Body	Body scanning; meditation about breathing; meditation about sounds; walking meditation; mindful yoga.
5–6	Thoughts/emotions	Meditation about thought flow, negative thoughts, and positive and negative emotions.
7–9	Interpersonal schemas	Meditation about distressing interpersonal experiences; meditation about decentering; accepting, compassion, and being well-disposed.

you have liked the other to do/say?"); (2) describe sensations/thoughts/emotions occurring there and then and here and now; and (3) try to adopt points of view different from their own. The instructors then try to help patients to become more compassionate toward themselves and others by stimulating the adoption of a more decentered and sympathetic position and explicitly thinking more benevolent ideas about oneself. To this end, the concluding part of the meditation is devoted to voluntarily eliciting thoughts involving accepting the self even in its least noble or desirable parts. The same thing is carried out in regard to accepting the other, but only after clarifying with patients that accepting does not signify passively submitting to or agreeing to what others do. Accepting means thoroughly understanding the existential conditions causing others' actions, including the contribution we ourselves give to their reactions.

Meditation about Distressing Interpersonal Experiences

In the initial interviews with patients before they are admitted to MIMBT, we evaluate the awareness acquired, during their personal therapies, of their own dysfunctional schemas.[1] Then the therapist summarizes a patient's situation by pointing out that the interpersonal schema → behavior in particular situations → rumination → suffering sequence and suggests mindfulness training with a view to the patient standing back more from his or her schemas and freeing him- or herself from the wearying and pointless ruminations that often dominate his or her mind. The patient thus has a clear idea, from the start, about what is going to be worked on and why and how this awareness constitutes a starting point for interpersonal meditation, which involves immersing oneself in relational situations that activate dysfunctional schemas. These forms of interpersonal meditation are the most original part of MIMBT.

Next we describe briefly one of these meditations—one that concerns distressing interpersonal experiences. Like all meditations, the exercise begins with the usual anchoring to the body and the senses: placing one's attention on posture, a rapid check of one's physical state, and concentrating on breathing. After letting their minds calm down and concentrate, participants are taken through the exploration of a distressing interpersonal situation experienced more or less recently and are asked to dwell on a single scene, to explore it in

[1] A favorable indicator for admission to a group could be a statement such as the following: "I know I'm living with a constant sense of being threatened, and this has been the case since I was a child. I'm so frightened about people overwhelming or dominating me that I tend to feel this anticipatory mistrust toward everyone. I know it's not always the case, that not everyone wants to take advantage of me, but every time that I'm with people I don't know or don't know very well, this tendency to be on the defensive gets triggered and so right from the start I start to see them as a potential danger." This statement contains evident references to dysfunctional schemas, and it is also possible to appreciate the patient's ability to grasp the basic aspects of his or her inner experience.

as detailed a manner as possible, and to focus on their emotional and mental states at that moment ("Let's recall how we felt, what thoughts crossed our minds, what physiological reactions we experienced, what we would have liked to do instinctively"). After this they are asked to switch their attention to the emotional and mental states of the other person in the scene, so as to favor the understanding of the other's perspective ("Now let's imagine how the other person might have felt, what could have passed through his mind, what he would have liked to do/say . . . "). Following this the patient is asked to go back to the initial "frame" and visualize it exactly as it is, as if it were an image from which one can stand back and which one can let go of. The goal is to train patients' ability to interrupt their ruminative thoughts and let go of the mental representations they have explored up to that moment and, at the same time, use their bodies and breathing like anchors, asking them to switch their attention to these in the here and now of meditation. The guided meditation ends by promoting a nonjudgmental, noncritical attitude of self-compassion and connectedness with the present moment ("Now that we've gone back into our body, in the here and now of real experience, let's try directing a loving and compassionate thought toward ourselves, even if we've been hurt or have hurt, been wrong, been weak, and so forth. Let's try to feel the others' presence in the room, all of them coming to grips with the task of taking care of the self and giving back to the self its sense of its value"). The steps for meditation on distressing interpersonal experiences are summarized in Table 13.2.

CASE EXAMPLE

Thirty-four-year-old Anna worked as a researcher. She sought therapy for social phobia and feared being judged inadequate and incapable of getting on with her work and expressing her ideas correctly. She imagined that she would

TABLE 13.2. Steps for Meditation on Distressing Interpersonal Experience

1. Focusing on the body (posture, breathing).
2. Recalling a distressing interpersonal situation; focusing on the scene; choice of "frame."
3. Focusing on the self: physiological response, emotions, thoughts; action tendencies; self's desires.
4. Focusing on the other: physiological response, emotions, thoughts (other's); other's desires (interpersonal schema).
5. Return to the initial frame; visualization of the scene and identification (sensations, emotions, and thoughts) at the present moment.
6. Imaginative detachment ("Let go of . . . ").
7. Return to the body (breathing).
8. Self-compassion and widespread awareness.

always be rejected, excluded, and alone. When in front of an audience, Anna sweated a lot, blushed, and felt dizzy. This made her anxious that she was about to fail. When thinking back over her past failures and especially looking ahead to those to come, she tended to ruminate. She adopted an avoidant coping strategy: She would postpone delivering articles and other publications, was standoffish with her colleagues, and stopped going out with her friends. She had been criticized at work for this, and she had few friends left. This reinforced her idea that she was a failure.

Anna suffered from obsessive–compulsive personality disorder. She was a perfectionist to the point of not completing jobs. She showed an excessive dedication to her work and to her productivity and was excessively conscientious and inflexible regarding morality, reluctant to work with others, and very rigid. She also had dependent and avoidant features. To make a decision, she needed excessive reassurance; she found it difficult to express disagreement and was reluctant to start work projects on her own; she was inhibited in her intimate relationships; and she saw herself as inept and inferior.

Her cognitive style tended toward intellectualizing, and she disregarded her emotions. Anna had difficulty recognizing her bodily feelings and labeling them in terms of emotions. She felt lacking in emotions and considered that that was a flaw she had. She aimed at a vague idea of well-being in which she would feel only positive emotions, which, however, she could not define.

Anna also had difficulty in grasping which thoughts triggered emotions and in understanding that her behavior was driven by emotions; for example, she could not grasp that avoidance was activated by shame at the idea of being judged negatively. She considered her ideas about her inadequacy to be irrefutable facts and lacked critical detachment.

Anna's Psychotherapy in Advance of the Mindfulness Group

Anna had been receiving metacognitive interpersonal therapy (MIT; Dimaggio et al., 2007, 2012, 2015; Dimaggio & Lysaker, 2010). During the first few months the focus was on translating somatic sensations into emotions, except for the sense of guilt that she had already recognized previously and that caused her to suffer. This focus made it possible for her to identify her anxiety as being linked to the fear of being wrong and being criticized. Her therapist then helped Anna to understand that her nonverbal signals—blushing, lowered glance, and unsteady voice—indicated shame. However, discovering that she felt inferior and ashamed activated some self-critical thoughts: "I shouldn't feel ashamed or inferior"; "I'm not capable of feeling better, of overcoming this sense of inferiority." Anna also saw that shortly after feeling ashamed and inferior, she entered reactive states in which her positive self-image resurfaced—"All things considered, I'm not really so horrible"—and she became angry because others did not acknowledge her qualities. The idea that others set high standards for her made her feel trampled on. Improved affect awareness made a longing for a partner who would nurture her, be warm, and take care of her emerge. She started to want to be free of her perfectionist standards and be accepted, even if imperfect. However, she was not succeeding.

Reformulation of the Schema

Once Anna became more able to describe her inner states, her therapist worked with her to reformulate her suffering in terms of pathogenic interpersonal schemas with the following structure (see Luborsky & Crits-Christoph, 1998): "Anna wished to feel recognized but imagined the other would criticize and reject her. Her reaction to this was to feel failure, frustration, sadness, and a sense of uselessness. She then tended to cope with such feelings by raising her standards or avoiding contacts." Thanks to the retracing of some memories from her development, Anna grasped that these ideas had a historical origin: When she used to display a wish to enjoy herself, relax, or devote her time to, for example, activities she found pleasurable, such as cooking or drawing, her mother reacted by underrating these activities and telling her to not waste time on nonsense rather than devoting herself to more "serious" things. At which point Anna started to doubt whether she really wanted what had, until a few seconds before, been important to her, and she progressively lost the ability to perceive what it was that she liked. At the same time, her mother gave her approval for her school performance and her intellectual side. Anna recalled that her father was detached and distracted, but he too was focused on her performance and on the idea that his daughter could still do better than she was achieving.

At this point the therapy goal became to achieve a critical distance from the schema, that is, understanding that, when she was gripped by these thoughts and emotions, she was not evaluating interpersonal relationships realistically but was driven by a rigid and stereotyped construction of events and was unable to see alternatives. To do this, her therapist proposed that Anna expose herself to critical judgments and that they jointly reevaluate events so as to see whether there were any interpretations as alternatives to the schema. Anna accepted this and started to find that she did not always commit mistakes in work tasks and that, if she did make a mistake, she was not despised or boycotted because of it. She noticed that her friends displayed affection and warmth toward her when she was in difficulty and that, if they seemed detached, it was a result of the coldness that she herself displayed. Thanks to this progress, her anxiety and ruminating began to decrease, and her avoidance diminished.

Nevertheless, her capacity to achieve a critical distance from her schemas was inconstant. Whereas in session or in relatively insignificant relationships, such as those with colleagues she saw sporadically or not very intimate friends, she managed to maintain or regain the critical distance from schemas with her more intimate friends, her superiors, or colleagues to whom she was more attached, the schemas returned, still in a rigid manner, and activated ruminations. Her social phobia remained intermittent. At this point the therapist proposed that Anna join a mindfulness group for personality disorder, with a view to strengthening her ability to distinguish between her schemas and reality, to interrupt her ruminating, to manage the emotions of guilt and shame in a more functional manner, to further reduce her anxiety, and to interpret others' intentions in a more realistic and multifaceted way.

Group Work

First Stage: Sessions 1–3

Anna gained awareness of how little she knew her body. During the body scan and mindful yoga she could not feel anything, and she criticized herself. During a group discussion, another patient pointed out to her that she was feeling inadequate and at fault because she was imposing the feeling of only positive sensations on herself. The instructors reminded her that the goal was to explore any state whatever, including a lack of sensations, uncritically. Anna stopped looking exclusively for positive emotions (which she did not, in any case, have), focused instead on tension, tachycardia, sweating, and a feeling of weight on her chest, and with curiosity tried to understand what they indicated.

Second Stage: Sessions 4–5

At this stage Anna realized that she had high expectations about her performance at mindfulness, and this helped her to grasp how much perfectionism dominated her mind.

Furthermore, when Anna realized that her mind produced a spontaneous thought flow, she tried taking certain negative thoughts less seriously and managed to arrive at considering them merely products of the mind and not facts. More precisely, she managed to see that during meditation even thoughts that she normally found very distressing and treated as true—such as "The others will think I'm not up to it," "I'll lose everything I've achieved," "I'll end up on my own with everyone pitying me"—were not a mirror image of reality but mental entities entering the field of consciousness, remaining there for a certain time, and then possibly leaving it to make room for other thoughts following the same cycle.

Anna also noticed that the more she tried to remain relaxed, the more her anxiety, linked to the thought "I must be up to it. I must show that I know, too, that I'm capable of it, too," increased ("Every time I try to maintain a positive thought or an emotion involving calmness, they immediately vanish"). She saw how pointless it was to avoid these thoughts: "I've tried to take these thoughts and put them away in a drawer but every time the drawer reopened and they flew out stronger than ever." Thanks to this realization, Anna was able to discover that her anxiety was being maintained by her failed attempts to crush negative thoughts and not by the fact that there were real reasons for worrying (Wells, 2008).

Third Stage: Sessions 5–8

At the end of the second stage, we were faced with a difficulty in helping Anna to detach herself from her schemas, which continued to be rigid in more intimate and significant situations. She interpreted her successes in therapy in the light of these perfectionist schemas: "Given that meditation comes easy to me, it means I'm not doing enough and ought to make more effort. There's sure to be something I haven't grasped and that's why it comes easy to me"; "I need to say something more interesting during group discussions; otherwise the others in the group will think I haven't understood anything."

Thoughts of this type, like the emotions of anxiety, shame, and guilt associated with them, appeared particularly resistant. To help the patient to overcome this obstacle, meditation on the schema turned out to be crucial. Thanks to it, in fact, Anna saw her schema from an observer position, and this gave her the possibility of achieving the awareness that "the idea that, if I don't say anything interesting, the others will consider me stupid and I'll feel useless is just my schema."

Through meditation on the schema, Anna looked back at a memory from a holiday with friends. During a moment of relaxation, a friend had talked about an event from American history. Anna realized how inadequate she had felt compared with her learned and superior friend and how this was the driving force behind her search for interesting subjects in order not to be judged "stupid" and sidelined.

This time Anna's comment was: "Finally I've managed to see that in reality what I was thinking and feeling was not real. As if I was looking at my mind from outside, I saw that it was just my schema, and so I was able to let go of it and go back to concentrating on breathing [recall that mindfulness meditation hinges on concentrating on breathing]."

At another moment in her meditation on the schema, Anna was asked to observe it "in the same way as we could observe water running when we're on a river bank," or "as we might observe what happens on the street when looking out of a window." At that moment Anna imagined an old house with an inner courtyard where she, "standing on the balcony," observed the coming and going of the shopkeepers who came to offer her their goods, with her being able to choose whether to accept them or not. The goods brought by the shopkeepers represented the parts of the schema that became activated in Anna, and at that moment she felt that the meditation was offering her the opportunity to choose whether to use a schema or behave freely.

Through the short commutation exercises included in her homework, Anna was able to train herself to maintain an awareness of the schema and to choose without complying with it. During a dinner with a girlfriend who was talking about her travels, Anna imagined that she was considered inferior by the friend. She told herself that what she was feeling and thinking was nothing other than the activation of her schema. She therefore chose to "not buy those goods from the shopkeeper" and thus to listen to her own emotional experience at that moment and then communicate it to her friend.

In the subsequent meditations on the schema, in which she was asked to imagine what the other person might think and feel in that situation, the idea that the other's mind did not necessarily contain what she believed began to take shape in the patient's mind. Remembering again the holiday episode during which a friend talked to her about American history, she said, "I had never stopped to think about it, but, if I'd been in his shoes, I can really say that he could have been engaged with what he was saying and he had pleasure being with me, instead of just thinking I didn't know anything about it."

Anna also imagined that the friend esteemed her, and she felt joy, richness, and personal worth. In her subsequent meditations, thanks not least to the group discussions in which she felt strengthened, she tried to familiarize herself with these positive experiences, which this time were not fantasies but real, and she managed to keep them going.

Her contact with this state of mind also was reinforced during a moment dedicated to the practice of compassion. During the practice, while she was again observing her proneness to criticize herself when she felt anxiety or shame or had negative thoughts, Anna started to make room for an attitude of compassion toward and acceptance of her emotions, the functioning of her mind, and her thoughts. At that moment she succeeded in slackening her self-criticism and started to be aware of a self-benevolent and well-disposed attitude. Following this, and not least thanks to practice at home, Anna felt that her guilt feelings "about not doing or not doing enough" were becoming lessened.

Lastly, the commutation exercises, employed at the stage at which Anna was gaining awareness of how her schema was activated, helped her to block the rumination process when it was triggered.

Once she had finished the mindfulness sessions, Anna felt less social anxiety in all her relationships, her guilt feelings had almost disappeared, and her ruminating became activated only sporadically, and she blocked it as soon as it arose. Her sense of personal dignity was intermittent, but, thanks to having experienced it, Anna succeeded in regaining it, sometimes without any particular effort and sometimes with more of an effort. A few months later, during individual therapy, she pointed out that her network of friends was much richer and her relations with her colleagues more relaxed. She started to have a romantic relationship.

CONCLUDING COMMENTS

The practice of mindfulness represents a wonderful support when tackling suffering, both of the day-to-day and the pathological kinds. In personality disorders the pathology mainly derives from learned interpersonal schemas that anticipate and react to unpleasant events and from mental habits (such as rumination) that produce further suffering. In personality disorders, particular dysfunctional interpersonal schemas and interpersonal rumination play a crucial role in generating, feeding, and maintaining suffering.

In adapting mindfulness programs to patients with personality disorder, we have tried to propose a short, economical, and potentially effective intervention. The aim is to supply patients with tools for more effectively freeing themselves from thoughts linked to interpersonal relationships that worry them. The core skills for a functional handling of emotional states are the same as in every other mindfulness program: voluntarily regulating attention and acquiring "online" awareness of the mental mechanisms that are the source of suffering and of the underlying schemas. Lastly, patients learn to accept and let go of distressing experiences and to make room for feelings of compassion, tolerance, and kindness toward themselves and others.

Unlike standard mindfulness, the program described here adopts several devices with the aim of maximizing the therapeutic alliance and the effectiveness with this particular clinical population. A summary follows:

1. Patients with personality disorders need to have undergone or be undergoing individual psychotherapy for a period of time sufficient to let them master the minimum skills needed for the training. In this way, at the time that they set about starting the training, the patients have already developed the basic cognitive skills (ability to recognize that in one's mind there are thoughts and emotions linked to specific autobiographical episodes; self-agency). These skills are needed to avoid meditation being seen as an unbearably frustrating experience.
2. Various stratagems are used to facilitate adhesion to the program: shorter meditations, room for inquiry, rapid commutation exercises, and emphasis on the practice of mindfulness in informal, noncoded daily life situations.
3. A psychoeducative module concentrating on the dimensions critical for patients with personality disorders is foreseen, including interpersonal rumination, pathogenic interpersonal schemas, and dysfunctional interpersonal cycles.
4. Specific meditation concentrating on the recalling of distressing interpersonal memories and the exploration of problematic mental states is adopted.
5. Patients are encouraged to stop any rumination that concentrates on being offended or on self-blame and to replace this with thoughts involving self-acceptance and self-compassion.

In the future we are going to need to prepare rigorous research designs to evaluate the results of this approach and whether it is more effective and tolerable than standard mindfulness programs and to analyze whether, other than its effect on the target symptoms, the program is also able to contribute to change in the self-pathology underlying the personality disorder—for example, by helping patients to question their schema-based interpretations and adopt a different attitude toward others, which would then improve their social lives.

REFERENCES

Alnæs, R., & Torgersen, S. (1988). The relationship between DSM-III symptom disorders (Axis I) and personality disorders (Axis II) in an outpatient population. *Acta Psychiatrica Scandinavica, 78*, 485–492.

Baer, R. A. (2003). Mindfulness training as a clinical intervention: A conceptual and empirical review. *Clinical Psychology: Science and Practice, 10,* 125–143.

Borkovec, T. D. (1994). The nature, functions, and origins of worry. In G. Davey & F. Tallis (Eds.), *Worrying: Perspectives on theory assessment and treatment* (pp. 5–33). Sussex, UK: Wiley.

Borkovec, T. D., Alcaine, O. M., & Behar, E. (2004). Avoidance theory of worry and generalized anxiety disorder. In R. G. Heimberg, C. L. Turk, & D. S. Mennin (Eds.), *Generalized anxiety disorder: Advances in research and practice* (pp. 77–108). New York: Guilford Press

Bowen, S., Chawla, N., & Marlatt, G. A. (2010). *Mindfulness-based relapse prevention for addictive behaviors: A clinician's guide.* New York: Guilford Press

Chapman, A. (2006). Dialectical behavior therapy: Current indications and unique elements. *Psychiatry, 3*(9), 62–68.

Chiesa, A., & Serretti, A. (2011). Mindfulness-based cognitive therapy for psychiatric disorders: A systematic review and meta-analysis. *Psychiatry Research, 187*(3), 441–453.

Dimaggio, G., & Lysaker, P. H. (2010). *Metacognition and severe adult mental disorders: From basic research to treatment.* London: Routledge.

Dimaggio, G., Montano, A., Popolo, R., & Salvatore, G. (2015). *Metacognitive interpersonal therapy for personality disorders: A treatment manual.* Hove, UK: Routledge.

Dimaggio, G., Salvatore, G., Fiore, D., Carcione, A., Nicolò, G., & Semerari, A. (2012). General principles for treating the overconstricted personality disorder: Toward operationalizing technique. *Journal of Personality Disorders, 26*, 63–83.

Dimaggio, G., Semerari, A., Carcione, A., Nicolò, G., & Procacci, M. (2007). *Psychotherapy of personality disorders: Metacognition, states of mind and interpersonal cycles.* London: Routledge.

Dugas, M. J., Freeston, M. H., Ladouceur, R., Rhéaume, J., Provencher, M. D., & Boisvert, J.-M. (1998). Worry themes in primary GAD, secondary GAD and other anxiety disorders. *Journal of Anxiety Disorders, 12*, 253–261.

Ehring, T., & Watkins, E. R. (2008). Repetitive negative thinking as a transdiagnostic process. *International Journal of Cognitive Therapy, 1*(3), 192–205.

Evans, S., Ferrando, S., Findler, M., Stowell, C., Smart, C., & Haglin, D. (2008). Mindfulness-based cognitive therapy for generalized anxiety disorder. *Journal of Anxiety Disorder, 22*(4), 716–721.

Fjorback, L. O., Arendt, M., Ornbøl, E., Fink, P., & Walach, H. (2011). Mindfulness-based stress reduction and mindfulness-based cognitive therapy: A systematic review of randomized controlled trials. *Acta Psychiatrica Scandinavica, 124*(2), 102–119.

Goldin, P., & Gross, J. (2010). Effects of mindfulness-based stress reduction (MBSR) on emotion regulation in social anxiety disorder. *Emotion, 10*(1), 83–91.

Kabat-Zinn, J. (1982). An outpatient program in behavioral medicine for chronic pain patients based on the practice of mindfulness meditation: Theoretical considerations and preliminary results. *General Hospital Psychiatry, 4,* 33–47.

Kabat-Zinn, J. (1990). *Full catastrophe living: Using the wisdom of your mind and body to face stress, pain, and illness.* New York: Delacorte.

Kearney, D. J., McDermott, K., Malte, C., Martinez, M., & Simpson, T. L. (2012). Association of participation in a mindfulness program with measures of PTSD, depression and quality of life in a veteran sample. *Journal of Clinical Psychology, 68*(1), 101–116.

Kerr, C. E., Sacchet, M. D., Lazar, S. W., Moore, C. I., & Jones, S. R. (2013). Mindfulness starts with the body: Somatosensory attention and top-down modulation of cortical alpha rhythms in mindfulness meditation. *Frontiers in Human Neuroscience, 7,* 12.

Kristeller, J. L., & Wolever, R. Q. (2011). Mindfulness-based eating awareness training for treating binge eating disorder: The conceptual foundation. *Eating Disorders, 19*(1), 49–61.

Linehan, M. M. (1993). *Cognitive-behavioral treatment of borderline personality disorder.* New York: Guilford Press.

Luborsky, L., & Crits-Christoph, P. (1998). *Understanding transference.* Washington, DC: American Psychological Association

Nolen-Hoeksema, S. (2000). The role of rumination in depressive disorders and mixed anxiety/depressive symptoms. *Journal of Abnormal Psychology, 109*(3), 504–511.

Papageorgiou, C., & Wells, A. (2009). A prospective test of the clinical metacognitive model of rumination and depression. *International Journal of Cognitive Therapy, 2*(2), 123–131.

Piet, J., & Hougaard, E. (2011). The effect of mindfulness-based cognitive therapy for prevention of relapse in recurrent major depressive disorder: A systematic review and meta-analysis. *Clinical Psychology Review, 31*(6), 1032–1040.

Schmidt, S., Grossman, P., Schwarzer, B., Jena, S., Naumann, J., & Walach, H. (2011). Treating fibromyalgia with mindfulness-based stress reduction: Results from a 3-armed randomized controlled trial. *Pain, 152,* 361–369.

Segal, Z. V., Williams, J. M. G., & Teasdale, J. D. (2002). *Mindfulness-based cognitive therapy for depression: A new approach to preventing relapse.* New York: Guilford Press.

Shapiro, S. L., Oman, D., Thoresen, C. E., Plante, T. G., & Flinders, T. (2008). Cultivating mindfulness: Effects on well-being. *Journal of Clinical Psychology, 64*(7), 840–862.

Siegel, D. (2007). *The mindful brain: Reflection and attunement in the cultivation of well-being.* New York: Norton.

Siegel, D. (2010). *Mindsight: The new science of personal transformation.* New York: Bantam Books.

Startup, H., Lavender, A., Oldershaw, A., Stott, R., Tchanturia, K., Treasure, J., et al.

(2013). Worry and rumination in anorexia nervosa. *Behavioural and Cognitive Psychotherapy*, *41*(3), 301–316.

Wanden-Berghe, R. G., Sanz-Valero, J., & Wanden-Berghe, C. (2011). The application of mindfulness to eating disorders treatment: A systematic review. *Eating Disorders*, *19*(1), 34–48.

Wells, A. (2008). *Metacognitive therapy for anxiety and depression*. New York: Guilford Press.

Wells, A., & Papageorgiou, C. (1998). Relationships between worry, obsessive-compulsive symptoms and meta-cognitive beliefs. *Behaviour Research and Therapy*, *36*(9), 899–913.

Wupperman, P., Neumann, C. S., Whitman, J. B., & Axelrod, S. R. (2009). The role of mindfulness in borderline personality disorder features. *Journal of Nervous and Mental Disease*, *197*(10), 766–771.

Zgierska, A., Rabago, D., Chawla, N., Kushner, K., Koehler, R., & Marlatt, A. (2009). Mindfulness meditation for substance use disorders: A systematic review. *Substance Abuse*, *30*(4), 266–294.

part five

TREATING INTERPERSONAL AND SELF FUNCTIONING

chapter 14

Treating Maladaptive Interpersonal Signatures

Nicole M. Cain and Aaron L. Pincus

Patients with personality disorders often seek psychotherapy for interpersonal problems or see their relationships as sources of their distress. Often these patients' interpersonal behaviors exacerbate other presenting anxiety, mood, or substance use symptoms and frustrate important others. Given the centrality of chronic disturbance in self–other processes and its painful consequences, it is not surprising that virtually all personality disorder theories (Lenzenweger & Clarkin, 2005), psychotherapeutic approaches (Magnavita, 2010), and the DSM-5 criteria for personality disorders (Skodol et al., 2011) emphasize, at least in part, interpersonal dysfunction. Inevitably, clinicians of all persuasions must effectively cope with the expectable threats to the therapeutic alliance, as well as the damage to patients' lives, caused by ingrained maladaptive relational patterns that are enacted inside and outside therapy. In this chapter, we aim to bring the contemporary integrative interpersonal model of personality psychopathology (Pincus, 2005a, 2005b; Pincus & Hopwood, 2012) and its treatment (Anchin & Pincus, 2010; Benjamin, 2003; Pincus & Cain, 2008) from bench to bedside by describing our therapeutic approach to maladaptive interpersonal functioning in personality disorders. First, we briefly review the assumptions of contemporary interpersonal theory and our use of interpersonal theory to inform the concept of an *interpersonal signature* for describing and understanding adaptive and maladaptive social behavior. The remainder of the chapter is devoted to the application of this framework to identifying and treating disturbed interpersonal relations.

CONTEMPORARY INTEGRATIVE INTERPERSONAL THEORY

Contemporary interpersonal theory (e.g., Benjamin, 2003; Horowitz et al., 2006; Kiesler, 1996; Pincus & Ansell, 2012) is based on four broad assumptions. First, the most important expressions of personality and psychopathology occur in phenomena involving more than one person (i.e., *interpersonal situations*). Pincus and Ansell (2003) defined the interpersonal situation as "the experience of a pattern of relating self with other associated with varying levels of anxiety (or security) in which learning takes place that significantly influences the development of self-concept and social behavior" (p. 210). The interpersonal situation is intimately tied to the genesis, development, maintenance, and mutability of personality and personality disorder through the continuous patterning and repatterning of interpersonal experience (social learning) in an effort to satisfy fundamental human motives (e.g., attachment and communion, autonomy and agency) in ways that increase security and self-esteem (positively reinforcing) and avoid anxiety (negatively reinforcing). Over time, this process gives rise to mental representations of self and others (Blatt, Auerbach, & Levy, 1997) and enduring patterns of adaptive or disturbed interpersonal relating (Benjamin, 1996; Horowitz, 2004; Pincus, 2005a).

Therefore, the second assumption is that interpersonal situations occur both between oneself and others and within the mind via the capacity for perception, mental representation, memory, fantasy, expectancy, and emotion. Variously referred to as *cognitive interpersonal schemas* (Marcotte & Safran, 2002), *internal working models* (Bowlby, 1969), *object relations* (Caligor & Clarkin, 2010), and *personifications* (Sullivan, 1953), at the core of these different conceptions of covert interpersonally related structures and processes is the view that developmental experiences within family and peer relationships, in dynamic interaction with biological temperament (Livesley, 2001), certain ingrained sensitivities, expectancies, and motives that give rise to disturbed interpersonal relations in patients with personality disorders. These representational structures, elaborated over the life span by one's interpersonal experiences and metacognitive processes (e.g., self-reflection), act as templates reflexively guiding and organizing one's network of perceptions, thoughts, feelings, and motivations in significant relationships (Anchin, 2002).

The third assumption is that agency and communion, core domains of human existence (Bakan, 1966; Wiggins, 2003), provide an integrative metastructure for conceptualizing interpersonal situations and their mental representations (Lukowitsky & Pincus, 2011; Pincus, 2005a). *Agency* refers to the condition of being a differentiated individual, and it is manifested in strivings for power and mastery that can protect and enhance one's differentiation. *Communion* refers to the condition of being part of a larger social entity and is manifested in strivings for intimacy, union, and solidarity with the larger entity. These metaconcepts form a superordinate structure, referred to as the *interpersonal circle* (IPC; Leary, 1957; Wiggins, 1996), which is used to derive descriptive and explanatory concepts of personality, mental health, and psychopathology at different levels of specificity (see Figure 14.1, top). At the broadest and most interdisciplinary level, agency and communion encompass the fundamental interpersonal motives, strivings, and values of human relations (Horowitz, 2004). Thus, when seeking to understand essential motivations in interpersonal situations, we may consider both the agentic and communal nature of the individual's personal strivings or current concerns (e.g., to be in control; to be close—*or their opposites*) and the specific behaviors enacted to achieve those goals. At a sharper level of resolution, the

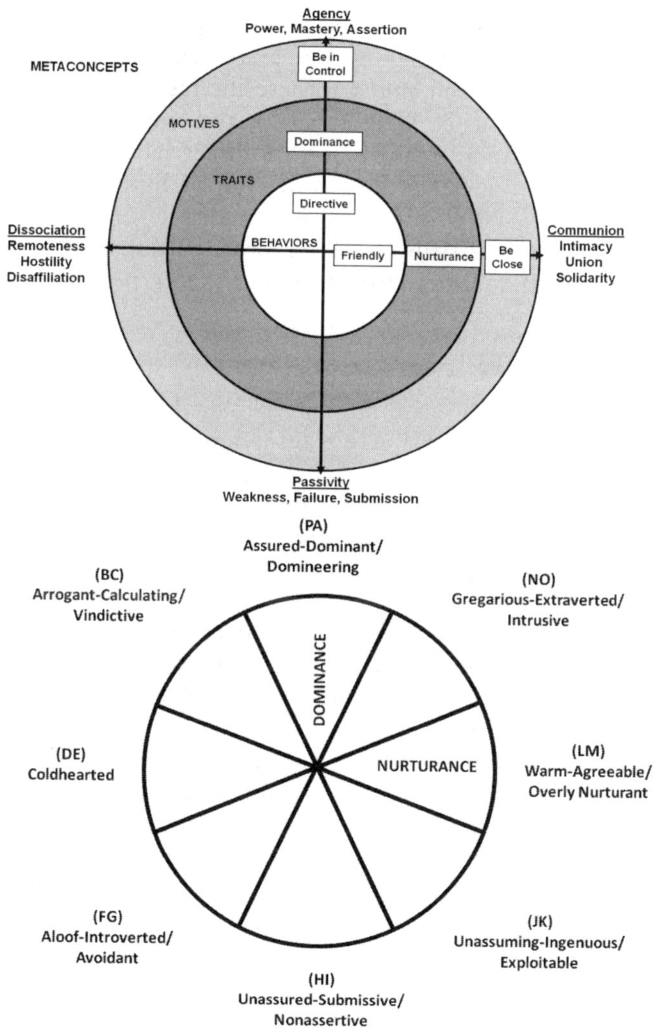

FIGURE 14.1. Agency and communion metaframework (top); interpersonal circle of traits/problems (bottom).

IPC provides conceptual coordinates for describing and measuring interpersonal traits and behaviors (Hopwood et al., 2011; Locke, 2010). Agentic and communal traits imply enduring patterns of perceiving, thinking, feeling, and behaving that describe an individual's relational tendencies aggregated across interpersonal situations—that is, one's interpersonal style. And, most specifically, the IPC classifies the nature and intensity of distinct interpersonal acts. Although the IPC has been empirically refined and extended over the years, its fundamental characteristics have been repeatedly validated. The most common instantiation of the IPC, at the intermediate level describing interpersonal traits and problems, is also presented in Figure 14.1 (bottom).

The final assumption of interpersonal theory is that interpersonal behavior is reciprocally influential in ongoing human transaction. The contemporary interpersonal approach is well suited to describe reciprocal social processes in psychopathology (Pincus & Wright, 2011), and empirical tests employing the agency-and-communion metaframework effectively model stability and variability in self–other social processes in samples both without (Fournier, Moskowitz, & Zuroff, 2009) and with personality disorders (Sadikaj, Russell, Moskowitz, & Paris, 2010). These self–other patterns, described by their agentic and communal qualities, are referred to as *interpersonal signatures*.

Interpersonal Signatures

The framework employed to examine interpersonal signatures is referred to in terms of adaptive and maladaptive transaction cycles (Kiesler, 1991), self-fulfilling prophecies (Carson, 1982), and vicious circles (Millon, 1996). Reciprocal relational patterns are socially reinforced through various transactional influences affecting self and other as they resolve, negotiate, or disintegrate the interpersonal situation. Interpersonal behaviors tend to pull, elicit, invite, or evoke "restricted classes" of responses from the other in a continual, dynamic transactional process. Carson (1991) referred to this as an interbehavioral contingency process in which "there is a tendency for a given individual's interpersonal behavior to be constrained or controlled in more or less predictable ways by the behavior received from an interaction partner" (p. 191). Thus interpersonal signatures are the consistent agentic and communal behavioral responses to the perceived agentic and communal characteristics of others in an interpersonal situation (Pincus, Lukowitsky, & Wright, 2010; Pincus, Lukowitsky, Wright, & Eichler, 2009; Pincus & Wright, 2011).

The IPC provides conceptual anchors and a lexicon to systematically describe interpersonal signatures (see Figure 14.2). The most basic of these processes is referred to as *interpersonal complementarity* (Carson, 1969; Kiesler, 1983). Interpersonal complementarity occurs when there is a match between the interpersonal goals of each person. That is, reciprocal patterns of activity evolve in which the agentic and communal needs of both persons are met in the interpersonal situation, leading to stability and likely recurrence of the pattern. Carson (1969) first proposed that complementarity could be

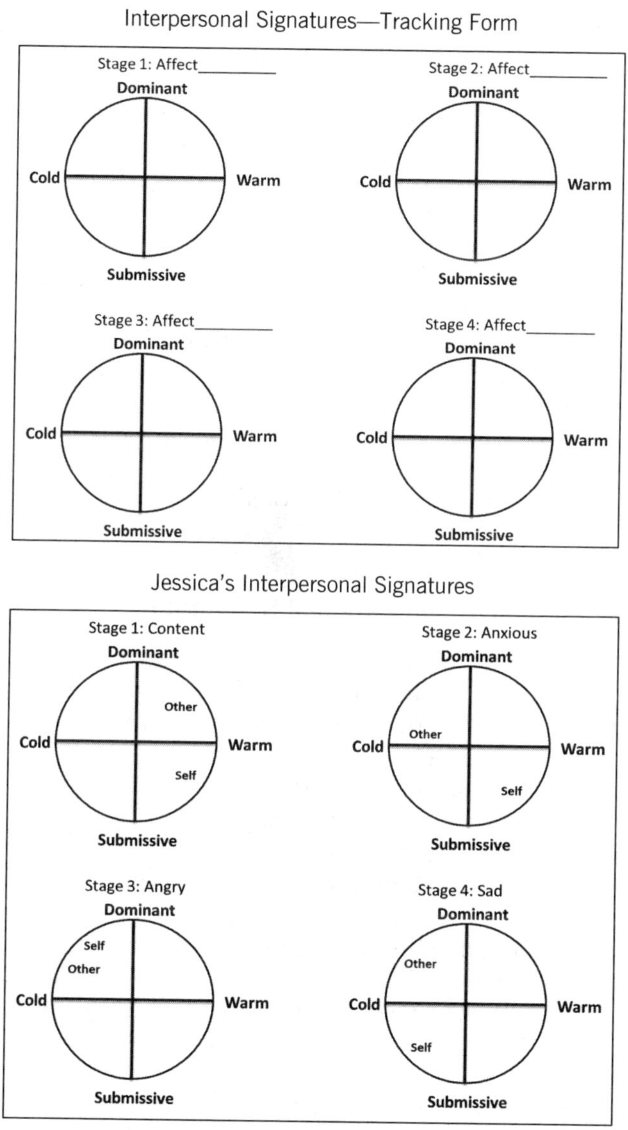

FIGURE 14.2. Tracking interpersonal signatures and associated affects (top); Jessica's interpersonal signatures (bottom).

defined via the IPC based on the social exchange of status (agency) and love (communion) as reflected in reciprocity for the vertical dimension (i.e., dominance pulls for submission; submission pulls for dominance) and correspondence for the horizontal dimension (friendliness pulls for friendliness; hostility pulls for hostility). Kiesler (1983) extended the principles of reciprocity and correspondence to complementary points along the entire IPC perimeter (e.g., hostile dominance pulls for hostile submission, friendly dominance pulls for friendly submission). Although complementarity is neither the only reciprocal interpersonal pattern that can be described by the IPC nor proposed as a universal law of interaction, empirical studies consistently find support for its probabilistic predictions (Sadler, Ethier, & Woody, 2011). A more precise phrasing of the final assumption of interpersonal theory is that complementarity should be considered a common baseline for the reciprocal influence of interpersonal behavior associated with healthy socialization. Deviations from complementary interpersonal signatures are more likely to disrupt interpersonal relations and may be indicative of pathological functioning (Fournier et al., 2009; Pincus et al., 2009; Roche, Pincus, Conroy, Hyde, & Ram, 2013). Common noncomplementary interpersonal signatures in psychotherapy with personality disorders include responding to therapist warmth with fear, suspicion, anger, or indifference; engaging in power struggles with the therapist for control; and chronic passivity in the face of all therapeutic efforts to mobilize the patient.

Interpersonal Signatures and Personality Disorders

Complementarity should not be conceived of as simply a behavioral stimulus–response chain of events. Rather, mediating internal psychological processes (e.g., each interactant's self–other schemas, the motives and needs embedded in these schemas, and their effects on subjective experience) influence the likelihood of complementary interpersonal signatures. An individual's chronic deviations from complementary reciprocal patterns of social behavior may be indicative of personality disorder, as they suggest impairments in: (1) recognizing the consensual understanding of interpersonal situations (e.g., psychotherapy), (2) adaptively communicating one's own interpersonal needs and motives, and (3) comprehending the needs of others and the intent of their interpersonal behavior (Anchin & Pincus, 2010; Pincus & Cain, 2008). In such cases, the individual pulls consistently and rigidly for responses that complement his or her own interpersonal behavior but has significant difficulty reciprocating with responses complementary to others' behavior. This reduces the likelihood that the agentic and communal motives of both persons will be satisfied in the interpersonal situation, creating disturbed interpersonal relations (Benjamin & Critchfield, 2010; Pincus 2005a; Pincus & Hopwood, 2012; Sullivan, 1953).

Normality, then, reflects the tendency or capacity to perceive self and other (i.e., interpersonal situations) in generally undistorted forms; that is, healthy individuals are generally able to accurately encode the agentic and communal "bids" proffered by others. All goes well, the interpersonal situation is resolved, and the relationship is stable. However, this is clearly not always the case in psychotherapy with patients with personality disorders.

Therapists generally attempt to work in their patients' best interest and promote a positive therapeutic relationship. Patients who are generally free of personality disorder typically enter therapy hoping for relief of their symptoms and are capable of experiencing the therapist as potentially helpful and benign. With complementary goals of seeking help and giving help (see also May, 1989), the therapist and patient are likely to develop a complementary interpersonal signature (i.e., a therapeutic alliance). Despite psychotherapists' taking a similar stance with patients with personality disorders, the beginning of therapy is often quite rocky, as the patients tend to view the therapists with fear, idealization, contempt, and so forth. Thus treatment often starts with noncomplementary interpersonal signatures, difficulties establishing a therapeutic alliance, and ongoing negotiation of the therapeutic relationship and frame.

What leads to patients' distorted perceptions of interpersonal situations, and subsequently, maladaptive interpersonal signatures? Psychodynamic, attachment, cognitive, and interpersonal theories converge in suggesting that dyadic mental representations are key influences on the perception and subjective elaboration of interpersonal input (Lukowitsky & Pincus, 2011). Individuals exhibit tendencies to organize their experience in certain ways (i.e., they have particular interpersonal schemas, expectancies, sensitivities, memories, fantasies, etc.), and we suggest that the best way to characterize these mediating social–cognitive–affective structures and processes is in terms of their agentic and communal characteristics. Interpersonal theory posits two main pathways by which one's schemas, expectancies, sensitivities, memories, and fantasies can distort the organization of interpersonal experience—one that is outside of awareness and one that is experienced consciously.

Parataxic Distortions

Sullivan (1953) proposed the concept of *parataxic distortion* to describe the mediation of social behavior by internal psychological processes and suggested that this occurs "when, beside the interpersonal situation as defined within the awareness of the speaker, there is a concomitant interpersonal situation quite different as to its principle integrating tendencies, of which the speaker is more or less completely unaware" (p. 92). The effects of unreflective, schema-driven distortions on interpersonal relations can occur in several forms, including chronic distortions of new interpersonal experiences (input), generation of rigid, extreme, and/or chronically non-normative interpersonal behavior (output), and dominance of self-protective motives (Horowitz, 2004; Horowitz et al., 2006), leading to the disconnection of interpersonal input and output.

We propose that healthy relations are promoted by the capacity to organize and elaborate incoming interpersonal input in generally undistorted ways, allowing for the agentic and communal needs of self and other to be mutually satisfied within the contextual norms of the situation. In psychotherapy, is the patient's perception of self and other relatively consistent with the therapist's perception of self and other (i.e., free of parataxic distortion)? In contrast, maladaptive interpersonal functioning is promoted when the perception of the interpersonal situation is, without apparent awareness, encoded in distorted or biased ways, leading to increased interpersonal insecurity and maladaptive interpersonal signatures (output) that disrupt interpersonal relations. In psychotherapy, this can be identified by a preponderance of noncomplementary interpersonal signatures between therapist and patient, as well as in patients' reports of their relationships with others. To account for the development and frequency of such distortions in personality pathology, interpersonal theory also outlines key maturational, motivational, and regulatory principles (see Benjamin, 2003; Horowitz, 2004; Pincus, 2005a; Pincus & Hopwood, 2012).

Self-Protective Motives

Beyond agency and communion, contemporary interpersonal theory identifies another class of interpersonal motives, referred to as *self-protective motives*, that can be described as arising "as a way of defending oneself from feelings of vulnerability that are related to relational schemas" that often take the form of "strategies people use to reassure themselves that they possess desired communal (e.g., likeable) and agentic (e.g., competent) self-qualities" (Horowitz et al., 2006, pp. 75–76). To the extent that a patient's early social learning occurred in a toxic developmental environment, the more likely they are to exhibit parataxic distortions of interpersonal situations, to feel threatened and vulnerable due to their characteristic ways of organizing interpersonal experience, and to engage in self-protective interpersonal behavior that is noncontingent with the behavior of others or the normative situational press (Pincus & Hopwood, 2012). The severity of personality pathology could be evaluated in terms of the pervasiveness of parataxic distortions and self-protective motives over time and situations. Severe personality pathology is often reflected in pervasive rigid or chaotic parataxic distortions. The former render the experience of most interpersonal situations functionally equivalent (and typically anxiety provoking and threatening to the self), whereas the latter render the experience of interpersonal situations highly inconsistent and unpredictable (commonly oscillating between secure and threatening organizations of experience).

Summary

We have briefly reviewed the assumptions of contemporary interpersonal theory with a specific focus on maladaptive interpersonal signatures, or the disturbed patterns of social perception and behavior that are at the core of personality pathology and its treatment. In the remainder of the chapter we present the clinical application of this approach.

TREATMENT STRATEGIES AND A CLINICAL EXAMPLE

There is no single interpersonal psychotherapy, but, rather, intervention techniques can be drawn from a variety of therapeutic approaches that view interpersonal processes as central to the development of pathology and to the patient's experience of distress (Anchin & Kiesler, 1982; Pincus & Cain, 2008). Based on contemporary interpersonal theory, the treatment of interpersonal signatures aims to promote new interpersonal awareness and learning, which leads to improved relational capacity and a reduction in symptoms. Appropriate intervention strategies are selected based on the core interpersonal processes that define a patient's pathology, as well as how that pathology is expressed within the interpersonal situation, the stage of therapy, the quality of the therapeutic relationship, and other relevant patient and therapist characteristics (Anchin & Pincus, 2010; Pincus & Hopwood, 2012).

Our approach to treatment integrates contemporary interpersonal theory with an object relations–based understanding of personality structure (Clarkin, Yeomans, & Kernberg, 2006; Pincus, 2005a). As noted earlier, interpersonal situations occur not only between self and other but also in the mind via social–cognitive–affective structures (i.e., schemas, object representations, internal working models) that transfer old interpersonal situations onto new situations through parataxic distortions. These internalizations reflect *if–then* propositions that characterize expectations and templates for new interpersonal situations (Pincus & Wright, 2011). Following object relations theory (Kernberg, 1975), these internalizations consist of a self-representation, an other-representation, and a linking affect. Thus treatment proceeds via an articulation of the internalizations of self and other associated with prominent interpersonal signatures and utilizes a sequence of clarifications, confrontations, and well-timed interpretations (Clarkin et al., 2006) to identify, challenge, and ultimately understand the etiology and maintenance of interpersonal signatures, thereby leading to increased interpersonal awareness and social learning.

Central to our therapeutic approach is the therapeutic relationship, which provides a proximal interpersonal situation through which to explore the patient's core interpersonal processes. The therapeutic relationship is both a vehicle for change and a context through which all intervention techniques are employed. This requires the therapist to be actively engaged in the therapeutic relationship as a *participant observer* (Anchin & Pincus, 2010; Pincus & Cain, 2008). The therapist is an active participant in the ongoing therapeutic relationship; therefore, his or her reactions to the patient often reflect the predominant interpersonal impacts of the patient's behavior on others. Importantly, the therapist is also an observer who is acutely attuned to interpersonal communication occurring in the patient's behavior, tone of voice, gestures, and symptoms. The therapist observes and reflects on what is occurring in the therapeutic relationship and begins to identify parataxic distortions that give rise to disturbed, noncomplementary relations between patient and therapist.

The parataxic distortion of current interpersonal situations as a function of early internalizations is a cardinal symptom of personality disorder pathology. Pervasive distortions in the organization of self–other experience render many interpersonal situations functionally equivalent for patients with personality disorder, eliciting generalized and rigid self-protective interpersonal patterns evoked by a small number of psychological triggers (e.g., others' coldness or others' control) to guide interpersonal schemas, motives, behavior, and/or expectancies (Pincus & Hopwood, 2012; Roche et al., 2013).

Case Example

To illustrate our treatment approach, we use material from the case of "Jessica," whose dysfunction and dissatisfaction with life can be operationalized in terms of her frustrated agentic, communal, and regulatory motives. Jessica is a married female in her mid-50s with a history of multiple psychiatric hospitalizations related to chronic suicidal ideation. The initial assessment phase with Jessica involved clarifying the nature and severity of her presenting pathology and the pervasiveness of her interpersonal problems across time, relationships, and situations. This initial assessment would take place over the first three sessions of treatment and would involve a thorough assessment of her views of herself and important others, her understanding of her symptoms, and a clinical and developmental history. During this assessment, the therapist is a participant observer, focusing simultaneously on (1) the patient's descriptions of self, other, relationships, and symptoms and (2) the nature of the unfolding therapeutic relationship in the here and now. The clinical data are used to confirm the presence and severity of symptom disorders and personality pathology and begin to identify the prominent interpersonal signatures and their developmental origins and current maladaptive expressions. Compatible approaches with these aims include the structural interview (Kernberg, 1984) and the interpersonal reconstructive therapy case formulation (Benjamin, 2003).

In terms of agency, Jessica consistently received negative reviews at work, and her boss had often threatened to fire her due to insubordination. She routinely refused to obey directions from her boss and complained that he was incompetent. In addition, she did not get along well with her coworkers, describing them as disrespectful and catty. Her coworkers often excluded her from lunchtime gatherings, leaving Jessica feeling sad and angry, which often manifested in tantrums of screaming and crying. She would lock herself in the bathroom for hours at a time during these fits, unable to complete her work. This led others to reject her and gossip about her behavior, which further contributed to her sense of alienation and decreased performance at work.

In terms of communion, Jessica had been married for over 25 years; however, this relationship was chaotic, with Jessica oscillating between idealization and devaluation of her husband. At times, she viewed him as distant, whereas at other times she viewed him as too controlling. Her husband had separated from her several times during their marriage and often threatened divorce. They had two sons, and Jessica reported loving feelings toward her sons but often devalued them. For example, she was dismissive of them when they did poorly at school, describing them as stupid or unmotivated. Her most recent psychiatric hospitalization occurred when her oldest son left for college. Jessica was unable to tolerate this separation and blamed her son for abandoning her for his academic pursuits. She reported no friendships, saying that no one seemed to like her. Jessica felt alienated and rejected by those around her and often commented that she had no one to turn to when she was upset. In terms of regulation, her emotions fluctuated wildly and were dominated by anger. Jessica often drank three or four glasses of wine after work each night to self-regulate and to feel less empty and alone. Her vacillating self-esteem was colored by an idealized image of herself coupled with self-doubt and self-criticism.

At the beginning of treatment, Jessica often idealized and devalued her therapist in a chaotic but not random manner. For example, she began most sessions by sitting in silence, arms folded, and staring out the window, waiting for her therapist to direct the session. In early sessions, her therapist would often begin by asking a seemingly neutral question (e.g., "Tell me what's on your mind"), and Jessica would respond warmly to the question, filling her therapist in on her week. As the session would continue, Jessica would become increasingly hostile and angry with her therapist, interpreting any silence on the part of her therapist as uninterest or withdrawal. A common exchange between Jessica and her therapist might go as follows:

JESSICA: You're not even listening to me anymore. Why aren't you saying anything?

THERAPIST: You perceive my silence to mean that I'm not listening to you.

PATIENT: You don't care about me! You sit there, wishing that I would just shut up and leave. (*Starts to gather her purse and coat on the couch around her.*)

THERAPIST: If I don't say anything, then it feels as though I don't care about you, and I am not interested in you.

PATIENT: You don't care! No one cares about me. People can't wait for me to go because they can't stand being around me.

Following an exchange like this, Jessica would often abruptly end sessions early, storming out of the office.

As a participant observer in the therapeutic relationship, Jessica's therapist was aware of complementarity and would question her experience of Jessica by asking herself, "What is this patient trying to evoke in me?" and/or "What am I feeling when I'm with this patient?" (Pincus & Cain, 2008). Through a thorough understanding of complementarity, the therapist can begin to anticipate and predict the effects of therapeutic behaviors (Anchin & Pincus, 2010; Benjamin, 2003). Specifically, any therapist behavior that complements the patient's pathological behavior would be predicted to relieve anxiety and build the alliance but also to reinforce the pathology. For example, if Jessica's therapist had continued to ask questions and follow up on information pertaining to Jessica's week, Jessica might have continued the session, feeling warm toward her therapist while continuing to rehash the week's minute details. However, this therapeutic stance would reinforce Jessica's pathology without identifying and understanding her parataxic distortions and maladaptive interpersonal signatures. Therapists must be aware that interventions that do not complement the patient's pathological behavior will likely increase anxiety and threaten the alliance but also provide new social learning that could promote change toward greater flexibility and adaptivity. Psychotherapy research suggests that it may be useful to sequence these strategies for optimal outcomes (Tracey, 2002). For example, Jessica's therapist may choose to initially follow Jessica's lead and take an admiring and submissive posture with her in order to develop the alliance. Once the alliance develops, it may be useful for her therapist to take an increasingly dominant position. Doing so would invite submissiveness on the part of Jessica (reciprocity principle). If her therapist can help Jessica to tolerate this in sessions, Jessica could generalize the capacity for submissiveness and cooperation to other relationships, becoming more flexible and less pathological in her interactions with others.

As treatment progresses with patients with personality disorders, the therapist utilizes a sequence of clarifications, confrontations, and well-timed interpretations to identify and explore parataxic distortions that may be occurring in the therapeutic relationship, as well as the relevant regulatory goal. For example, in the initial stages of treatment, the therapist may be curious about how the patient perceives him or her and ask to hear more about the patient's perceptions and distortions, thus clarifying how the patient views the therapist at any given point in session. As the therapy progresses, the therapist begins to gently point out and confront the discrepancies between the proximal interpersonal situation (e.g., the therapeutic relationship) and the internal interpersonal situation (i.e., the patient's parataxic distortions), understanding that this will stress the therapeutic relationship and evoke anxiety in the patient. Finally, in the later stages of therapy, the therapist begins to link the patient's distorted view of self and other in the therapeutic relationship to early internalizations via interpretation. The timing of the interpretation phase is quite important. Depending on the type and severity of personality disorder pathology, it may take the therapist quite some time to begin interpreting the links between the patient's views of self and other, her or his early relationships, and her or his symptoms and functional impairments. And occasionally developmental origins of interpersonal distortions will not be a focal element of treatment. When employed, the goal of these interpretations is to help the patient better mentalize his or her interpersonal patterns, improving self- and affect regulation. If interpretations are made too quickly, the patient may feel too vulnerable or attacked or criticized, evoking self-protective motives and impulses to terminate treatment prematurely, thus losing the opportunity for mentalization.

Developmental Antecedents, Toxic Learning Environments, and Past Social Learning

Once the therapist identifies and articulates the patient's interpersonal signatures, then he or she systematically begins to link these interpersonal signatures via interpretation to developmental antecedents, toxic early environments, and past social learning in an effort to understand the etiology and maintenance of these characteristic patterns of relating to others. Benjamin's (2003) developmental learning and loving (DLL) theory argued that attachment itself is the fundamental motivation that catalyzes social learning processes. Benjamin proposed three developmental "copy processes" that describe the ways in which early interpersonal experiences are internalized as a function of achieving either secure or insecure attachment. The first is *identification*, which is defined as "treating others as one has been treated." To the extent that individuals strongly identify with early caretakers, there will be a tendency to act toward others in ways that copy how important others have acted toward the developing person. This mediates the selection of interpersonal output and may lead to repetition of such behavior regardless of agentic and communal goals and behaviors of actual others, that is, noncomplementary patterns. The second is *recapitulation*, which is defined as "maintaining a position complementary to an internalized other." This can be described as reacting "as if the internalized other is still there and in control." In this case, new interpersonal input is likely to be distorted such that the proximal other is experienced as similar to the internalized other, or new interpersonal input from the proximal other may simply be ignored and behavior may recapitulate old patterns with the dominant internalized other. The third is *introjection*, which is defined as "treating the self as one has been treated." By treating oneself in introjected ways, security and esteem are maintained despite noncomplementary behavior in relations with others.

Pincus and Ansell (2003) extended the catalysts of social learning beyond attachment motivation by proposing that "reciprocal interpersonal patterns develop in concert with emerging motives that take developmental priority" (p. 223). These developmentally emergent motives may begin with the formation of early attachment bonds and felt security, but then separation–individuation and the experiences of self-esteem and additional unfolding motives may become priorities. Interpersonal patterns can also be associated with traumatic learning that leads to self-protective motives, as well as coping strategies for impinging events, such as early loss of an attachment figure, childhood illness or injury, and neglect or abuse. Identifying the developmental and traumatic catalysts for internalization and social learning allows greater understanding of current interpersonal signatures. For example, in terms of achieving adult attachment relationships, some individuals have developed hostile strategies such as verbally or physically fighting in order to elicit some form of interpersonal connection, whereas others have developed submissive strategies such as avoiding conflict and deferring to the wishes of the other in order to be liked and elicit gratitude. A person's social learning history will significantly influence his or her ability to accurately organize new interpersonal experiences.

Returning to the case of Jessica, it is important to note the toxic developmental learning history underlying her interpersonal signatures. Jessica's father was an alcoholic who paid little or no attention to her. When he did notice her, he did so in an aggressive and verbally abusive manner, telling her that she was stupid or unattractive. Her mother was depressed and withdrawn, sometimes being hospitalized for months at a time, leaving Jessica alone with only her father's verbal tirades as attention. Her father's drinking and her mother's mental illnesses were family secrets, and the family went to great lengths to keep these from the outside world. This limited Jessica's ability to form a secure attachment or a stable identity and impaired her regulatory capacity.

A Clinical Illustration of Interpersonal Signatures

Jessica's core maladaptive interpersonal signatures involved a communal conflict related to her developmental experiences with her parents, especially with her father, and centered around her attachment needs for attention and care from others. Specifically, her internalizations were dominated by the thought "If he ignores me, then he doesn't care" and its opposite, "if he is abusive, then he does care." The need to be cared for and attended to and the maladaptive signatures associated with it led Jessica to recapitulate her chaotic and stormy relationship with her father in new interpersonal situations. In other words, Jessica was highly sensitive to rejection, and she experienced all sorts of interpersonal behavior from others as functionally equivalent (signs of impending abandonment). She protected herself from a sense of connectedness with others via provocative hostility and aggression when she sensed abandonment. This led to an insecure adult attachment style and a chronically frustrated communal motive—a miserable but familiar experience for Jessica.

Jessica often recapitulated this same pattern with her therapist. Driven by her core interpersonal expectancy that others would abandon or reject her, she commonly interpreted her therapist's silence as uninterest and would become angry and lash out. To illustrate how Jessica's interpersonal signatures would be explored and understood in psychotherapy, we have plotted Jessica's maladaptive interpersonal signatures onto the IPC (see Figure 14.2, bottom panel). In stage 1, as her therapist inquires about what may be on her mind, Jessica begins by being warm and submissive (discloses what's on her mind) and perceives her therapist as warm and dominant (interested and caring). She feels content and begins to relate relatively superficial details about her week. Her therapist uses clarification to further understand the psychological content of Jessica's narrative. In stage 2, her therapist may show less interest in the *content* of her speech or may begin to confront discrepancies in Jessica's narrative. Although this is done therapeutically to avoid reinforcing superficial conversation, Jessica often organizes her experience of self and other in automatic, unreflective, schema-driven ways (i.e., parataxic distortion) and perceives withdrawal of therapist interest, which is not objectively present. Regardless of reality, Jessica now experiences herself as warm and her therapist as cold, creating noncomplementary instability and anxiety in their relationship. Jessica becomes anxious and feels vulnerable, folding her arms in front of her and pulling her purse close. In stage 3, Jessica must protect herself from the perceived withdrawal and now attempts to provoke the other's involvement by angrily accusing her therapist of lack of interest. Her therapist may try to interpret this shift in the therapeutic relationship as an effort to provoke an angry engagement and link this to the relationship with her father. The therapist must anticipate that this interpretation could lead to further dysregulation in the patient. For example:

JESSICA: (*yelling*) Why do I bother coming here? You don't care about me and you don't listen to me. Why do I pay for this? You're just a terrible therapist who silently counts her money, laughing all the way to the bank.

THERAPIST: There's been a shift in how you perceive me. As I've become more silent, you've become angrier and angrier with me. I wonder if your anger is an attempt to provoke a reaction from me, maybe wanting more attention from me similar to how it was with your father. You felt that he ignored you until he became angry with you.

JESSICA: (*yelling*) Like I said, no one cares! You're a jerk and he's a jerk! Therapy is a waste of my time!

This exchange could lead to a noncomplementary power struggle, in which both Jessica and her therapist are cold and dominant and Jessica becomes angry, both identifying with her father and recapitulating their familiar relational dynamic. Her therapist is now at risk of enacting the habitual cold dominant role with Jessica. If this dynamic continues, it will lead to Jessica's stage 4 experiences of sadness and withdrawal. In stage 4 of Figure 14.2 (bottom panel), the other withdraws emotionally and/or responds in kind and angrily rejects Jessica. Jessica feels abandoned, lonely, and sad (i.e., cold/submissive) and the interpersonal situation has returned to stable complementarity, but it does not turn out well for Jessica. She may end the session early by leaving or by becoming so withdrawn that she is unable to participate in treatment. Her therapist has become the rejecting other she fears, and both have missed an opportunity to mentalize the interpersonal situation in a therapeutically useful way (Hopwood, Wright, Ansell, & Pincus, 2013).

To avoid this hostile enactment, it is important for Jessica's therapist to (1) be sensitive to moments when the patient is likely to perceive, particularly through parataxic distortion, withdrawal or uninterest, (2) be cautious not to withdraw or express uninterest without realizing it, and (3) interpret evidence of anxiety as related to the patient's parataxic distortions. However, these maladaptive interpersonal signatures are often strongly entrenched in patients with personality disorders via internalization and thus are inevitable in many interpersonal situations, meaning that the third and fourth stages are somewhat out of the therapist's control. In other words, it is likely that Jessica would perceive her therapist as withdrawing even if she objectively was not. It is important for the therapist to avoid verbally sparring with Jessica and to use the experience of stage 3 to help Jessica mentalize this dynamic as it occurs and develop an awareness of her parataxic distortion, or her tendency to identify with and recapitulate an old attachment relationship, and of the broader links between her current and past interpersonal situations.

Depending on the type and severity of the personality disorder, the process of identifying interpersonal signatures and linking these signatures to developmental antecedents may progress quite slowly, and it is possible that the therapist may not get to the developmental antecedents at all. For example, the patient may end treatment before the developmental and traumatic catalysts for internalization and social learning are fully identified. However, by focusing on linking present symptoms and impairments to past social learning, the patient's will to change may be evoked and new social learning can occur both inside and outside of treatment. Similar to Benjamin's (2003) interpersonal reconstructive therapy, the goal of our treatment approach is to support the growth-oriented part of the patient that is ready, willing, and able to change her or his maladaptive interpersonal signatures. It is often the case that with a patient with personality disorder, the more regressive part of the patient is dominant early on in the therapy. It then becomes the primary task of the therapist to form an alliance with the growth-oriented part of the patient from the very beginning of the therapy and to engage that part of the patient in the process of new social learning within the context of the therapeutic relationship.

The therapist encouraged new interpersonal learning for Jessica by helping her to observe their interaction more objectively and to link it to other interpersonal situations, past and present, through a series of well-timed clarifications, confrontations, and interpretations. The therapist also clarified that she was not angry with Jessica and would not abandon her by modeling a judicious use of interpersonal warmth during the volatile third stage of her recurring pattern. Doing so reduced the likelihood that the process would end with Jessica's demoralization and withdrawal from treatment. This alternative ending to the interpersonal situation strengthens Jessica's capacity to develop insight. Fully engaging in a recurrent, alternative relational process with her therapist provided Jessica with a clearer understanding of what her maladaptive interpersonal signatures are for and where they came from. This new insight can evoke her will to change and to continue to develop new and more adaptive interpersonal signatures (Anchin & Pincus, 2010; Benjamin, 2003; Hopwood et al., 2013; Pincus & Hopwood, 2012).

CONCLUDING COMMENTS

We argue that contemporary interpersonal theory can play a central role in advancing the treatment of personality pathology because of its particular focus on agentic and communal aspects of relational functioning, the reciprocal nature of relational behavior, the identification of maladaptive interpersonal signatures associated with distorted perceptions of self and other and the self-protective motives they evoke, and the role of interpersonal copy processes in healthy and abnormal personality development. As DSM-5 now emphasizes self and interpersonal dysfunction as the core features of personality disorder (Criterion A), it is even more important to employ an integrative interpersonal framework for identifying, describing, and treating the disturbed interpersonal relations found in personality disorders (Pincus, 2011; Wright, 2011).

REFERENCES

Anchin, J. C. (2002). Relational psychoanalytic enactments and psychotherapy integration: Dualities, dialectics, and directions: Comment of Frank (2002). *Journal of Psychotherapy Integration, 12*, 302–346.

Anchin, J. C., & Kiesler, D. J. (1982). *Handbook of interpersonal psychotherapy*. New York: Pergamon Press.

Anchin, J. C., & Pincus, A. L. (2010). Evidence-based interpersonal psychotherapy with personality disorders: Theory, components, and strategies. In J. J. Magnavita (Ed.), *Evidence-based treatment of personality dysfunction: Principles, methods, and processes* (pp. 113–166). Washington, DC: American Psychological Association.

Bakan, D. (1966). *The duality of human existence: Isolation and communion in Western man*. Boston: Beacon Press.

Benjamin, L. S. (1996). *Interpersonal diagnosis and treatment of personality disorders* (2nd ed.). New York: Guilford Press.

Benjamin, L. S. (2003). *Interpersonal reconstructive therapy: An integrative, personality-based treatment for complex cases*. New York: Guilford Press.

Benjamin, L. S., & Critchfield, K. L. (2010). An interpersonal perspective on therapy alliance and techniques. In J. C. Muran & J. P. Barber (Eds.), *The therapeutic alliance: An evidence-based guide to practice* (pp. 123–149). New York: Guilford Press.

Blatt, S. J., Auerbach, J. S., & Levy, K. N. (1997). Mental representations in personality development, psychopathology, and the therapeutic process. *Review of General Psychology, 1*, 351–374.

Bowlby, J. (1969). *Attachment and loss: Vol 1. Attachment*. New York: Basic Books.

Caligor, E., & Clarkin, J. F. (2010). An object relations model of personality and personality pathology. In J. F. Clarkin, P. Fonagy, & G. O. Gabbard (Eds.), *Psychodynamic psychotherapy for personality disorders: A clinical handbook* (pp. 3–35). Arlington, VA: American Psychiatric Association Press.

Carson, R. C. (1969). *Interaction concepts of personality.* Chicago: Aldine.

Carson, R. C. (1982). Self-fulfilling prophecy, maladaptive behavior, and psychotherapy. In J. C. Anchin & D. J. Kiesler (Eds.), *Handbook of interpersonal psychotherapy* (pp. 64–77). New York: Pergamon Press.

Carson, R. C. (1991). The social–interactional viewpoint. In M. Hersen, A. Kazdin, & A. Bellack (Eds.), *The clinical psychology handbook* (2nd ed., pp. 185–199). New York: Pergamon Press.

Clarkin, J. F., Yeomans, F. E., & Kernberg, O. F. (2006). *Psychotherapy for borderline personality: Focusing on object relations.* Washington, DC: American Psychiatric Publishing.

Fournier, M., Moskowitz, D. S., & Zuroff, D. (2009). The interpersonal signature. *Journal of Research in Personality, 43,* 155–162.

Hopwood, C. J., Ansell, E. A., Pincus, A. L., Wright, A. G. C., Lukowitsky, M. R., & Roche, M. J. (2011). The circumplex structure of interpersonal sensitivities. *Journal of Personality, 79,* 707–740.

Hopwood, C. J., Wright, A. G. C., Ansell, E. B., & Pincus, A. L. (2013). The interpersonal core of personality pathology. *Journal of Personality Disorders, 27,* 270–295.

Horowitz, L. M. (2004). *Interpersonal foundations of psychopathology.* Washington, DC: American Psychological Association.

Horowitz, L. M., Wilson, K. R., Turan, B., Zolotsev, P., Constantino, M. J., & Henderson, L. (2006). How interpersonal motives clarify the meaning of interpersonal behavior: A revised circumplex model. *Personality and Social Psychology Review, 10,* 67–86.

Kernberg, O. F. (1975). *Borderline conditions and pathological narcissism.* New York: Jason Aronson.

Kernberg, O. F. (1984). *Severe personality disorders: Psychotherapeutic strategies.* New Haven, CT: Yale University Press.

Kiesler, D. J. (1983). The 1982 interpersonal circle: A taxonomy for complementarity in human transactions. *Psychological Review, 90,* 185–214.

Kiesler, D. J. (1991). Interpersonal methods of assessment and diagnosis. In C. R. Snyder & D. R. Forsyth (Eds.), *Handbook of social and clinical psychology* (pp. 438–468). New York: Pergamon Press.

Kiesler, D. J. (1996). *Contemporary interpersonal theory and research: Personality, psychopathology, and psychotherapy.* Hoboken, NJ: Wiley.

Leary, T. (1957). *Interpersonal diagnosis of personality.* New York: Ronald Press.

Lenzenweger, M. F., & Clarkin, J. F. (Eds.). (2005). *Major theories of personality disorder* (2nd ed.). New York: Guilford Press.

Livesley, W. J. (2001). Conceptual and taxonomic issues. In W. J. Livesley (Ed.), *Handbook of personality disorders* (pp. 3–38). New York: Guilford Press.

Locke, K. D. (2010). Circumplex measures of interpersonal constructs. In L. M. Horowitz & S. Strack (Eds.), *Handbook of interpersonal psychology* (pp. 313–324). Hoboken, NJ: Wiley.

Lukowitsky, M. R., & Pincus, A. L. (2011). The pantheoretical nature of mental representations and their ability to predict interpersonal adjustment in a nonclinical sample. *Psychoanalytic Psychology, 28,* 48–74.

Magnavita, J. J. (2010). *Evidence-based treatment of personality dysfunction: Principles, methods, and processes.* Washington, DC: American Psychological Association.

Marcotte, D., & Safran, J. D. (2002). Cognitive–interpersonal psychotherapy. In F. W. Kaslow (Ed.), *Comprehensive handbook of psychotherapy: Integrative/eclectic* (Vol. 4, pp. 273–293). Hoboken, NJ: Wiley.

May, R. (1989). *The art of counseling* (rev. ed.). New York: Gardner Press.

Millon, T. (1996). *Disorders of personality: DSM-IV and beyond.* Hoboken, NJ: Wiley.

Pincus, A. L. (2005a). A contemporary integrative interpersonal theory of personality disorders. In M. F. Lenzenweger & J. F. Clarkin (Eds.), *Major theories of personality disorder* (2nd ed., pp. 282–331). New York: Guilford Press.

Pincus, A. L. (2005b). The interpersonal nexus of personality disorders. In S. Strack (Ed.), *Handbook of personology and psychopathology* (pp. 120–139). Hoboken, NJ: Wiley.

Pincus, A. L. (2011). Some comments on nomology, diagnostic process, and narcissistic personality disorder in the DSM-5 proposal for personality and personality disorders. *Personality Disorders: Theory, Research, and Treatment, 2,* 41–53.

Pincus, A. L., & Ansell, E. B. (2003). Interpersonal theory of personality. In T. Millon & M. Lerner (Eds.), *Handbook of psychology: Personality and social psychology* (Vol. 5, pp. 209–229). Hoboken, NJ: Wiley.

Pincus, A. L., & Ansell, E. B. (2012). Interpersonal theory of personality. In J. Suls & H. Tennen (Eds.), *Handbook of psychology: Vol. 5. Personality and social psychology* (2nd ed., pp. 141–159). Hoboken, NJ: Wiley.

Pincus, A. L., & Cain, N. M. (2008). Interpersonal psychotherapy. In D. C. S. Richard & S. K. Huprich (Eds.), *Clinical psychology: Assessment, treatment, and research* (pp. 213–245). San Diego, CA: Academic Press.

Pincus, A. L., & Hopwood, C. J. (2012). A contemporary interpersonal model of personality pathology and personality disorder. In T. A. Widiger (Ed.), *Oxford handbook of personality disorders* (pp. 372–398). New York: Oxford University Press.

Pincus, A. L., Lukowitsky, M. R., & Wright, A. G. C. (2010). The interpersonal nexus of personality and psychopathology. In T. Millon, R. F. Krueger, & E. Simonsen (Eds.), *Contemporary directions in psychopathology: Scientific foundations for DSM-5 and ICD-11* (pp. 523–552). New York: Guilford Press.

Pincus, A. L., Lukowitsky, M. R., Wright, A. G. C., & Eichler, W. C. (2009). The interpersonal nexus of persons, situations, and psychopathology. *Journal of Research in Personality, 43,* 264–265.

Pincus, A. L., & Wright, A. G. C. (2011). Interpersonal diagnosis of psychopathology. In L. M. Horowitz & S. Strack (Eds.), *Handbook of interpersonal psychology* (pp. 359–381). Hoboken, NJ: Wiley.

Roche, M. J., Pincus, A. L., Conroy, D. E., Hyde, A. L, & Ram, N. (2013). Pathological narcissism and interpersonal behavior in daily life. *Personality Disorders: Theory, Research, and Treatment, 4*(4), 315–323.

Sadikaj, G., Russell, J. J., Moskowitz, D. S., & Paris, J. (2010). Affect dysregulation in individuals with borderline personality disorder: Persistence and interpersonal triggers. *Journal of Personality Assessment, 92,* 490–500.

Sadler, P., Ethier, N., & Woody, E. (2011). Interpersonal complementarity. In L. M. Horowitz & S. Strack (Eds.), *Handbook of interpersonal psychology* (pp. 123–142). Hoboken, NJ: Wiley.

Skodol, A. E., Clark, L. A., Bender, D. S., Krueger, R. F., Morey, L., Verheul, R., et al. (2011). Proposed changes in personality and personality disorder assessment and diagnosis for DSM-5: Part I. Description and rationale. *Personality Disorders: Theory, Research, and Treatment, 2,* 4–22.

Sullivan, H. S. (1953). *The interpersonal theory of psychiatry.* New York: Norton.

Tracey, T. J. G. (2002). Stages of counseling and therapy: An examination of complementarity and the working alliance. In G. S. Tryon (Ed.), *Counseling based on process research: Applying what we know* (pp. 265–297). Boston: Allyn & Bacon.

Wiggins, J. S. (1996). An informal history of the interpersonal circumplex tradition. *Journal of Personality Assessment, 66,* 217–233.

Wiggins, J. S. (2003). *Paradigms of personality assessment.* New York: Guilford Press.

Wright, A. G. C. (2011). Quantitative and qualitative distinctions in personality disorder. *Journal of Personality Assessment, 93,* 370–379.

chapter 15

Promoting Radical Openness and Flexible Control

Thomas R. Lynch, Roelie J. Hempel, and Lee Anna Clark

Mental health is often equated with self-control—the ability to inhibit various urges, impulses, behaviors, or desires. Indeed, the capacity for self-control is highly valued by most societies, and failures in self-control characterize many of the personal and social problems afflicting modern civilization—including substance abuse, criminal activities, domestic violence, financial difficulties, teen pregnancy, smoking, and obesity (Baumeister, Heatherton, & Tice, 1994; Moffitt et al., 2011). However, too much self-control can be equally problematic. Excessive self-control is associated with social isolation, poor interpersonal functioning, perfectionism, rigidity, lack of emotional expression, and severe and difficult-to-treat mental health problems, such as anorexia nervosa, chronic depression, and obsessive–compulsive personality disorder (Asendorpf, Denissen, & van Aken, 2008; Chapman & Goldberg, 2011; Eisenberg, Fabes, Guthrie, & Reiser, 2000; Lynch & Cheavens, 2008; Meeus, Van de Schoot, Klimstra, & Branje, 2011; Zucker et al., 2007). The preceding observations address prior limitations in the literature regarding the development and maintenance of two broad classes of psychopathology: *undercontrolled* and *overcontrolled* disorders, which largely parallel the well-established division between internalizing and externalizing disorders first introduced by Achenbach and colleagues (Achenbach, 1966; Crijnen, Achenbach, & Verhulst, 1997). Personality researchers have supported the utility of these broad approaches via the identification of a robust hierarchical structure of *personality dimensions* with clear links to social functioning and psychological disorder (Digman, 1997; Krueger, Caspi, Moffitt, Silva, & McGee, 1996; Markon, Krueger, & Watson, 2005). Whereas undercontrolled, impulsive, dramatic, emotionally expressive children have been shown to be more likely to develop externalizing disorders (Eisenberg et al., 2000; Kendler, Prescott, Myers, & Neale, 2003; Krueger, 1999), overcontrolled, emotionally constricted, risk-averse children are more likely to develop internalizing disorders and become socially isolated adults (Asendorpf et al., 2008; Asendorpf & van Aken, 1999; Caspi, 2000; Chapman & Goldberg, 2011; Eisenberg et al., 2000; Markon et al., 2005; Meeus et al., 2011; Robins, John, Caspi, Moffitt, & Stouthamer-Loeber, 1996). These observations have clear treatment implications: (1) We should not assume that patient capabilities for effective emotional responding already exist but emphasize the need for skills-based approaches, and (2) disorders of undercontrol and emotional dysregulation are likely to benefit from interventions designed to enhance constraint or inhibitory control, whereas disorders of emotional overcontrol are likely to benefit from interventions designed to relax inhibitory control and increase flexible responding.

The aim of this chapter is to provide a brief overview of the theoretical foundation and therapeutic stance for treating personality disorders of overcontrol and related disorders that is based on 19 years of research informed by experimental, longitudinal, and correlational research, including two randomized controlled trials (RCTs) of refractory depression with comorbid obsessive–compulsive personality dysfunction (Lynch, Morse, Mendelson, & Robins, 2003; Lynch, Trost, Salsman, & Linehan, 2007), one noncontrolled trial with adult inpatients with anorexia nervosa (Lynch et al., 2013), and an ongoing large multisite RCT (Lynch, *www.reframed.org.uk*). A secondary aim of this chapter is to briefly introduce a transdiagnostic neuroregulatory model of personality and socioemotional functioning that provides the foundation for interventions, including a novel treatment target linking the communicative functions of emotional expression to the formation of close social bonds (Lynch, in press; Lynch et al., 2013; Lynch, Hempel, & Dunkley, in press).

OVERCONTROLLED PERSONALITY DISORDERS

A quick examination of the fifth edition of the *Diagnostic and Statistical Manual of Mental Disorders* (DSM-5; American Psychiatric Association, 2013) reveals that personality disorders involve pervasive and long-standing problems with emotion/impulse control and interpersonal relationships. What is less obvious, however, is that these two features can be demarcated further into two basically opposite forms of self-regulation. Problems in emotion/impulse control can involve difficulties with either undercontrol (disinhibition) or overcontrol (rigid inhibition), and interpersonal problems can involve either chaotic/angry/intense (undercontrol) or distant/aloof/cautious (overcontrol) relationships. The core commonalities of personality disorder characterized by overcontrol (i.e., paranoid, obsessive–compulsive, and avoidant styles) are (1) a strong desire to control one's environment; (2) restrained emotional expression; (3) limited social interaction and problems with close relationships (due to mistrust, aloofness, distancing, fear or rejection or criticism); and (4) cognitive and behavioral rigidity.

We define overcontrol (OC) as the confluence of three temperamental and environmental "forces"—two internal and one external. OC becomes a severe problem when all three influences—specifically, high threat sensitivity (negative affectivity, NA), low reward sensitivity (positive affectivity, PA), and salient family/environmental pressures—are extreme (Lynch & Cheavens, 2008; Lynch et al., in press). For people with OC, the social influence or "nurture" component of their model involves a family/environmental history emphasizing mistakes as *intolerable* and sociobiographic feedback that self-control is *imperative*. The key sociobiographic difference between the biosocial theory for OC disorders and the biosocial theory for borderline personality disorder (BPD) (Crowell, Beauchaine, & Linehan, 2009; Linehan, 1993) is that, whereas the sociobiographic environment of BPD intermittently reinforces impulsive behaviors and/or extreme displays of emotion, the sociobiographic environment of OC reinforces avoidance of risk, masking inner feelings, following rules, and appearing calm or controlled. The transaction between the nature and nurture components of this model results in the maladaptive self-control style of OC. This maladaptive coping style is hypothesized to be reinforced intermittently via negative and positive reinforcement (e.g., reductions in arousal, increased nurturance, and/or praise), and, as such, OC coping becomes increasingly rigid over time. OC is hypothesized to involve core skill deficits associated with (1) *emotional awareness and expression*—manifested by minimization of distress, inhibited expression, and/or disingenuous expression (e.g., smiling when distressed), (2) *forming intimate relationships*—manifested by aloof/distant relationships and low empathy/validation skills, and (3) *receptivity and openness*—manifested by high risk aversion, avoidance of novelty, and automatic discounting of critical feedback. Finally, overcontrolled tendencies (as well as undercontrolled) are considered dimensional in nature; thus individuals are expected to fall on a spectrum from lesser to greater resemblance of each type.

Interestingly, despite strong evidence that OC personality disorders (e.g., obsessive–compulsive, paranoid, and avoidant) are common and figure prominently in poor treatment response for Axis I disorders (e.g., Fava et al., 2002; Fournier et al., 2008; Morse & Lynch, 2004), personality disorder research has focused overwhelmingly on dramatic–erratic or undercontrolled personality disorders (e.g., borderline, antisocial; Tyrer, Mitchard, Methuen, & Ranger, 2003). Our contention is that a major reason so many individuals fail to respond to interventions even when delivered adequately is that the majority of treatment approaches assume that categories of disorders are homogeneous in nature and that self-control or emotion regulation are linear (i.e., one can never have too much self-control). Our approach considers it important to account for the dynamic and cyclical transactions occurring between perceptual (i.e., appraisal of a situation as being safe, novel, threatening, rewarding, or overwhelming) and regulatory (i.e., self-control tendencies) factors—positing a quadratic (inverted U) model suggesting that both extremes of chronic *undercontrol* and *overcontrol* are most likely to be treatment resistant. Major depressive disorder exemplifies this challenge. It is frequently diagnosed in the context of a wide range of comorbid conditions and has high prevalence rates among both undercontrolled and overcontrolled styles of personality functioning (Corruble, Ginestet, & Guelfi, 1996). An estimated 40–60% of unipolar depressed patients meet criteria for comorbid personality disorder (see, e.g., Fava et al., 2002; Klein et al., 1995; Riso et al., 2003), and OC personality disorders are the most common—that is, paranoid, avoidant, and obsessive–compulsive personality disorders (Candrian et al., 2008; Fava et al., 2002; Fournier et al., 2009).

Based on our own research (Clark, 2005; Clark & Watson, 2008; Krause, Mendelson, & Lynch, 2003; Lynch, Robins, Morse, & Krause, 2001; Lynch, Schneider, Rosenthal, & Cheavens, 2007; Rosenthal, Cheavens, Lejuez, & Lynch, 2005; Watson, Clark, & Harkness, 1994) and recent findings from personality and neurobiobehavioral studies (Beauchaine, 2001; Gray & McNaughton, 2000; Porges, 1995), we have developed a transdiagnostic neuroregulatory model of personality and socioemotional functioning that is designed to address the aforementioned limitations (see Figure 15.1). According to this model, personality is conceptualized to involve relatively stable perceptual and regulatory response patterns that are moderated by differing sociobiographic experiences (e.g., family environment, trauma experiences, reinforcement history) and differing genetic/temperamental predispositions (i.e., threat sensitivity, reward sensitivity, and disinhibition vs. constraint).

Our neuroregulatory model informs treatment approaches for OC. The model parses emotion regulation into three transacting temporal components: (1) *neuroceptive tendencies (sensory-perceptual regulation)*, the degree to which incoming stimuli are perceived as safe, novel, threatening, rewarding, or overwhelming; (2) *response tendencies (central-cognitive or internal regulation)*, the degree to which the evolutionarily disposed autonomic nervous system (ANS) is activated and modified via top-down central-cognitive regulation strategies involving cortical brain regions associated with language, memory, and executive control; and (3) *self-control tendencies (response selection or external regulation)*, the degree to which individuals yield to versus inhibit these response tendencies—most often manifested via facial expressions, gestures, and actions. Separating external regulation from internal regulation

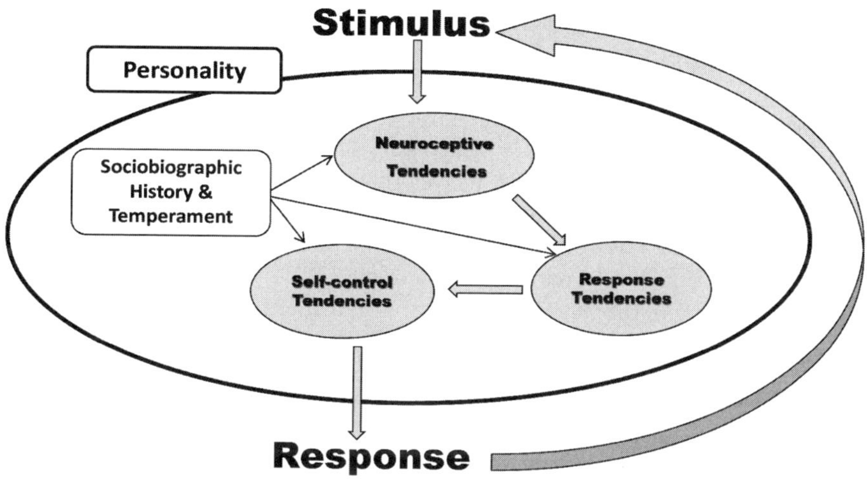

FIGURE 15.1. A neuroregulatory model of personality and socioemotional functioning.

helps explain why a person can "feel" hostility *inside* yet *not* display any "overt" signs of hostility on the *outside*.

The ANS plays a significant role in our model; a very brief summary is presented here. The model proposes that the organism's natural set point is calm-readiness. However, whenever novelty or an "associative mismatch" occurs—meaning current sensory inputs are discrepant with what would be predicted based on stored representations (Gross, 2006)—a quick and oftentimes unconscious evaluative process ensues. The primary function of this evaluative process is to assign valence/significance to novel, discrepant, and/or mismatched stimuli. The model proposes that there are five evolutionarily derived "neuroceptive tendencies" that influence our perception of the environment and our behavioral/emotional responses—specifically safe, novel, threat, reward, or overwhelming threat/reward. Stimuli can be internal (e.g., sensations, thoughts), external (e.g., dog bark), or contextual (e.g., time of day). The neuroceptive process can involve automatic bottom-up appraisals (i.e., quick primary appraisals occurring most often without conscious awareness) or top-down appraisals (i.e., secondary appraisals involving language/memory that are accessible to conscious awareness).

Neuroceptive appraisal processes are hypothesized to differ between individuals as a function of personality. Once a stimulus is neuroceptively evaluated (most often in milliseconds), automatic evolutionarily prepared *response tendencies* are elicited. Response tendencies involve images, thoughts, sensations, and urging components and are what most people refer to as "feelings." Response tendencies can be modified. For example, top-down processes might "agree" with a primary bottom-up appraisal of a pending reward by labeling a crowd of people in a city street as a "parade" rather than a "riot," thereby increasing excitatory-approach response tendencies. Importantly, a response tendency is a *propensity for action*, not the action itself. For example, when we neuroceptively evaluate the environment as safe, the ventral vagal complex (VVC) of the parasympathetic nervous system (PNS) is activated. Because this system is connected to the cranial nerves that control the muscles of the face, neck, middle ear, and vocal cords, the activation of this system allows us to be receptive to our environment, to respond to novel stimuli, and to communicate more effectively with others. Porges (2001) has termed this system the *social engagement system*. However, when there is a potential threat or reward in the environment, the PNS-VVC withdraws and the sympathetic nervous system (SNS), which facilitates flight, fight, and positive approach behaviors (Beauchaine, 2001; Gray & McNaughton, 2000; Löw et al., 2008; Porges, 2001), is activated. Finally, when a threat or reward is perceived as overwhelming and inescapable, the SNS withdraws and the dorsal vagal complex of the PNS is activated. Activation of this system facilitates behaviors that evolutionarily are adaptive for conservation of metabolic resources when SNS response tendencies are ineffective and can lead to shutting down, immobilization, numbing, lowered pain sensitivity, and fainting (Porges, 1995, 2001; Schauer & Elbert, 2010). Importantly, whether or not a response tendency is expressed depends on one's "self-control tendencies"—a core component of personality (see Figure 15.1).

Self-control tendencies can be effortless and quick (in milliseconds) and can occur without conscious awareness, or they can involve higher-order processes that are effortful and/or require conscious intention. Thus self-control involves *complex regulatory functions* that fundamentally permit or restrict the expression of a response tendency. For example, top-down processes might agree with the primary bottom-up appraisal of threat or reward and act upon its associated response tendency, leading to enhanced emotional responding and further activation of SNS motivational systems (disinhibition), or they might disagree with the primary appraisal, leading to inhibition (constraint) of the response tendency. Behavioral responses depend on the degree to which a person yields to or inhibits these response tendencies, suggesting that a person's characteristic style of self-control may be particularly relevant clinically (i.e., one's personality).

TARGETING OC TENDENCIES

Our neuroregulatory model argues that optimal self-control is an emergent capacity that requires "receptivity" or "openness" to changing environmental contingencies—that is, self-control is influenced by "gating parameters," how incoming stimuli are evaluated or perceived (neuroceptive tendencies). We contend that a necessary prerequisite for flexible control involves being receptive to discrepant or disconfirming stimuli (e.g., feedback suggesting that behavioral change is needed). Indeed, our approach suggests a developmental pathway from self-control to higher-order self-regulation, meaning that the "best" self-control emerges when individuals have learned well how to cope with their own temperament and its interaction with the environment. Thus, whereas one can have "too much self-control," by definition it's impossible to have "too much self-regulation," because a well-regulated person adjusts in whatever way needed for optimal performance. The gating parameters for OC are hypothesized to bias the evaluation of stimuli—metaphorically, and perhaps actually as well, an individual with OC tendencies is more likely to notice the thorns than the flowers when walking in a rose garden. Although the individual perceives OC as keeping him- or herself safe from possible dangers, the consequence for the individual is greater experiences of anxiety and other negative emotions and less frequent experiences of safety, joy, and other positive emotions.

Maladaptive OC is considered a problem of emotional loneliness—not emotion dysregulation. Individuals with OC tendencies may not necessarily avoid contact with others—for example, they may attend social events out of a sense of duty or obligation. However, they lack the core skills and biotemperamental propensities needed to form strong, intimate bonds with others. The emphasis on the development of a strong therapeutic alliance is considered essential when working with patients with OC because it provides the foundation for corrective environmental feedback that discounts prior negative experiences associated with the formation of intimate relationships. The primary goals of the orientation and commitment stage of therapy are to help the patient begin to understand how his or her OC style of coping is related to the problems he or she is seeking treatment for (e.g., depression, anxiety, restricted eating, interpersonal difficulties), to orient the patient to the demands of treatment, and to establish a therapeutic relationship. This normally requires approximately four sessions. During this early phase of treatment, therapists should search for nonpejorative ways to describe the OC style, being mindful that strong desires to avoid making a mistake or appear out of control may make self-identification difficult for some patients with OC. The goal is to "spark" an appreciation for self-inquiry and the patient's insight that OC both solves and creates problems for him or her while linking these insights to important goals identified by the patient. This process includes collaborative discussions focused on helping the patient self-identify the ways in which OC manifests for him or her. We have found the questions in Table 15.1 clinically useful as a means of facilitating these discussions.

However, OC threat hypersensitivity combined with tendencies to mask inner feelings can make the task of gaining genuine commitment or willingness to consider change a daunting enterprise. For example, therapists may find patients with OC tendencies readily agreeing and committing to treatment principles and expectations early on, only to later discover extreme ambivalence, strong aversion, or anger directed toward the treatment or the therapist that appears suddenly and without apparent warning. Moreover, the

TABLE 15.1. Questions to Ask in Identifying an OC Style

"How might you describe yourself?"

1. "Do you believe it is important to 'do things properly' or 'right'?"
2. "Are you a perfectionist?"
3. "Are you cautious and careful about how you do things?"
4. "Do you prefer order and structure? Are you organized?"
5. "Do you like to plan ahead? Do you think before acting?"
6. "Are you able to delay gratification? Are you able to easily inhibit an impulse?"
7. "Do you consider yourself conscientious? Are you dutiful?"
8. "Are you quiet, restrained, or reserved by nature?"
9. "Is it hard to impress you?"
10. "Does it take time to get to know you?"
11. "Are you likely to not reveal your opinion immediately until you get to know someone better?"

naturally avoidant and risk-averse nature of OC, particularly when it comes to interpersonal conflict, makes extreme escape behaviors highly probable when alliance ruptures occur—manifested most frequently by patient dropout or refusals to reengage with the therapist. Thus, early in treatment, declarations of commitment, affirmations of agreement, and/or positive reports of acceptability by patients should be viewed as "possibilities" rather than truths. Therapeutic alliance ruptures are essential to address when treating OC (life-threatening behavior would be considered the most essential). This means that the relationship with a patient with OC takes precedence over other behavioral responses that on the surface appear therapy interfering or noncompliant. Thus stopping and assessing potential alliance ruptures is considered more important than covering scheduled material. Once a potential alliance rupture is addressed and/or repaired (this can take a few minutes), the therapist then returns to the primary focus for that session.

Our experience suggests that therapists should expect their first alliance rupture to occur by about the sixth session and, if this and similar ruptures are repaired, to anticipate a solid working alliance to develop by about the 14th session. However, these should be considered broad principles rather than rules. Five OC treatment themes are typically addressed during the early phases of treatment: inhibited emotional expression, overly cautious and hypervigilant behavior, rigid and rule-governed behavior, aloof/distant relationships, and envy and bitterness. Individualized and behaviorally specific treatment targets derived from these themes are then mutually agreed to be relevant by both the therapist and patient and then typically monitored on a daily basis via diary cards. Following is a transcript of a session demonstrating how to "pull" an individualized treatment target from a discussion about one of the OC themes with a 54-year-old female patient with

OC tendencies who had a long-standing history of chronic depression and obsessive–compulsive personality disorder.

THERAPIST: So, one of the things you are saying is that you have . . . more or less . . . always considered yourself a perfectionist. How do you think this might have impacted your relationships with others? [Uses the patient's self-report of perfectionism as a link for introducing the path to flexible-mind OC theme "decrease aloof and distant relationships."]

PATIENT: Hmmm . . . I don't really know for sure. My sis always says I am a stickler for details . . . and it does seem to annoy her. (*pause*) I know that I'm definitely considered a control freak at work . . . but I see this as a virtue.

THERAPIST: OK . . . so something about being a control freak . . . controlling things . . . being highly organized . . . perhaps structured . . . something about this, you think may be upsetting to others? [Keeps focused on topic, ignores comment about control being a virtue, and globally describes behaviors that may be linked to the theme of aloof and distant interpersonal relationships.]

PATIENT: Not upsetting . . . they just don't seem to like it.

THERAPIST: What do you think they don't like about it? [Helps the patient refine the target.]

PATIENT: I don't know . . . maybe they're jealous (*slight smile; pause, looking at the therapist*) . . . I guess it is annoying to have someone telling you what to do . . . it is my job . . . but not really for my sister . . . I just think most people don't know how to keep things organized.

THERAPIST: So what you're saying is that you think that sometimes people find it annoying when you tell them what to do or how to organize things? [Keeps focused on topic of perfectionism by ignoring the comment about jealousy—though the therapist notes the use of this word for possible later targeting around envy and bitterness; instead, therapist summarizes a behaviorally specific description of how perfectionism might be linked to the patient's interpersonal relations and asks for confirmation from the patient.]

PATIENT: Yeah, that's it.

THERAPIST: So maybe what we could do . . . is start to monitor how often you tell others what to do or try to organize things—and see if you find it linked to annoyance on other people's part. How do you think their annoyance is manifested? [Uses the patient's own words in describing the target to be monitored and then asks for clarification as to how the patient knows others are annoyed.]

PATIENT: Hmm . . . that's a good question . . . (*pause*) . . . my sis just tells me . . . she'll say things like "I already know what to do" or "All right, already, I see your point! Stop trying to fix me!" Things like that . . . (*pause*) . . . but at work it's more subtle . . . sometimes people just walk away . . . they don't respond to my email . . . even after I've sent it four times! It's really frustrating because my job is to make sure that the policy and procedures for quality control are followed . . . people just don't understand the importance of this.

THERAPIST: It sounds like you're not appreciated for your work. (*The patient nods affirmation.*) . . . Maybe we can look at how being appreciated is linked to all of this. For now, though, I am thinking that perhaps we start out small . . . and just start to look for times that you organize or tell others what to do and then see if we can make sense of it. Would you be willing to do this? [Notices that appreciation may be a core issue for the patient but remains focused on target of linking perfectionism to interpersonal functioning.]

PATIENT: Yeah . . . that sounds OK to me . . . and now that you say it . . . I am definitely not appreciated.

THERAPIST: OK . . . how about this. What if we put on the diary card under overt behaviors . . . something like "telling others what to do" ranked 0–5 . . . with a 0 meaning that it didn't happen at all that day . . . say a 3 means that you were telling people what to do fairly often that day . . . and a 5 means that you were really a control freak that day. (*pause*) We could also monitor under private behaviors "feeling unappreciated" . . . again on a 0–5 scale . . . and then see if we find feeling unappreciated is linked to days you bossed others or told them what to do a lot. What do you think about this? [Uses the patient's words to describe the target, orients the patient on how to rate the behavior, and then adds one additional target—feeling unappreciated—because the patient had identified it is relevant.]

In the preceding scenario, it is important to notice that the therapist was careful not to introduce too many targets, despite there being a number that showed up during the discussion (e.g., jealousy, possible envy, or anger/resentment). Moreover, assuming that anger or envy are already targeted or will be targeted in the near future, then how anger or envy may be linked to "telling others what to do" can be highlighted in future sessions during diary card review. Once three to four individualized targets have been identified, defined, and placed on a diary card, the therapist should determine which OC theme on the path to flexible-mindedness should take priority (e.g., aloof and distant relationships) and identify the relevant individualized targets linked to that theme, and then loosely rank-order the remaining OC themes and targets in the same manner.

Importantly, our therapeutic stance emphasizes the prosocial nature of OC as a means to gain commitment for change. For example, *individuals who desire to meet or exceed expectations* are essential for the survival of our species, and high standards are needed in order for communities to flourish. Thus the role of the therapist treating OC may be best described as that of "tribal ambassador"—one who recognizes the personal sacrifices made by the individual with OC to meet or exceed expectations and warmly welcomes him or her to "rejoin the tribe." As ambassador, the therapist signals kindness, cooperation, and acceptance rather than fixing, correcting, restricting, or improving. The overall message is: "Welcome home, you have worked hard and deserve a rest" (see Table 15.2 for a summary).

RADICAL OPENNESS

We posit that emotional well-being involves three overlapping elements or capacities: openness, flexibility, and social connectedness. The term *radical openness* represents the confluence of these three core features. As a state of mind, it entails a willingness to surrender prior preconceptions about how the world should be in order to adapt to an ever-changing environment, and the new skills and approaches outlined in this chapter are derived from these basic principles (see Lynch, in press; Lynch et al., in press). Radical openness (RO) posits that *we are unable to see things as they are, but that instead we see things as we are.* From this perspective, "facts" or "truth" can often be misleading, partly because "we don't know what we don't know," because things are constantly changing, and because there is a great deal of experience occurring outside of our conscious awareness. Thus radical openness requires a willingness to doubt or question our inner convictions or intuitions without falling apart or mindlessly giving in. Rather than seeking equanimity, wisdom, or a sense of peace, radical openness encourages *self-inquiry* into

TABLE 15.2. Therapeutic Stance with OC Personality Disorders

- Therapist recognizes that patients with OC need to let go of always striving to perform better or try harder.
- The therapist is less directive and encourages independence of action or opinion in the patient.
- The therapist encourages engagement rather than avoidance of conflict and learning from corrective feedback.
- The major focus is on RO skills and establishing social connectedness.
- The therapist recognizes therapeutic alliance ruptures as opportunities for growth.
- The emphasis is on self-inquiry and self-discovery rather than impulse control.
- The therapist appreciates that the lives of patients with OC are miserable even though this may not always be apparent.
- The therapist rewards candid disclosure and uninhibited expression of emotion.

our habitual response patterns and a willingness to reveal to others what we discover—a process we call "outing oneself" (Lynch, in press; Lynch et al., in press). Outing one's personality quirks or weaknesses to another person goes opposite to OC tendencies to mask inner feelings; therefore, the importance of this when treating OC cannot be overstated. Finally, self-inquiry begins by asking, "Is there something to learn here?"

SOCIAL SIGNALING AND BIOTEMPERAMENTAL DEFICITS

Our approach links neurophysiology and the communicative functions of emotion to the formation of close social bonds. Although the majority of emotion theories emphasize that emotions function to *motivate actions* and *communicate intentions,* we extend existing models by positing that, in humans at least, emotions also function to facilitate the formation of strong social bonds essential for species survival (via micro-mimicry of facial expressions; Lynch, in press; Lynch et al., in press; Schneider, Hempel, & Lynch, 2013). For example, incongruence between felt experience and displayed behavior makes it more likely that others will perceive the incongruent person as untrustworthy or inauthentic (e.g., Boone & Buck, 2003; English & John, 2013; Mauss et al., 2011); it signals lack of predictability or trustworthiness (Boone & Buck, 2003; Kernis & Goldman, 2006; Reis & Patrick, 1996), making social connectedness less likely and depressive experiences more likely (Mauss et al., 2011). Consequently, we postulate that individuals' OC self-control efforts—designed to sidestep social difficulties—function to create the consequence they most desire to avoid, that is, people prefer not to interact with them and see them as inauthentic, leading to increased social ostracism and depression. Following is a transcript of a session with a 51-year-old male with chronic depression and comorbid obsessive–compulsive and avoidant personality disorders. During the session a therapist discusses the importance of open and vulnerable expression as a means for enhancing social connectedness.

THERAPIST: I'm aware of imagining that you are starting to consider that some of the ways you learned to cope with your anxiety and other emotions—not only when you were young, but now as an adult—kept you safe but also had some downsides too. Am I sensing things correctly?

PATIENT: Hmmm . . . I think I am beginning to understand this more . . . I always was a wallflower, don't think it, don't show it . . . stayed out of trouble . . . but I also felt different from the other kids. I was an outsider . . . always looking in . . . and angry that others seemed to find it easy. It was a . . . oh, wait . . . it *is* a lonely existence. (*Pause, smiles.*) Eventually I just assumed I was better off without relationships.

THERAPIST: Being on the outside—hmmmm, yeah, not much fun. (*Pause.*) Also, you mentioned that you learned to not show your feelings to others—that way you couldn't be hurt. What is sort of interesting; is that there is now research clearly showing that hiding feelings and not expressing our emotions can actually lead to being socially ostracized. Have you ever heard about anything like that?

PATIENT: Nope, I eventually came to the conclusion that everyone was fake and phony.

THERAPIST: Perhaps true—at least some of the time (*chuckles*). (*Pause.*) Though it is also true that not everyone feels on the outside of the tribe—at least not all of the time. Do you think it's possible that your habit not to express vulnerable feelings to others may have inadvertently impacted your relationships?

PATIENT: Yeah, I hate to admit it . . . my blank face is my suit of armor.

THERAPIST: Sometimes though, it might be nice to take off the armor . . . after all, it must get hot in there sometimes. (*Slight chuckle; pause.*) What is really strange, though, is that research shows that open expression and self-disclosure, instead of making people run away, is actually perceived as a safety signal by others. That is, we tend to trust those who freely express their emotions—particularly when the situation calls for it. It seems that when we take our armor off, others feel that it is safe to take theirs off, too—and then we can all have a picnic! (*Laughs.*)

PATIENT: (*smiling*) Yeah, I see your point—I guess it would be hard to eat a sandwich with a helmet on. (*Chuckles.*)

THERAPIST: I am glad we are discussing this . . . because this is one of the things we believe may be keeping you stuck in some way—both with your depression and anxiety, but also making you feel like an outsider. Would you be willing to consider working on changing this in some way?

PATIENT: What, you want me to just start expressing myself—willy-nilly?

THERAPIST: (*sensing a potential alliance rupture*) No, certainly not! And don't you dare start! (*Smiling.*) Actually, though—perhaps just a little bit . . . with the understanding that open expression will not involve us simply having you go out and express emotions without awareness or consideration . . . on the contrary; effective emotional expression is always context dependent. What I would like to start working with you on is the idea of learning how to take off your armor when the situation might call for it. I think in some ways, you've been doing this already in our relationship. How does this feel to you?

PATIENT: A bit scary.

THERAPIST: (*soft tone of voice*) Yeah, makes sense—it's hard to change habits . . . what is most important is that we work at a pace that makes sense to you . . . and we not lose the essence of who you are . . . meaning you have a style of your own, and we don't want to change everything . . . that just doesn't make sense. How are you feeling now . . . right in this moment?

Thus treatment goals directly target both the *transmit* and *receive* features of the patient's emotional communication. Interventions are carefully sequenced—that is, therapists should work to first increase social safety and reduce defensive arousal prior to encouraging patients to experiment with new skills or approaches designed to enhance intimate relationships. This is operationalized via two key strategies: First, we reduce SNS mediated defensive arousal by teaching skills designed to activate the PNS-VVC social safety system—based on research showing neuroinhibitory relationships between the PNS and SNS and polyvagal theory (Berntson, Cacioppo, & Quigley, 1991; Porges, 1995). When used prior to social interactions, PNS-VVC activation makes it more likely for free expression of emotion to occur, as this system innervates our "social muscles." Activation of the social safety system functions to communicate openness and receptivity, thereby making it more likely for interacting partners to feel similarly and to consider the communication trustworthy and authentic. Second, specific social skills designed to compensate for overlearned emotion inhibition and consequent aloof/distant relationships are taught—for example, how to share personal information, to discriminate whether someone desires more intimacy, to express vulnerable emotions, and to validate others.

A growing literature suggests that this approach has utility (Linehan, Bohus, & Lynch, 2007; Lynch & Cheavens, 2008; Porges, 2001). For example, several studies have found that meditation (Murata et al., 2004; Takahashi et al., 2005; Tang et al., 2009; Wu & Lo, 2008), relaxing music (Peng, Koo, & Yu, 2009; White, 1999), and stress and affect management programs (Bradley et al., 2010; McCraty, Barrios-Choplin, Rozman, Atkinson, & Watkins, 1998) all can increase PNS activity and decrease self-reported stress. In addition, conjuring positive emotions, such as loving kindness, compassion, and acceptance, can down-regulate the psychophysiological effects of negative emotions that activate flight-or-fight behaviors and increase social affiliation (Fredrickson & Levenson, 1998; Fredrickson, Mancuso, Branigan, & Tugade, 2000). Finally, more objective techniques to increase PNS activity without direct emotional or psychological intervention also can be applied. The presentation of acoustic stimuli to increase neural innervation to the muscles of the middle ear (a component of the PNS-VVC social safety system) has been reported to improve social behavior in children with autism by increasing eye gaze, facial expressivity, and social interaction with others (Porges, 2001). Essentially, we contend that biotemperamental predispositions matter when treating OC. Individuals with OC unintentionally bring mood states into social situations that function to isolate them from others. We target biotemperamental biases by changing physiology first—prior to targeting modification of thoughts or social behavioral responses. Moreover, skills emphasize the tribal nature of our species—informed by theory positing that emotional well-being is often highly influenced by our visceral experience of social connectedness.

CONCLUDING COMMENTS

The treatment approaches outlined in this chapter are designed for a spectrum of disorders that share similar genotypic–phenotypic features linked to excessive self-control or overcontrol. We conceptualize the fundamental problem of OC as *emotional loneliness*—not lack of contact but lack of connection with others *that is secondary to social-signalling deficits and low openness*. Two assumptions are a core part of successful treatment: (1) Patients with OC are prosocial despite often appearing aloof or distant, and (2) patients with OC need to let go of always trying to perform better or try harder. Moreover, we theorize that the temperamental and expressive deficits of OC are seminal in creating negative social transactions that function to maintain psychological distress and mitigate the efficacy of otherwise potentially helpful strategies unless dealt with first. The OC tendency to mask inner feelings makes matters worse: Research shows that social ostracism is exacerbated by the chronic inhibition of emotional expression (e.g., Gross & John, 2003). Though their self-control efforts are designed to avoid social difficulties, their OC coping style creates the very thing they desire desperately to avoid; that is, people prefer to not interact with them and see them as inauthentic. Our approach significantly differs from other existing treatment approaches, most notably by linking the communicative functions of emotional expression to the formation of close social bonds via skills targeting social signaling and changing neurophysiological arousal. The strategies outlined in this chapter represent only a subset of approaches that are part of a comprehensive treatment manual (Lynch, in press; Lynch et al., in press).

Finally, RO is not something that can be grasped solely via intellectual means; for example, patients with OC are unlikely to believe it is socially acceptable for an adult to play, relax, admit fallibility, or openly express emotions unless they see their therapist model it first. Thus we encourage therapists to practice what they "preach"—based on the assumption that therapists need to be capable in using the approaches that they recommend in their daily lives if they are to be effective teaching them.

REFERENCES

Achenbach, T. M. (1966). The classification of children's psychiatric symptoms: A factor-analytic study. *Psychological Monographs: General and Applied, 80*(7), 1–37.

American Psychiatric Association. (2013). *Diagnostic and statistical manual of mental disorders* (5th ed.). Arlington, VA: Author.

Asendorpf, J. B., Denissen, J. J. A., & van Aken, M. A. G. (2008). Inhibited and aggressive preschool children at 23 years of age: Personality and social transitions into adulthood. *Developmental Psychology, 44*(4), 997–1011.

Asendorpf, J. B., & van Aken, M. A. (1999). Resilient, overcontrolled, and undercontrolled personality prototypes in childhood: Replicability, predictive power, and the trait-type issue. *Journal of Personality and Social Psychology, 77*(4), 815–832.

Baumeister, R. F., Heatherton, T. F., & Tice, D. M. (1994). *Losing control: How and why people fail at self-regulation.* San Diego, CA: Academic Press.

Beauchaine, T. P. (2001). Vagal tone, development, and Gray's motivational theory: Toward an integrated model of autonomic nervous system functioning in psychopathology. *Development and Psychopathology, 13*(2), 183–214.

Berntson, G. G., Cacioppo, J. T., & Quigley, K. S. (1991). Autonomic determinism: The modes of autonomic control, the doctrine of autonomic space, and the laws of autonomic constraint. *Psychological Review, 98*(4), 459–487.

Boone, R. T., & Buck, R. (2003). Emotional expressivity and trustworthiness: The role of nonverbal behavior in the evolution of cooperation. *Journal of Nonverbal Behavior, 27*(3), 163–182.

Bradley, R. T., McCraty, R., Atkinson, M., Tomasino, D., Daugherty, A., & Arguelles, L. (2010). Emotion self-regulation, psychophysiological coherence, and test anxiety: Results from an experiment using electrophysiological measures. *Applied Psychophysiology and Biofeedback, 35*(4), 261–283.

Candrian, M., Schwartz, F., Farabaugh, A., Perlis, R. H., Ehlert, U., & Fava, M. (2008). Personality disorders and perceived stress in major depressive disorder. *Psychiatry Research, 160*(2), 184–191.

Caspi, A. (2000). The child is father of the man: Personality continuities from childhood to adulthood. *Journal of Personality and Social Psychology, 78*(1), 158–172.

Chapman, B. P., & Goldberg, L. R. (2011). Replicability and 40-year predictive power of childhood ARC types. *Journal of Personality and Social Psychology, 101*(3), 593–606.

Clark, L. A. (2005). Temperament as a unifying basis for personality and psychopathology. *Journal of Abnormal Psychology, 114*(4), 505–521.

Clark, L. A., & Watson, D.. (2008). Temperament: An organizing paradigm for trait psychology. In O. P. John, R. W. Robins, & L. A. Pervin (Eds.), *Handbook of personality psychology: Theory and research* (3rd ed., pp. 265–286). New York: Guilford Press.

Corruble, E., Ginestet, D., & Guelfi, J. D. (1996). Comorbidity of personality disorders and unipolar major depression: A review. *Journal of Affective Disorders, 37*(2–3), 157–170.

Crijnen, A. A., Achenbach, T. M., & Verhulst, F. C. (1997). Comparisons of problems reported by parents of children in 12 cultures: Total problems, externalizing, and internalizing. *Journal of the American Academy of Child and Adolescent Psychiatry, 36*(9), 1269–1277.

Crowell, S. E., Beauchaine, T. P., & Linehan, M. M. (2009). A biosocial developmental model of borderline personality: Elaborating and extending Linehan's theory. *Psychological Bulletin, 135*(3), 495–510.

Digman, J. M. (1997). Higher-order factors of the Big Five. *Journal of Personality and Social Psychology, 73*(6), 1246–1256.

Eisenberg, N., Fabes, R. A., Guthrie, I. K., & Reiser, M. (2000). Dispositional emotionality and regulation: Their role in predicting quality of social functioning. *Journal of Personality and Social Psychology, 78*(1), 136–157.

English, T., & John, O. P. (2013). Understanding the social effects of emotion regulation: The mediating role of authenticity for individual differences in suppression. *Emotion, 13*(2), 314–329.

Fava, M., Farabaugh, A. H., Sickinger, A. H., Wright, E., Alpert, J. E., Sonawalla, S., et al. (2002). Personality disorders and depression. *Psychological Medicine: A Journal of Research in Psychiatry and the Allied Sciences, 32*(6), 1049–1057.

Fournier, J. C., DeRubeis, R. J., Shelton, R. C., Gallop, R., Amsterdam, J. D., & Hollon, S. D. (2008). Antidepressant medications v. cognitive therapy in people with depression with or without personality disorder. *British Journal of Psychiatry, 192*(2), 124–129.

Fournier, J. C., DeRubeis, R. J., Shelton, R. C., Hollon, S. D., Amsterdam, J. D., & Gallop, R. (2009). Prediction of response to medication and cognitive therapy in the treatment of moderate to severe depression. *Journal of Consulting and Clinical Psychology, 77*(4), 775–787.

Fredrickson, B. L., & Levenson, R. W. (1998). Positive emotions speed recovery from the cardiovascular sequelae of negative emotions. *Cognition and Emotion, 12*, 191–220.

Fredrickson, B. L., Mancuso, R. A., Branigan, C., & Tugade, M. M. (2000). The undoing effect of positive emotions. *Motivation and Emotion, 24*(4), 237–258.

Gray, J. A., & McNaughton, N. (2000). *The neuropsychology of anxiety: An enquiry into the functions of the septo-hippocampal system.* Oxford, UK: Oxford University Press.

Gross, J. J., & John, O. P. (2003). Individual differences in two emotion regulation processes: Implications for affect, relationships, and well-being. *Journal of Personality and Social Psychology, 85*(2), 348–362.

Gross, L. (2006). How the human brain detects unexpected events. *PLoS Biology, 4*(12), e443.

Kendler, K. S., Prescott, C. A., Myers, J., & Neale, M. C. (2003). The structure of genetic and environmental risk factors for common psychiatric and substance use disorders in men and women. *Archives of General Psychiatry, 60*(9), 929–937.

Kernis, M. H., & Goldman, B. M. (2006). A multicomponent conceptualization of authenticity: Theory and research. In M. P. Zanna (Ed.), *Advances in experimental social psychology* (Vol. 38, pp. 283–357). San Diego, CA: Elsevier Academic Press.

Klein, D. N., Riso, L. P., Donaldson, S. K., Schwartz, J. E., Anderson, R. L., Ouimette, P. C., et al. (1995). Family study of early-onset dysthymia: Mood and personality disorders in relatives of outpatients with dysthymia and episodic major depression and normal controls. *Archives of General Psychiatry, 52*(6), 487–496.

Krause, E. D., Mendelson, T., & Lynch, T. R. (2003). Childhood emotional invalidation and adult psychological distress: The mediating role of emotional inhibition. *Child Abuse and Neglect, 27*(2), 199–213.

Krueger, R. F. (1999). Personality traits in late adolescence predict mental disorders in early adulthood: A prospective-epidemiological study. *Journal of Personality, 67*(1), 39–65.

Krueger, R. F., Caspi, A., Moffitt, T. E., Silva, P. A., & McGee, R. (1996). Personality traits are differentially linked to mental disorders: A multitrait–multidiagnosis study of an adolescent birth cohort. *Journal of Abnormal Psychology, 105*(3), 299–312.

Linehan, M. M. (1993). *Cognitive-behavioral treatment of borderline personality disorder.* New York: Guilford Press.

Linehan, M. M., Bohus, M., & Lynch, T. R. (2007). Dialectical behaviour therapy for pervasive emotion dysregulation: Theoretical and practical underpinnings. In J. J. Gross (Ed.), *Handbook of emotion regulation* (pp. 581–605). New York: Guilford Press.

Löw, A., Lang, P. J., Smith, J. C., & Bradley, M. M. (2008). Both predator and prey: Emotional arousal in threat and reward. *Psychological Science, 19*(9), 865–873.

Lynch, T. R. (in press). *Radically open dialectical behavior therapy for disorders of overcontrol.* New York: Guilford Press.

Lynch, T. R., & Cheavens, J. S. (2008). Dialectical behavior therapy for comorbid personality disorders. *Journal of Clinical Psychology, 64*(2), 154–167.

Lynch, T. R., Gray, K. L., Hempel, R. J., Titley, M., Chen, E. Y., & O'Mahen, H. A. (2013). Radically open-dialectical behavior therapy for adult anorexia nervosa: Feasibility and outcomes from an inpatient program. *BMC Psychiatry, 13*, 293. Available at *www.biomedcentral.com/1471-244X/13/293.*

Lynch, T. R., Hempel, R. J., & Dunkley, C. (in press). Remembering our tribal nature: Radically open-dialectical behavior therapy for disorders of overcontrol. *American Journal of Psychotherapy.*

Lynch, T. R., Morse, J. Q., Mendelson, T., & Robins, C. J. (2003). Dialectical behavior therapy for depressed older adults: A randomized pilot study. *American Journal of Geriatric Psychiatry, 11*(1), 33–45.

Lynch, T. R., Robins, C. J., Morse, J. Q., & Krause, E. D. (2001). A mediational model relating affect intensity, emotion inhibition, and psychological distress. *Behavior Therapy, 32*(3), 519–536.

Lynch, T. R., Schneider, K. G., Rosenthal, M. Z., & Cheavens, J. S. (2007). A mediational model of trait negative affectivity, dispositional thought suppression, and intrusive thoughts following laboratory stressors. *Behaviour Research and Therapy, 45*(4), 749–761.

Lynch, T. R., Trost, W. T., Salsman, N., & Linehan, M. M. (2007). Dialectical behavior therapy for borderline personality disorder. *Annual Review of Clinical Psychology, 3*, 181–205.

Markon, K. E., Krueger, R. F., & Watson, D. (2005). Delineating the structure of normal and abnormal personality: An integrative hierarchical approach. *Journal of Personality and Social Psychology, 88*(1), 139–157.

Mauss, I. B., Shallcross, A. J., Troy, A. S., John, O. P., Ferrer, E., Wilhelm, F. H., et al. (2011). Don't hide your happiness!: Positive emotion dissociation, social connectedness, and psychological functioning. *Journal of Personality and Social Psychology, 100*(4), 738–748.

McCraty, R., Barrios-Choplin, B., Rozman, D., Atkinson, M., & Watkins, A. D. (1998). The impact of a new emotional self-management program on stress, emotions, heart rate variability, DHEA and cortisol. *Integrative Physiological and Behavioral Science, 33*(2), 151–170.

Meeus, W., Van de Schoot, R., Klimstra, T., & Branje, S. (2011). Personality types in adolescence: Change and stability and links with adjustment and relationships: A five-wave longitudinal study. *Developmental Psychology, 47*(4), 1181–1195.

Moffitt, T. E., Arseneault, L., Belsky, D., Dickson, N., Hancox, R. J., Harrington, H., et al. (2011). A gradient of childhood self-control predicts health, wealth, and public safety. *Proceedings of the National Academy of Sciences of the USA, 108*(7), 2693–2698.

Morse, J. Q., & Lynch, T. R. (2004). A preliminary investigation of self-reported personality disorders in late life: Prevalence, predictors of depressive severity, and clinical correlates. *Aging and Mental Health, 8*(4), 307–315.

Murata, T., Takahashi, T., Hamada, T., Omori, M., Kosaka, H., Yoshida, H., et al. (2004). Individual trait anxiety levels characterizing the properties of Zen meditation. *Neuropsychobiology, 50*(2), 189–194.

Peng, S. M., Koo, M., & Yu, Z. R. (2009). Effects of music and essential oil inhalation on cardiac autonomic balance in healthy individuals. *Journal of Alternative and Complementary Medicine, 15*(1), 53–57.

Porges, S. W. (1995). Orienting in a defensive world: Mammalian modifications of our evolutionary heritage: A polyvagal theory. *Psychophysiology, 32*(4), 301–318.

Porges, S. W. (2001). The polyvagal theory: Phylogenetic substrates of a social nervous system. *International Journal of Psychophysiology, 42*(2), 123–146.

Reis, H. T., & Patrick, B. C. (1996). Attachment and intimacy: Component processes. In E. T. Higgins & A. W. Kruglanski (Eds.), *Social psychology: Handbook of basic principles* (pp. 523–563). New York: Guilford Press.

Riso, L. P., Blandino, J. A., Penna, S., Dacey, S., Grant, M. M., Du Toit, P. L., et al. (2003). Cognitive aspects of chronic depression. *Journal of Abnormal Psychology, 112*(1), 72–80.

Robins, R. W., John, O. P., Caspi, A., Moffitt, T. E., & Stouthamer-Loeber, M. (1996). Resilient, overcontrolled, and undercontrolled boys: Three replicable personality types. *Journal of Personality and Social Psychology, 70*(1), 157–171.

Rosenthal, M. Z., Cheavens, J. S., Lejuez, C. W., & Lynch, T. R. (2005). Thought suppression mediates the relationship between negative affect and borderline personality disorder symptoms. *Behaviour Research and Therapy, 43*(9), 1173–1185.

Schauer, M., & Elbert, T. (2010). Dissociation following traumatic stress: Etiology and treatment. *Zeitschrift für Psychologie/Journal of Psychology, 218*(2), 109–127.

Schneider, K. G., Hempel, R. J., & Lynch, T. R. (2013). That "poker face" just might lose you the game!: The impact of expressive suppression and mimicry on sensitivity to facial expressions of emotion. *Emotion, 13*(5), 852–866.

Takahashi, T., Murata, T., Hamada, T., Omori, M., Kosaka, H., Kikuchi, M., et al. (2005). Changes in EEG and autonomic nervous activity during meditation and their association with personality traits. *International Journal of Psychophysiology, 55*(2), 199–207.

Tang, Y., Ma, Y., Fan, Y., Feng, H., Wang, J., Feng, S., et al. (2009). Central and autonomic nervous system interaction is altered by short-term meditation. *Proceedings of the National Academy of Sciences, 106*(22), 8865–8870.

Tyrer, P., Mitchard, S., Methuen, C., & Ranger, M. (2003). Treatment-rejecting and treatment-seeking personality disorders: Type R and Type S. *Journal of Personality Disorders, 17*(3), 263–267.

Watson, D., Clark, L. A., & Harkness, A. R. (1994). Structures of personality and their relevance to psychopathology. *Journal of Abnormal Psychology, 103*(1), 18–31.

White, J. M. (1999). Effects of relaxing music on cardiac autonomic balance and anxiety after acute myocardial infarction. *American Journal of Critical Care, 8*(4), 220–230.

Wu, S.-D., & Lo, P.-C. (2008). Inward-attention meditation increases parasympathetic activity: A study based on heart rate variability. *Biomedical Research, 29*(5), 245–250.

Zucker, N. L., Losh, M., Bulik, C. M., LaBar, K. S., Piven, J., & Pelphrey, K. A. (2007). Anorexia nervosa and autism spectrum disorders: Guided investigation of social cognitive endophenotypes. *Psychological Bulletin, 133*(6), 976–1006.

chapter 16

Treatment of Violence-Prone Individuals with Psychopathic Personality Traits

Stephen C. P. Wong

Psychopathy is characterized by a constellation of personality traits pertaining mainly to the affective and interpersonal domains. Psychopathic and violence-prone individuals are challenging to treat. Despite advances in the assessment and treatment of personality disorders, in the assessment and prediction of recidivism and violence, and in offender rehabilitation,[1] there is, as yet, no generally acceptable treatment approach for violence-prone adults with psychopathic traits.[2] An integration of these areas of research and practice may shed light on the effective treatment of adults to reduce risk of aggression and violence. This is the goal of this chapter.

ASSESSMENT OF PSYCHOPATHY

Psychopathy is a psychological construct underpinned by a number of personality traits that, taken together, are often described as a personality disorder.

[1] *Offender rehabilitation* refers to services provided to offenders to reduce the risk of or actual reoffending. The services may vary from formal clinical interventions to offender case management processes and so forth.

[2] *Offender* is used as a generic term to refer to those who have had contact with or are held by law in the criminal justice or forensic mental health systems.

The point of departure of the current conception of psychopathy is Cleckley's (1941) description of the construct. This emphasizes affective deficits, such as shallow affect, lack of remorse and shame, callousness and lack of empathy, and dysfunctional social functioning, such as egocentricity, manipulativeness, unwillingness to accept responsibility, insincerity, lying, and antisociality (Cleckley, 1941; Hare, 2003). The most widely used and researched method of assessment is the Psychopathy Checklist—Revised (PCL-R[3]; Hare, 2003), a 20-item symptom construct rating scale. The PCL-R broadly comprises two correlated factors: Factor 1 (F1), which taps interpersonal and affective traits, and Factor 2 (F2), which represents unstable behaviors, including impulsivity, persistent antisocial and criminal behaviors, and a poorly regulated and unstable lifestyle. However, the number of factors indicative of psychopathy continues to be debated (Cooke & Michie, 2001; Hare, 2003; Patrick, 2006). There are other systems and tools to conceptualize and assess psychopathy, such as that of Lilienfeld and Fowler (2006) and Blackburn (1993). For the purpose of this chapter, the PCL-R is used as the operational definition of psychopathy.

DEFINITION OF VIOLENCE

A problem encountered when evaluating, predicting, and treating violent behavior associated with personality disorder is the lack of a universally accepted definition of violence; the term is used broadly to describe various actions resulting in physical or psychological harm to people. Moreover, definitions have changed over time and with technological developments. For example, cyberbullying, or bullying over the Internet, with no direct physical or even visual contact, has been deemed a form of violence (Kowalski, Limber, Patricia, & Agatston, 2007). Most violent behaviors are also illegal and criminal, except, for example, acts of war. For researchers, defining violence as "behaviors that can or are expected to lead to significant physical or psychological harm" (see Wong & Gordon, 2006, p. 288) would probably suffice as a working definition. However, the definition of the criterion or outcome variable for treatment can range from self- or third-party reports of violence to informal or formal contact with mental health or criminal justice agencies to formal adjudications, convictions, and incarceration; the base rate also varies accordingly. There are also different types of violent behaviors, such as nonsexual, sexual, and domestic violence, and different corresponding treatment approaches, as is discussed later. Violence reduction, of necessity, is a broad term that refers to the reduction of the severity and/or frequency of violent behaviors against others (see Di Placido, Simon, Witte, Gu, & Wong, 2006; Yang, Wong, & Coid, 2010). This definition of violence excludes self-harming

[3]The PCL—Screening Version (PCL-SV) is included in discussions of the PCL-R.

and suicidal behaviors. The criterion variable for violence reduction treatment should be set according to the specific goal of the treatment and the practicality of data collection.

A BRIEF OVERVIEW OF PSYCHOPATHY TREATMENT LITERATURE

Although there is extensive therapeutic nihilism regarding the treatment of psychopathy, there are in fact few well-designed studies. A narrative review by Wong (2000) found that few studies used clearly defined assessment criteria, provided an adequate description of the treatment approach, or used control groups with appropriate outcome measures. One of the best designed studies reported treatment that was considered unsuitable for individuals with psychopathy even by the studies' authors (Rice, Harris, & Cormier, 1989): Treatment involved participants operating the program and even prescribing medication to each other. Little wonder that treatment appears to actually increase violence recidivism (Rice et al., 1989; Rice, Harris, & Cormier, 1992). Subsequently, Salekin (2002) reported a meta-analysis based on 42 studies and concluded that there was a significant mean rate of successful intervention. However, Harris and Rice (2006) pointed out multiple methodological problems with the meta-analysis. Many of the studies Salekin included were completed before the development of objective measures of psychopathy; hence, only four studies used the PCL-R, and few included a control group. Harris and Rice also questioned the methodologies used to constitute a comparison group. Another systematic review also pointed out the poor state of the psychopathy treatment literature (D'Silva, Duggan, & McCarthy, 2004). In essence, Salekin's and D'Silva and colleagues' analyses included so few well-designed studies that it is difficult to draw any meaningful conclusion about which treatment approach is more efficacious.

A more recent review (Salekin, Worley, & Grimes, 2010) included a few new studies with positive results but highlighted both the lack of good consistent evidence on treatment efficacy and the lack of theories to guide treatment. They mentioned a "mental model" for the treatment of psychopathy in youth but no provided no details. A further review (Polaschek, 2014) also pointed out the lack of empirical support for the commonly held belief that offenders with psychopathy are "untreatable" and highlighted more recent positive outcome studies. Despite recent optimism, a clearly articulated model for the treatment of psychopathy is still lacking.

Psychopathy is a personality disorder, but most, if not all, individuals with psychopathy come into contact with the forensic mental health or the criminal justice systems not because of their disorder but because of their criminality and violence. It is not against the law to have a personality disorder! Their releases from various forms of involuntary detentions or civil commitments, almost without exception, are contingent on reducing their risk of violence and antisocial behaviors. As such, one of the objectives of their treatment and management should be concerned with the reduction of violence, and this is the treatment objective used in this chapter.

TREATMENT OF PERSONALITY DISORDER: THE GENERIC–SPECIFIC FACTORS

In terms of the treatment of personality disorder generally, systematic reviews and evaluation research, some based on randomized controlled trials, show that some treatments are effective (e.g., Linehan, 1993). Although this chapter cannot discuss this literature in detail, Livesley (2003, 2007a, 2007b) concluded that most therapies have comparable efficacy (see also Livesley, Dimaggio, & Clarkin, Chapter 1, this volume). This suggests that all effective therapies share some common or generic factors that account for the observed changes. These generic factors include the establishment of a therapeutic alliance or a positive and supportive engagement between therapists and clients (Beck, Freeman, Davis, & Associates, 2004; Livesley, 2007b).

Despite these commonalities, most therapies address a limited number of problems, and none is sufficiently comprehensive to cover the broad range of problems usually found among those with personality disorders. Some treatments are more focused on issues with emotional dysregulation, others on modifying maladaptive cognitive schemas and the like. A problem-based selection of what works for whom means the identification of specific problems, which are then matched with the appropriate treatments; this has been referred to as the "specific factors" approach in personality disorder treatment (Livesley, 2007a, 2007b).

The generic–specific model of treatment is highly congruent with Palmer's (1996) distinction between nonprogrammatic (generic) and programmatic (specific) factors in offender rehabilitation and reduction of recidivism. Nonprogrammatic factors included the appropriate matching of staff–offender interaction styles and staff personality characteristics such as interpersonal sensitivity, openness, warmth, and so forth. Programmatic factors included target interventions such as prosocial skills training, cognitive-behavioral skills training, education, vocational training, family interventions, and so forth, essentially the specific factors.

The evidence also supports the importance of the interaction between service providers and offenders in determining reoffending rates: Where there was positive mutual regard between staff and youth offenders, only 10% of those participants failed, compared with 40% of those with low mutual regard (Jesness, Allison, McCormick, Wedge, & Young, 1975, pp. 153–154, as cited in Palmer, 1996). The association between positive regard and recidivism was more likely a consequence of differences in the caseworkers' behavior toward the clients than of common client characteristics. The nonspecific factor of client positive regard for staff potentiated whatever specific treatment effects were present and contributed about as much to outcome as did type of treatment (Jesness, 1975, p. 759; as cited in Wong & Hare, 2005, p. 49).

The risk–need–responsivity (RNR) framework is one of the most widely used models in offender rehabilitation work (see Andrews & Bonta, 2010). After reviewing the results of 70 meta-analyses on offender rehabilitation, McGuire (2008, p. 2591) concluded that the RNR was currently the best validated model for offender rehabilitation. The RNR principles are intended for offender rehabilitation in general, but some have estimated that as much as 50% of the male offender population can be considered as suffering from some form of personality disorder, primarily antisocial personality disorder (APD) (Fazel & Danesh, 2002). As well, Andrews and Bonta (2010) have suggested that RNR principles are relevant to the treatment of personality disorder in general and APD in particular in that personality disorder can be considered as a responsivity consideration.

The RNR approach proposes that intensity of treatment should match the clients' risk level—the *risk* principle. The *need* principle stipulates that the individual's criminogenic needs—that is, the thoughts, feelings, and behaviors that cause or closely associate with violence or criminality, such as criminal attitudes and peer groups and so on—must be identified and targeted in treatment. The need principle guides the identification of targets and processes of intervention, that is, what to treat. The *responsivity* principle posits that treatment methods must accommodate the clients' idiosyncratic characteristics, such as their learning styles, readiness for treatment, cultural backgrounds, and so forth. For example, Andrews and Bonta (1994) underscored the importance of the relationship between correctional workers and offenders as being "open, flexible, and enthusiastic . . . wherein people feel free to express their opinions, feelings and experiences." Other qualities include respect, caring, attentiveness, and expression of understanding, including modeling prosocial and disapproving antisocial behaviors, and so forth (see Andrews & Bonta, 1994, p. 410). Paul Gendreau (1996), writing about the principle of effective intervention with offenders within the RNR framework, noted that staff should relate to offenders in interpersonally sensitive and constructive ways; be firm but fair, strong but understanding, and caring. The relevant interpersonal skills should include clarity in communication, warmth, humor, openness, and the ability to manage professional boundaries in order to work collaboratively with participants, to foster good working alliances, and to model prosocial behaviors so as to be an effective source of positive reinforcement for program participants.

The responsivity principle within the RNR framework for offender rehabilitation is similar in many ways to the generic factor within the generic–specific framework for the treatment of personality disorder; similarly, the need and risk factors have many similarities with specific factors. Given the significant crossover between Livesley's (2007b) framework on the treatment of personality disorder and Andrews and Bonta's (2010) RNR framework on offender rehabilitation, it may be possible to integrate the treatment of psychopathy, a personality disorder, with reduction in violence and reoffending, a key requirement in offender rehabilitation.

PSYCHOPATHY, VIOLENCE, AND VIOLENCE REDUCTION TREATMENT

Extensive empirical evidence, including the results of meta-analyses, link psychopathy (assessed using the PCL-R) with criminality and violence; high-scoring individuals exhibit more violence and aggression in prospective follow-up studies (Walters, 2003; Walters, Wilson, & Glover, 2011; Yang et al., 2010). Although PCL-R total score can predict violence, the factor scores (F1 and F2) differ in their effectiveness in predicting violence. Recent meta-analyses showed that the chronic antisocial and unstable behaviors captured by F2 significantly predicted violence recidivism (with an AUC of about .65), whereas psychopathic personality traits, assessed by F1, predicted violence no better than chance with an area under the curve (AUC) of .56 with a 95% confidence interval overlapping with .5. The results were replicated in both ethnic groups in a recent study of a large sample (n = 435) of non-Aboriginal and Aboriginal male Canadian federal offenders (Olver, Neumann, Wong, & Hare, 2013). The lifestyle and antisocial factors (Factor 2) each significantly predicted violent and nonviolent recidivism among Aboriginal and non-Aboriginal groups, with corresponding AUC values of .65 and .77, respectively). By contrast, the interpersonal or affective factors (Factor 1) did not significantly predict any of the recidivism criteria for either ethnic offender group. The results were also replicated recently in a group of Belgian male offenders with learning disabilities (Pouls & Jeandarme, 2014). A group of mixed-gender Swedish forensic psychiatric patients and offenders assessed with the PCL—Screening Version (Douglas, Strand, Belfrage, Fransson, & Levander, 2005) showed similar results. In a 24-year follow-up of a group of Canadian male offenders, again F1 did not significantly predict nonviolent, violent, or general recidivism, but F2 and total scores predicted marginally to moderately well at 3-, 5-, 10-, and 20-year follow-up (Olver & Wong, 2014). A further meta-analysis again showed that for sexual, violent, and violent-plus-sexual recidivism in a sex offender sample, F1 did not significantly predict all three recidivism outcomes, whereas F2 and total scores did (Hawes, Boccaccini, & Murrie, 2013). Research now has consistently showed that F2 rather than F1 predicts reoffending measured in different offender samples, with different outcomes and over different follow-up periods. While F1 and F2 may not individually predict recidivism, there could be interaction effects, that is, high F1 or F2 could potentiate recidivism predicted by the other factor. A recent meta-analysis failed to show significant interactions between F1 and F2 (Kennealy, Skeem, Walters, & Camp, 2010).

The evidence suggests that when treating violent offenders with psychopathy it is important to decompose the disorder into its components (see also Clarkin & Livesley, Chapter 4, this volume). Violence reduction treatment should be primarily directed at F2 characteristics linked to violent reoffending, and that a primary focus on F1 features (unrelated to violence) is unlikely to be effective; treatments attempting to change F1 personality, even if effective, are unlikely to reduce violence. However, this does not mean that F1 features can be ignored; an extensive literature indicates that F1 traits are closely linked to treatment-interfering and noncompliance behaviors and poor treatment performance, such as dropout. Offenders with psychopathy assessed using the PCL-R were resistant to and unmotivated toward treatment, showed little treatment improvement, and had high dropout rates (Ogloff, Wong, & Greenwood, 1990). In a sample of offenders with personality disorders treated in a high-security forensic mental health setting, higher PCL-R scores were associated with poorer therapeutic improvements (Hughes, Hogue, Hollin, & Champion, 1997). Similarly, in female substance abusers, higher PCL-R scores were associated with higher treatment attrition, noncompliance with drug tests, and inconsistent program attendance. At least two studies have examined the treatment responses as a function of F1 and F2 scores. Hobson, Shine, and Roberts (2000) showed that Factor 1 traits are strongly associated with treatment-interfering behaviors. In a recent study of male sex offenders participating in a cognitive-behaviorally based treatment, F1 and, in particular, the affective or Facet 2 of F1, together with being unmarried, uniquely predicted program attrition (Olver & Wong, 2011).

The overall results suggest that treatment directed at changing the F1 core psychopathic personality traits is unlikely to reduce violence, whereas treatment directed at changing chronic antisocial and poorly regulated behaviors—that is, F2 characteristics—is more likely to bring about reductions in violence. However, it is essential to contain treatment-interfering behaviors related to F1.

The literature on whether F1 and F2 are changeable on their own or with treatment is scant. Harpur and Hare (1994) showed that the magnitude of F2 decreased substantially with age (from a Factor 2 score of 13 to 4, a reduction of 67% from the late teens to the 60s)—a finding similar to the well-known age–crime curve (see U.S. Department of Justice, 1997)—whereas F1 remained quite constant over the same age bands. Such a decrease of F2 with age also signals that psychopathy, as measured by the PCL-R total score, can decrease through the reduction in F2 rather than F1 features. F2, given its strong links with recidivism, can be conceptualized as a proxy of an extended pattern of antisocial behaviors. The offender rehabilitation literature shows that treatments such as skill-based and behavioral methods reduce reoffending and antisocial behaviors.

The next section sets forth a model for the violence reduction treatment of individuals with psychopathic personality traits.

A MODEL FOR VIOLENCE REDUCTION TREATMENT OF INDIVIDUALS WITH PSYCHOPATHIC TRAITS

The treatment of violence-prone individuals with psychopathic traits can be conceptualized within a two-component model based on the PCL-R two-factor notion of psychopathy, the generic–specific framework in the treatment of personality disorder, and the RNR principles in offender rehabilitation (also see Wong, 2013; Wong, Gordon, Gu, Lewis, & Olver, 2012; Wong & Olver, 2015). Within this model, the objective of treatment is to reduce the risk of violence and antisocial behaviors rather than to effect changes in the core psychopathic personality features, that is, F1 characteristics.

Component 1 of the model is termed the *interpersonal component* (IC) that corresponds to PCL-R F1 interpersonal and affective features. The treatment implications of IC emphasize that it is important to engage and motivate the individual, to establish therapeutic alliance, to carefully manage and contain treatment-interfering behaviors, and to maintain professional boundaries such that the treatment program can be delivered as planned, that is, to maintain program integrity. The IC for treating psychopathy is analogous to the generic factor proposed for the treatment of personality disorder in general (Livesley, 2007b) and is closely aligned with the responsivity principle of the RNR model of offender rehabilitation (Andrews & Bonta, 2010).

Component 2 of the model is termed the *criminogenic component* (CC) and corresponds to F2 of the PCL-R. The treatment implications of CC are that effective treatment should be directed toward the individual's problem areas or criminogenic needs that are closely associated with violence and antisocial behaviors. Addressing these problem areas should reduce the risk of future violence. The CC is analogous to the specific factor proposed by Livesley (2007b) in the treatment of offenders with personality disorder and with the risk and need principles of the RNR model for offender rehabilitation (Andrews & Bonta, 2010). The model is discussed in more detail next.

Component 1: The Interpersonal Component

The treatment implications of the IC are to engage offenders in a functional working relationship or alliance in order to motivate them to engage in treatment and to manage treatment-interfering behaviors. Each of these interrelated issues is discussed in this section.

Motivating the Unmotivated

Psychopathy is almost synonymous with the lack of motivation to change; some may say there is no better example of an oxymoron than that of a treatment-motivated psychopath! Individuals with psychopathy should not be expected to be *intrinsically* motivated to change, as, by definition, those who refuse to accept responsibility for their actions, see themselves as superior, and show little empathy (essentially F1 traits) are unlikely to have an intrinsic need for change. There may be *extrinsic* reasons for wanting to change, such as the opportunity for release, reduced security, or other short-term personal benefits. These externally based or, in some cases, "talking the talk" motivations, which may appear to be disingenuous, shallow, or insincere, are quite frequently what one has to work with, at least at the beginning. As such, intrinsic motivation for change should not be stipulated as a prerequisite for entry into treatment (also see Livesley, 2007a, p. 219); otherwise, we can easily put people with psychopathy into a Catch-22 situation: If they have no intrinsic motivation to change, they cannot be accepted for treatment, and, without treatment, they will likely not be intrinsically motivated. Being intrinsically or sincerely motivated for treatment is tantamount to expressing a willingness to collaborate and work with the treatment providers to address entrenched personal problems; to form a functional interpersonal working relationship with the therapist to work on issues that may be deeply threatening or alien to oneself. The psychopathic personality traits are the antithesis of such undertakings, and, if a person with psychopathy, in fact, were so motivated, he or she would have already made significant personality changes for the better. As such, taking people with psychopathy into treatment only when they are intrinsically motivated is tantamount to offering treatment only to those who have already improved and may not require treatment. One of the IC treatment objectives is to work with the individual to develop some intrinsic motivation for prosocial behaviors by starting with extrinsic motivation.

Motivational interviewing techniques, as described by Miller and Rollnick (2012), are often used to facilitate the treatment engagement of resistant and unmotivated clients by attending to four key principles: expressing empathy, developing discrepancies, rolling with resistance, and supporting self-efficacy. The approach is useful in working with individuals with psychopathy who appear to be unmotivated and resistant, who project blame, and who are argumentative and constantly playing one-upmanship. Expressing empathy may not come easily to some therapists because of the horrendous acts that some individuals with psychopathy have committed. Maintaining one's professionalism may alleviate some personal reactions and help maintain objectivity. Developing discrepancy is often the key to opening the door ever so slightly for the person to see his or her self-defeating behaviors. The following vignette illustrates how the four principles of motivational interviewing can be applied in a therapy session with an offender with psychopathy.

THERAPIST: So, what do you want to get out of the program?

OFFENDER: Nothing, there is nothing I want from this "Mickey Mouse" program that I don't already know and I don't want to be in it anyways. I know the research too; many guys who'd been through it still get back into trouble, right? [arrogant; testing and pulling for an argument]

THERAPIST: Mm, well, didn't you say you want to get a lower security classification? [Trying to convince the offender of the usefulness of the program at this point will likely precipitate an argument, and is therefore counterproductive.]

OFFENDER: They'd never give it to me anyways. They are too stupid to do those classifications right and they only do them right for guys they like. The system is all screwed up and you can never get a fair deal. You have seen how it works, right? Well, I am not lying, am I? [again, pulling for an argument]

THERAPIST: Well, if you say so. [Roll with resistance and avoid argumentation.] But I can understand it is frustrating to keep getting stuck and don't feel you can get out of it. [express empathy] Just curious, what happened in your last reclassification meeting? [priming for information to show how the offender might have been sabotaging himself]

OFFENDER: I told that SOB to put that piece of paper where it belongs; you know what I mean? You should look at his face when I said that, ha ha! Teach him a lesson or two, right? Well, I don't care and so what. There is always next time.

THERAPIST: Yeah, it is frustrating getting turned down three times in a row, isn't it? [express empathy and support] Well, ... mmm, but, how is all that helping you get what you want? [develop discrepancy: wanting security reduction but repeatedly shooting himself in the foot]

OFFENDER: I know what you mean but that is what he deserved. He asked for it, so, what can I do? [not my fault, but he is not shutting the door completely]

THERAPIST: Yeah, that hasn't worked for you; [avoid argument, express support without denigrating the established process] maybe try something different, you know. Say, the other day you were pretty cool telling that guard what you want when he wasn't too keen on getting it for you. [support self-efficacy] Something like that may work, you know. Think about it, and we can talk about that next time we meet. [Don't push too hard too fast; the door may have cracked open slightly for the seed to be planted.]

Motivation, or getting buy-in, at best, is achieved by building on small gains. Given the many adversities these individuals have experienced and the reinforcement they received for their dysfunctional behaviors, buy-in is not something that can be achieved in one step. How many of our own New Year's resolutions go by the wayside? Rolling with resistance and avoiding argumentation are particularly useful approaches with offenders with psychopathy, who are highly adapt in drawing the therapist into meaningless debates, thereby gaining control of the situation and side-stepping relevant issues. As in judo or tai chi, by rolling with resistance, the destructive forces can be dissipated not by opposing or pushing back—that is, by confrontation (at least early in therapy)—but by skillfully redirecting them away in a harmless way. The inexperienced therapist may be drawn into an argument and waste much time and energy trying to win that argument, which is not the goal. The goal for the therapist is to redirect challenges and provocations by keeping the treatment goal in mind and then trying to find a way to get individuals with psychopathy to try new behaviors (e.g., being assertive rather than aggressive in the security review meeting) that, hopefully, help the offender to attain goals he failed to achieve with more dysfunctional behaviors (e.g., arguing with the security officer). Although the reinforcement contingencies are similar to what one would use when working with offenders without psychopathy, the approaches needed to manage therapeutic interactions with individuals with psychopathy can be quite different. When the working alliance is tenuous, resistance is best managed by stepping back (rolling with resistance) and trying another approach or simply planting a seed that can be taken up later. Within a more robust alliance, a more direct approach can be tried. The therapist must be very goal oriented, find the path of least resistance to get to the goal, and avoid the many traps and distractions on the way.

Building Working Alliances

As is the case when treating all forms of personality disorder, a good alliance is essential in treating psychopathy (Wong & Hare, 2005) but, unfortunately, difficult to achieve. The concept of working alliance can be decomposed into three domains: bond, task, and goal (Bordin, 1994, 1994; Wong & Hare, 2005, pp. 19–20). In treatment, the therapist and client work collaboratively on shared treatment *tasks* (specific factors) to reach the agreed-on and shared *goals* (specific factors), sustained by positive affective regard or *bond* (generic factors) between them. The bond is often considered key to a good alliance. However, those with high F1 Facet 2 callous unemotional traits have difficulty maintaining affective bonds. Sometimes, their superficial verbalization of affective words—saying they are "so sorry" but without the affective "music" or genuine felt affective responses (see McCord & McCord, 1964)—in individual or group therapy (e.g., empathy training) can reinforce the perception of the individual's lack of sincerity and inability to engage and signal that treatment is not progressing. Staff may conclude that treatment has failed and reject any further therapeutic work with the individual, leading to treatment termination. Olver and Wong (2010) reported that the affective facet of the PCL-R and marital status uniquely predicted treatment dropout in a sex offender program with a number of offenders with psychopathy. Such therapeutic nihilism can readily become a self-fulfilling prophecy.

The difficulty that the individual with psychopathy has in bonding with the therapist should not be taken as a litmus test of treatment failure or noncompliance. Therapists can still work collaboratively with the individual to set goals and to work on tasks needed to reach the goals within a respectful and professional relationship. Also, even those with relatively high PCL-R scores may not fit the callous unemotional prototype often attributed to them. Though not common, it is possible to have a PCL-R total score of 32 (about the 91st percentile and deemed by most to be quite psychopathic) with all eight F1 items scoring 1, indicating uncertainty about whether the items can be applied to the individual. This is another reason that it is important to read both the PCL-R total and the F1 and F2 scores carefully before making statements about the individual's F1 psychopathic traits.

The tasks and goals are discussed in detail under the CC, or Component 2, as they pertain to problem areas linked to violence and antisocial behaviors. For example, the interpersonally intimidating and aggressive responses shown to the security officer in the vignette can be replaced and moderated by more assertive and appropriate behaviors (tasks) to achieve the goal of lowering a security classification.

Containing Treatment-Interfering Behaviors and Maintaining Professional Boundaries

Working with forensic clients presents a special challenge in maintaining professional boundaries. Many offenders grew up in chaotic families and social environments, and many have experienced physical or sexual abuse (boundary violations) that deprived them of appropriate role models for how to set limits and maintain interpersonal boundaries. Such difficulties are magnified in individuals with psychopathy by their Facet 1 interpersonally exploitative traits such as lying, conning, manipulation, narcissism, and failure to take responsibility for their actions (see Wong & Hare, 2005, pp. 19–20). They tend to play staff members against each other, spread rumors and innuendoes, and intimidate staff members and other program participants. When staff members feel lied to, preyed upon, intimated, and victimized, they may question or blame one another and lose focus on treating the individual. These are serious treatment-interfering behaviors that can evoke strong negative reactions from staff, leading to staff splitting, boundary violations, and even the demoralization of the treatment team, thus compromising treatment integrity, that is, the delivery of treatment as designed. An important task for therapists when treating psychopathy is to manage their own reactions; in essence, to inoculate themselves against treatment-interfering behaviors. Working on building and repairing the alliance requires the therapist to manage such reactions.

The reactions to treatment-interfering behaviors, together with the inability to engage offenders with psychopathy in treatment, may lead to feelings of despair, hopelessness, helplessness, inadequacy, or personal failure among staff. The externalization of these feelings may lead to the use of highly punitive means to regain control of the situation, showing hostile reactions such as lashing back in anger, engaging in battles of will, or, in some cases, falling prey to the machinations of the person with psychopathy, such as becoming his or her mouthpiece or forming unprofessional liaisons with him or her and avoiding meaningful therapeutic contact. All these instances of boundary violations are obviously the antithesis of good treatment. However, from the perspective of the individual with psychopathy, they may be desired outcomes, reflecting an intentional or unintentional desire to exploit treatment. Staff members have to recognize and manage such behaviors. Ways to promote a collaborative working relationship while minimizing the likelihood of boundary violation are discussed next (see Bowers, 2002; Doren, 1987; Wong & Hare, 2005).

The key in managing these problems is to maintain objectivity, be nonjudgmental, and avoid labeling or demonizing psychopathy. It often helps to try to separate the person from his or her behaviors; most people with psychopathy do not fit the extreme prototype often used to illustrate psychopathy. Not all individuals with psychopathy are serial killers or sexual sadists. Indeed, psychopathic personality can be viewed as a maladaptive variant of common personality traits (Widiger, Simonsen, Sirovatka, & Regier, 2006). The behaviors characterized by F1 are those that brought the individual into treatment and not reasons for discharging them from treatment. The ideas that psychopathy is untreatable or that treatment can make psychopathy worse are not supported empirically.

To counteract the interpersonal manipulation and staff splitting, it is best for staff to work as a cohesive team rather than individually; this decreases individual vulnerability to manipulation and machination. A small, highly cohesive team of three or four members can usually provide the range of interventions needed. This approach lessens the chance of staff splitting and provides opportunities for mutual support and debriefing. It allows staff members to work through any negative feelings engendered by psychopathic behaviors with colleagues rather expressing them toward the individual—a process that Bower (2002) called reciprocal emotional pumping. The support engendered in this way increases staff resiliency and personal resolve in one's work. For those managing clients with psychopathy in solo practices, it is advisable to seek supervision and debriefings from competent colleagues on a routine basis.

It is key to recognize and repair staff splitting proactively by being aware of deviations from the group's or one's usual clinical practices and be willing to point them out within the team in a constructive and caring manner. Staff may wish to form a buddy system (dyads or triads) for the purpose of monitoring one another's behaviors on boundary issues. Teams should always follow explicit and structured treatment plans and be mindful of deviation from usual practices. This requires open lines of communication within the team and regular discussions of each person's perception of the individual's treatment plan and progress. Staff members also need to be acutely aware of typical maneuvers used by individuals with psychopathy, such as convincing a staff member to keep small secrets—a conditioning tactic that is often the beginning of a slippery slope. The limits of confidentiality have to be clearly articulated and agreed to by all staff members and shared with the offender. Goals should be revisited and reset at preset intervals to avoid drifts from established goals. Any changes should be gradual. When treating these individuals, one should be cautious about dramatic improvements. These kinds of precautions can go some way toward maintaining treatment integrity and motivating the individual to engage in interventions to reduce the risk of violence. These interventions are discussed next as part of Component 2 of the model.

Component 2: Criminogenic Component

The CC of the model entails identifying and treating specific problems of the individual with psychopathy that are the causes of, or closely associated with, violence.

What to Treat?

The CC is linked to F2. Although research suggests that F2 predicts violence and that items such as "parasitic lifestyle" or "lacking in long-term goals" can change, it should be noted that that F2 was not developed to guide violence reduction treatment and that some items, such as "early behavioral problems" and "juvenile delinquency," are unchangeable. To capture the underlying variance of F2 for treatment purposes, it is essential to identify, preferably using a risk-assessment tool, dynamic or changeable risk predictors that are proxies of F2 whose reduction through treatment can decrease violence and antisociality. For example, the Violence Risk Scale (VRS; Wong & Gordon, 1999–2003, 2006) was developed as a dynamic risk-assessment and treatment-planning tool based on the RNR principles. The measure has 6 static and 20 dynamic risk predictors to assess risk of violence (risk principle), treatment targets (need principle), and treatment readiness (responsivity principle) and to measure risk change. Ratings of dynamic predictors (0, 1, 2, 3) indicate the strength of association between the predictor (such as criminal attitude) and violence. Examples of the dynamic predictors include antisocial attitudes and beliefs (e.g., loathing of law-abiding behaviors, justification of antisocial behaviors), emotion dysregulation (e.g., excessive anger, irritability), violent lifestyle (e.g., gang affiliation), aggressive interpersonal interaction style, substance use, and so forth.

The individual's readiness for treatment for each treatment target is then assessed using a modified version of the stages-of-change model (Prochaska, DiClemente, & Norcross, 1992) to establish a pretreatment baseline measure (e.g., at the contemplation stage before treatment). At the conclusion of treatment, the stage of change for each treatment target is reassessed (e.g., now at the action stage after treatment). Risk reduction is indicated by progression through the stages of change (e.g., from contemplation to action) and is translated into a quantitative reduction in violence risk. The pretreatment stage of change can be used to guide the selection of appropriate intervention strategies matched to the level of treatment readiness; the posttreatment risk level and the stage of change can be used to guide posttreatment risk management (Wong & Gordon, 2004).

The sum of 20 VRS dynamic items correlates strongly with F2 ($r = .80$, $p < .001$), thus capturing the F2 variance that predicts violent recidivism (AUC = .75; Wong & Gordon, 2006). As an illustration, a VRS assessment yields an individualized set of dynamic risk factors that specify the thoughts (rationalizing violent behaviors), feelings (anger), behaviors (interpersonal aggression), living conditions (access to intoxicants and/or negative peers), and so on that may put the individual at risk for reoffending and violence, and these become treatment targets. Figure 16.1 is a profile of the 20 VRS dynamic items showing the percentages of individuals who had identified the item as a treatment target in samples of general offenders and individuals with psychopathy. Although individuals with psychopathy have more VRS risk factors identified as treatment targets than general offenders, the types of risk factors endorsed by the two groups are similar, so the treatment targets for the two groups are largely the same. Changes in VRS dynamic predictors in a community sample of offenders with psychopathy (mean PCL-R = 26) participating in a violence reduction treatment are linked to reduction in violent recidivism (Lewis, Olver, & Wong, 2012; Olver, Lewis, & Wong, 2013). These findings are discussed in more detail later in the chapter. Although dynamic risk-assessment tools offer a systematic way to identify treatment needs, a combination of dynamic risk assessment and clinical case formulation is the preferred approach because individuals, especially those with more extreme scores, often have atypical treatment needs that are not identified by specialized risk-assessment tools.

How to Treat?

The term *treatment* is used broadly to refer to interventions conceptualized and delivered in a systematic manner to alleviate certain problematic conditions and that are empirically supported or rationally derived. This includes empirically supported psychotherapies, pharmacotherapy, highly structured and module-based programs delivered by nonclinically trained staff, such as prison or correctional officers, and also general counseling, casework, education, and occupational training used in offender rehabilitation to reduce reoffending that have been shown to be effective (Lipsey, 2009). The effectiveness of psychodynamic therapy and cognitive-behavioral and skill-based interventions is discussed because these approaches are most frequently reported in the literature (Salekin, 2002; Salekin et al., 2010; Wong, 2000).

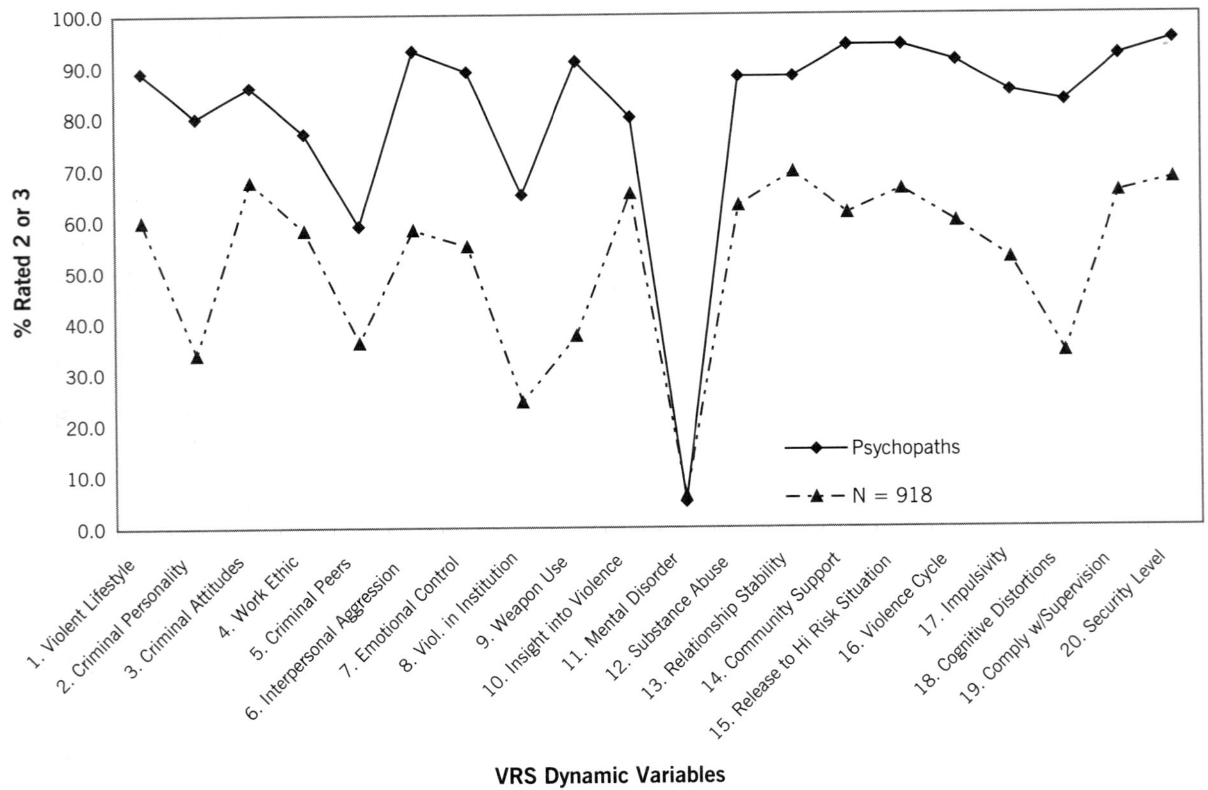

FIGURE 16.1. Dynamic risk profile assessed using the VRS. From Wong and Gordon (2006). Copyright 2006 by the American Psychological Association. Adapted by permission.

PSYCHODYNAMIC THERAPY

Gabbard (2004, p. 2) defined long-term psychodynamic psychotherapy as "a therapy that involves careful attention to the therapist–patient interaction, with thoughtfully timed interpretation of transference and resistance embedded in a sophisticated appreciation of the therapist's contribution to the two-person field." The effectiveness of any treatment is best evaluated by randomized controlled trials (RCTs). However, real-world applicability can be limited by the strict experimental controls and requirements of RCTs (Rothwell, 2005), so evaluation of treatment efficacy should not be limited to RCTs, as was pointed out by Hollin (2008). Unfortunately, few studies have evaluated the efficacy of psychodynamic therapy for psychopathy or APD. Leichsenring's (2010) review of 11 RCTs of psychodynamic psychotherapy for personality disorder noted that most were of borderline and cluster C personality disorders or a heterogeneous group of personality disorders and that none were of psychopathy or APD. Leichsenring and Leibing's (2003) earlier meta-analysis comparing the effectiveness of psychodynamic psychotherapy and cognitive-behavioral therapy (CBT) for personality disorders noted no significant differences. Only one study (Woody, McLellan, Luborsky, & O'Brien, 1985) investigated the outcome of a sample of drug addicts with APD, but offending behaviors were not used as outcomes.

The National Institute for Health and Care Excellence (NICE; 2009) treatment guidelines for APD with comments on the treatment of psychopathy based on review of the literature on treatment efficacy rather than any particular theoretical approach recommend a cognitive-behavioral group-based approach to reducing offending behaviors; no mention was made of the use of psychodynamic treatment approaches. The guidelines also suggest modifying and adapting the treatment approach to the needs of the individual, including treating comorbid disorders, adjusting treatment intensity to the client's needs, and monitoring progress, similar to the RNR principles. Providing strong and consistent staff support is also deemed particularly important. The guidelines suggest that pharmacological interventions should not be routinely used to treat APD or associated behaviors such as aggression, anger, and impulsivity.

The relevance of psychodynamic therapy also needs to be considered in the context of Stone's (2010) discussion of limiting or unfavorable factors in the treatment of personality disorder with psychodynamic therapy. He listed 10 factors that are likely to adversely affect treatment: (1) poor reflective capacity or concreteness of thought; (2) ego fragility; (3) poor empathic capacity; (4) impulsivity, especially if aggravated by substance abuse; (5) arrogance, grandiosity, contemptuousness, entitlement, and exploitativeness; (6) lying, deceitfulness, callousness, conning, and lack of remorse; (7) dismissive attachment style; (8) bitterness, indiscretion, shallowness, vindictiveness, sensation seeking; (9) controlling and taking pleasure in the suffering of others; and (10) marked rigidity of personality. Most of these attributes characterize psychopathic personality, including the majority of F1 features, suggesting substantial obstacles to using dynamic psychotherapy to treat psychopathy. However, even if F1 features could be addressed successfully, treatment is unlikely to reduce future violence because F1 features are not linked to violence.

COGNITIVE AND COGNITIVE-BEHAVIORAL/SKILL-BASED THERAPY

Cognitive therapies tend to take a more "pragmatic" approach to treating psychopathy and APD than some other therapies. For example, "rather than attempting to build a better moral structure through the induction of affect such as anxiety or shame (changing personality), cognitive therapy of APD can be conceptualized as improving moral and social behavior through enhancement of cognitive functioning" (Beck et al., 2004, p. 168). from essentially being self-serving and self-centered to taking into account others' feelings or perspectives—an enlightened self-interest approach. These improvements may lead to a lessened number of institutional misconducts or repeated reinstitutionalization. Beck and colleagues (2004) also acknowledged the importance of skill development to address deficits in perspective taking, impulse control, emotional regulation, frustration tolerance, communication and assertiveness, consequential thinking, and, of course, cognitive restructuring. In the treatment of psychopathy, cognitive therapy, CBT, and skill-based approaches have many common attributes. As such, these treatment approaches are considered together.

An extensive literature, including meta-analyses and narrative reviews (see Andrews et al., 1990; Gendreau & Ross, 1979; Lipsey, 2009; Lipsey & Wilson, 1998), often referred to as the "what works" literature as a rejoinder to the "nothing works" notion put forth by Martinson (1974), shows consistent positive evidence on the efficacy of some treatments to reduce reoffending, criminality, and antisocial behaviors among offenders, which include many with APD (50–80%; Fazel & Danesh, 2002; Hare, 2003) and psychopathy (4.5–15%; Hare, 2003). Of particular relevance is McGuire's (2008) review of 70 meta-analyses of offender treatment outcome studies between 1985 and 2007 and additional studies with primary data. McGuire concluded that "there is sufficient evidence currently available to substantiate the claim that personal violence can be reduced by psychosocial interventions" (p. 2577) and that "emotional self management, interpersonal skills, social problem solving and allied training approaches show mainly positive effects with a reasonably high degree of reliability" (p. 2591). Earlier meta-analyses also supported McGuire's overall results. A meta-analysis of 154 treatment comparisons of adult and young offenders found significantly larger effect sizes (phi = 0.30) in recidivism reduction for what was deemed "appropriate" treatment, that is, behaviorally oriented, delivered to high-risk cases, provided in well-structured programs, and focused on criminogenic needs (Andrews et al., 1990).

A more recent meta-analysis compared different types of counseling and skill-building approaches among juvenile offenders based on 548 independent study samples reported between 1958 and 2002 (Lipsey, 2009). The counseling approaches included individual, mentoring, family, family crisis, group, peer, mixed, and mixed with referral and skill building, including behavioral, cognitive-behavioral, social skills, challenge, academic, and job-related skills. Overall, there was no statistical difference in recidivism effects between the two approaches or between the different subtypes of intervention within each approach. Behavioral and cognitive-behavioral approaches led to a 20% reduction in recidivism rates compared with a 13% reduction for other approaches. Mentoring and group counseling showed a more than 20% reduction of recidivism compared with 13% or less in the rest. Statistically speaking, however, these differences were not significant. The author acknowledged that the lack of power because of the limited sample size and the use of random effect analyses models may have made it difficult to establish differential effects (Lipsey, 2009, p. 142). Treatment efficacy was reduced for juveniles with aggressive or violent histories, suggesting that caution should be exercised in generalizing these findings to adult offenders with psychopathic traits.

Overall, the meta-analytic evidence favors using a cognitive-behavioral skill-based treatment approach to reduce the risk of recidivism. Although the evidence suggests that no one treatment approach within the CBT skills-based framework is clearly better than another, it does not imply that one should not use a rationally derived process to justify the inclusion or exclusion of aspects of treatment that are better suited to different offender need profiles or management requirements. For example, for offenders with more serious substance abuse and/or gang affiliation problems and for offenders in prisons versus those in the community, the treatment program should be adjusted accordingly. One should attend to the research evidence but at the same time be sensitive to the demands of the individual, the group, or the treatment situation in order to make appropriate adjustments to the content and delivery of the program. One size just doesn't fit all. No violence reduction program meets the needs of all individuals. This is not surprising given the early state of psychopathy treatment and continued debate about psychopathy assessment. However, from my viewpoint, many existing treatments have useful components that could contribute to a more general program—most notably, the learning of cognitive and behavioral skills through didactic instructional and experiential methods, including modeling, role playing, performance feedback, and generalization training, as exemplified by aggression replacement training (Goldstein, 2004), along with relapse prevention (Laws, 1998; Marlatt & Gordon, 1985) and motivational interviewing techniques. Multisystemic therapy illustrates another feature of a general program, the importance of providing treatment "24 hours a day and seven days a week" (Henggeler, Schoenwald, Borduin, Rowland, & Cunningham, 1998, p. 43). Although the 24/7 notion is not always practical, the idea is that treatment and the generalization of new learning to the everyday environment should be part of program design. Organizing treatment based on the RNR principles is also key. The RNR principles and their theoretical underpinning, the psychology of criminal conduct (Andrews & Bonta, 2010), also highlight the importance of supporting prosocial endeavors (see the good life model, Ward & Brown, 2004; but also see Andrews, Bonta, & Wormith, 2011, for comments on the model) besides reduction of antisocial and violence behaviors. The violence reduction program (see Wong & Gordon, 2013) attempts to combine all these features within one program; evaluations of its effectiveness have generated some encouraging results, as discussed later.

There are similarities and differences in treatment approaches for different types of violent behavior, such as nonsexual, sexual, and domestic violence. Component 1 treatment approaches are applicable to treating all types of violent behaviors because they address cross-cutting similarities. The difference lies in Component 2 treatment that is specific to type of violence. For example, with sexual violence, considerable attention should be paid to assessing and treating sexual deviancy, in addition to treatment for general criminality and violence. The two-component model integrates the literature on the assessment of psychopathy, the treatment of personality disorder especially for offenders with personality disorders, and the rehabilitation of offenders to reduce reoffending—the "what works" literature. Because this treatment often takes place in highly secure and complex environments, delivery can be challenging, even with a well-conceptualized program.

ORGANIZING TREATMENT DELIVERY

The organizational dynamics of the secure forensic mental health or prison settings in which treatment usually takes place are often complex, involving multiple disciplines with goals that are not always complementary; for example, security and treatment goals are often at odds. Three factors stand out as special challenges that can adversely affect treatment integrity: the organization of the multidisciplinary team, the coordination of different components of the treatment program, and the management support of the program.

The Multidisciplinary Team

Although a multidisciplinary team approach can enrich treatment by providing diverse professional perspectives and expertise, it has to be implemented in a collaborative and focused manner. The team that includes all disciplines should share and support a clearly articulated and conceptualized treatment model. The challenge here is that the treatment of psychopathy is still controversial, and a treatment model supported by all disciplines is often lacking. As a result, the multidisciplinary approach may result in a diversity of opinions as to what treatments should be used and how they should be delivered. As psychologist Donald R. Gannon has said, "Where facts are few, experts are many." In the worst-case scenario, different disciplines work in silos with little communication between them, delivering a myriad of interventions each purporting to be effective in achieving some discipline-specific goal. As a result, treatment participants may be given confusing or conflicting messages. Open disagreements and jockeying for resources or recognition among disciplines—turf wars—provide opportunities for the individual with psychopathy to divide and conquer. Staff splitting and manipulations will exacerbate the problem; staff members might feel demoralized, isolated, lacking in direction, or burned out, increasing the likelihood of boundary violation.

To counter such a divisive approach, it is essential that teams adopt a common evidence-based and clearly articulated treatment model accepted by all disciplines. Clear treatment goals should be set and ways of achieving such goals articulated, ideally in the form of written treatment plan shared with the offender. Professional expertise and decision making should be exercised in an integrated manner to achieve treatment goals. All staff members involved in treatment delivery should commit to such goals and speak with one voice: All roads should lead to Rome, essentially delivering treatment in a highly integrated manner.

An example of an effective multidisciplinary approach is multisystemic therapy (MST), a social-ecological, evidence-based intervention to reduce antisocial behavior among high-risk youth (Henggeler et al., 1998). MST mobilizes different positive social influences in the youth's natural environment, such as family, school, home, and community, allowing participants to access a comprehensive array of services to address their specific physical, emotional, social, and educational needs. MST utilizes a multidisciplinary team with professions that complement one another. The team is carefully coordinated and provided with strong and consistent clinical supervision to ensure coherent service delivery.

One of the major challenges within a multidisciplinary team in a custodial environment is integrating treatment and security requirements, both of which are represented in most teams. Within a prison or forensic mental health facility, treatment has to be delivered within a safe and secured environment. Understandably, security staff does not have the same work objectives as treatment staff, and, at times, they may work at odds with one another. Resolving conflicts between the security and the treatment requirements is always challenging because the two disciplines differ in background, training, and work objectives. However, unless the two disciplines are well coordinated, offenders can be caught in the middle, compromising treatment delivery and integrity, as illustrated by the following vignette.

TREATMENT STAFF MEMBER: Tom, you got mad and hit your roommate. You know that is not right. You know what the consequences are, Tom.

OFFENDER: Yeah, but I hit him because he showed no respect and yelled at me. OK, OK, so I need to go to the quiet room to chill out. I'll do that, but when can I come out? I really hate that room; you know I can freak out just being in that room for too long.

TREATMENT STAFF MEMBER: I know. No one likes that room, and it's good you go voluntarily. That is definitely better than last time, Tom. Well, you have to keep yourself together for *x* hours, as we have agreed to. After that, you can come out for up to *y* minutes so we can see how you are doing. Is that OK?

OFFENDER: OK.

OFFENDER: (*later, to a security staff member*) I have been keeping myself together for *x* hours. I was told I can come out for a while. If I stay in much longer, I can freak out; I just can't stand the room.

SECURITY STAFF MEMBER: You are doing fine in there and, if you are going to freak out, then you should stay there longer. Can't let you out if you are going to freak out, that is the rule, and that is what we have to do to maintain security.

OFFENDER: But I only freak out if I stay in the room for a long time.

The treatment and security staff members were both trying to do their jobs, but obviously the lack of coordination of treatment and security requirements resulted in conflicting messages for the offender. This could be easily resolved by having the offender let out after *x* hours but under the supervision of security, with the understanding that inappropriate behaviors would result in returning to the quiet room and that continued appropriate behaviors may lead to being released from segregation. This arrangement must be agreed to by all parties involved, preferably in writing so there is no misunderstanding among staff. The behavioral contingencies must be rationally derived, clearly articulated, and consistently implemented by staff. Positive behaviors must be reinforced in a consistent manner. Staff training, supervision, and continued support are essential in maintaining consistency in program implementation, an essential aspect of program integrity.

This is a simple illustration of the potential conflict between treatment and security needs, which requires proactive negotiation by program designers to establish procedures to accommodate both requirements. Other approaches to integrate security and treatment functions effectively include the collaboration between security and clinical leads in the selection of appropriate security staff to work with offenders with psychopathy. Security staff should receive additional training on psychopathy, personality disorder, and the treatment program so that they are aware of the program's goals and objectives. The security staff's role within the treatment program should be clearly defined such as to support and reinforce positive prosocial behaviors and to point out negative behaviors. Security sanctions, when necessary, should not be in conflict with good clinical practice, as illustrated by the vignette.

A Multi-Intervention Approach

Most program participants have multiple criminogenic needs (see Figure 16.1) requiring multiple interventions. This requirement is handled differently in different programs. With some programs, each need, such as substance use, antisocial attitudes, and dysfunctional social relationships and networks, is treated using separate intervention modules, which require offenders to move from one module or intervention to the next to address all their problems. Alternatively, individuals may attend several different established therapies (such as dialectical behavior therapy and schema-focused therapy) or several therapy groups developed locally to address specific problems. This can lead to disjointed and poorly coordinated treatment. Staff members delivering the different therapies may have limited communication with one another and become therapy-focused rather than program objective–focused. Sometimes, these problems are complicated further by using outside therapists who have limited connection with staff involved in day-to-day management to deliver specific forms of treatment. The myriad of interventions are often poorly integrated; different terminologies are used to describe the same problem and intervention, and there is a lack of clarity as to how the different interventions could contribute to the overall treatment objectives. In such sliced-salami-like treatment approaches, in which the whole is often obscured by its individual parts, offenders may find it difficult to integrate the many sources of information available to them. Sequencing of the interventions becomes unwieldy, unresponsive to the needs of the offender, and time-consuming, thus increasing program costs. For example, if anger control is an issue but the module is scheduled next to last, such intervention cannot be provided to the offender as needed and in a timely manner. The multidimensional approach may also be complicated when treatment objectives become discipline-specific rather than program-specific. For example, occupational and recreational therapies may be incorporated into the overall program in a discipline-specific way—as learning to engage in constructive recreation activities—rather than in a program-specific way, as learning to engage in constructive recreational activities to bring about the reduction in reoffending risk.

When offenders have multiple problems, it is best that treatment target them together rather than one by one. An eclectic combination of different interventions, if required, should be integrated in treatment delivery. An eclectic approach does not "mean that multiple interventions can be delivered as separate and unrelated modules. A curriculum approach that assigns patients to an array of modules tailored to their individual problems is inappropriate because it offers little opportunity to . . . bring about the integration needed to address core self and interpersonal problems" (Livesley, 2007b, p. 33).

Management and Organizational Support

Successful implementation of a treatment program that is part of a larger organization requires support from the parent organization. Harris and Smith (1996), synthesizing the work of other commentators (Ellickson & Petersilia, 1983; Petersilia, 1990; also see Wong & Hare, 2005), identified three conditions for successful program implementation. First, the more closely the goals of the program and the parent organization are aligned, the better the chance of success. Second, all levels of the system need to be committed to the program, from external stakeholders to senior governance of the institution to program manager to line staff. The program must also have a clear line of authority: There should be no ambiguity about who is in charge. Third, appropriate resources must be consistently made available to the program. Ellickson and Petersilia (1983) found that better implemented programs and those that are better adapted to the structure of the organization have a higher likelihood of success, a conclusion supported by several meta-analyses and reviews (Andrews et al., 1990; Lipsey, 2009; Lipsey & Cullen, 2007; Lipsey & Wilson, 1998). At times, a somewhat less efficacious but better implemented program outperformed a more efficacious but less well-implemented program. As Lipsey (2009) put it after a review of the efficacy of different juvenile programs, "It does not take a magic bullet program to impact recidivism, but only one that is well made and well aimed" (p. 145). In essence, KISS (*K*eep *I*t *S*imple, *S*tupid), but do it well! However, Andrews and colleagues (1990) have argued that simplicity, though important, needs to follow certain rules. The more the program adheres to RNR principles, the larger the effect size is in relation to recidivism reduction, a relationship that holds for programs showing high, medium, and low levels of program integrity. At the same time, programs with higher integrity have larger effect sizes than those with lower integrity (Andrews & Bonta, 2010, p. 396).

A systematic assessment of the integrity of correctional rehabilitation programs can be carried out using the Correctional Program Assessment Inventory (CPAI; Gendreau & Andrews, 1994, as cited in Andrews & Bonta, 2010), which evaluates eight domains indicative of program integrity: (1) organizational culture, reflecting the agency's goals, ethical standards, outreach and self-evaluations; (2) program implementation/maintenance; (3) management and staff characteristics; (4) offender risk and need assessment practices; (5) program adherence to RNR characteristics; (6) staff interpersonal and relationship skill levels; (7) interagency communication; and (8) pre- and postprogram evaluation of outcomes. CPAI scores can be used to evaluate the association between program integrity and reoffending. Lowenkamp (2004, as cited in Andrew & Bonta, 2010, pp. 405–406), in a survey of community correctional facilities including both halfway houses and community correctional facilities with a total of 13,221 offenders, found that the total CPAI score correlated positively with the effect sizes of recidivism (0.41). Overall, the evidence suggests that program integrity is important to ensure efficacy.

ASSESSING TREATMENT EFFECTIVENESS

After all is said about choosing the appropriate treatment model and optimizing delivery, the remaining question is "Does it work?" That is, does treatment decrease the risk of future violence? The question can be answered by assessing the association of violence risk changes in treatment with reduction in violence recidivism in the community.

From Talking the Talk to Walking the Walk

In custodial settings, the antisocial behaviors of offenders with psychopathy can take on very different appearances or even go underground due to close monitoring and punishments for such behaviors. The literature is rife with examples of how people with psychopathy can con and manipulate their way through treatment by giving the appearance of having been rehabilitated. Hence, going from talking the talk to walking the walk and evaluating the authenticity of changes is a challenge. For example, a child molester who used the Internet to lure his victims may resort to viewing and masturbating to images of children in magazines, and the person with psychopathy who swindled and defrauded others may turn into a jailhouse lawyer. The presence of these *offense analogue behaviors*, or *OABs,* suggest that the underlying criminogenic factor is unchanged. Treatment should target these OABs as proxies of underlying criminological factors with the goal of replacing them with *offense reduction behaviors*, or *ORBs,* that is, their prosocial, adaptive counterparts. For example, promoting a change from using interpersonally intimidating and aggressive behaviors (OABs, such as in the vignette with the security officer) to using negotiations and problem-solving strategies (ORBs; see Gordon & Wong, 2010). It is unusual for OABs to simply disappear without being replaced by something else, as OABs serve to satisfy certain needs for people with psychopathy. OABs can be temporarily suppressed to achieve situational demands, such as to look good or to secure specific rewards, but sustained prosocial changes are unlikely unless they are replaced by consistent, generalizable prosocially adaptive alternatives. Careful observation of both OABs and ORBs is needed to assess legitimate and lasting changes in risk. The temporary suppression of OABs without establishing corresponding ORBs may account for the enigma that some individuals with psychopathy may be viewed by staff as being good citizens in custody but then go on to commit seemingly inextricably serious crimes on release to the community.

Treatment Outcome Evaluations

Recent studies with more stringent controls have examined the responses of offenders with psychopathy to contemporary treatment approaches. Olver and Wong (2009) used a dynamic risk-assessment tool, the Violent Risk Scale—Sex Offender version (VRS-SO) to measure risk changes in treatment of an adult male PCL-R assessed sex offender with psychopathy treated in a CBT- based sex offender treatment program, not unlike the treatment model described earlier, that has been shown to be effective in reducing sexual and violent recidivism (Nicholaichuk, Gordon, Gu, & Wong, 2000; Olver, Wong, & Nicholaichuk, 2009). Treatment improvements operationalized as reduction in risk assessed with the VRS-SO were associated with reduction in sexual and violent recidivism in the community in a 10-year follow-up after controlling for sexual offender risk, PCL-R scores, and length of follow-up. Similar results were obtained in a separate study for high-risk nonsexual violent offenders with mean PCL-R ratings of 26 that were treated in a violence reduction–focused program based on the RNR model using CBT approaches. A 4-year follow-up in the community showed that reduction in risk was associated with reduction in violent recidivism (Lewis et al., 2012; Olver et al., 2013). The objective of both studies was to determine whether risk changes for treated offenders are linked to recidivism change and, as such, no control group was used.

Treatment and control groups were used to assess the effects of participating in a treatment program for about 9 months, similar to that used in the Lewis and colleagues (2012) study (PCL-R = 28; $n = 32$ for both groups), with a case-matched control design (Wong et al., 2012). Both groups were matched for PCL-R total, F1 and F2 scores, length of follow-up, risk level, age, and past criminal histories. No significant differences were observed between violent and nonviolent recidivism rates, but those in the treated group who reoffended received much shorter sentences, suggesting that they committed less serious offenses than their untreated counterparts. The results suggest that treatment may reduce the seriousness of reoffending, thus supporting a harm reduction effect, and that a larger dose of treatment, that is, longer treatment length, is likely needed for such participants. Although more studies are necessary, these results suggest cautious optimism about the possibility of reducing violence and aggression in offenders with psychopathy.

The treatment programs reported in various studies showing positive treatment outcomes are based on the RNR principles with general or sexual violence reduction as the overall program goals (Di Placido et al., 2005; Lewis et al., 2012; Olver & Wong, 2009; Wong et al., 2012). Criminogenic needs (thoughts, feelings, and behaviors linked to violence) are identified as treatment targets using dynamic risk-assessment tools, and treatment methods are based on a combination of cognitive-behavioral approaches and careful monitoring of OAB and ORBs, as well as working alliances between the staff and offenders. Psychopathic personality traits (F1 characteristics) are treated as responsivity issues within the RNR model. The objective of treatment is not to change these F1 personality traits in order to reduce the risk of violence. The programs are also described in detail elsewhere (see Olver & Wong, 2013; Wong & Gordon, 2013; Wong, Gordon, & Gu, 2007).

CONCLUDING COMMENTS

Despite the very poor literature on the treatment of psychopathy, the general consensus among most researchers is that, though treatment of offenders with psychopathy may be quite challenging, they are *not* untreatable and that evidence-based treatment approaches *do not* make them worse. Advances in the assessment of psychopathy, risk assessment, and offender rehabilitation have pointed to testable approaches that can be applied systematically in the treatment of offenders with psychopathic traits to reduce their risk of violent reoffending. This chapter outlined one such approach with some positive treatment outcome results. Although it is far too early to say the puzzle has been solved, it is fair to say that the essential pieces of the puzzle can be identified. More clinical and research efforts will be required to finally put together and evaluate an integrated treatment model for offenders with psychopathy. It is hoped that theoretically sound and well-designed interventions for people with psychopathy and other similarly challenging offenders could be implemented, maintained, and accepted by forensic authorities as essential requirements of good clinical practice in managing these individuals just as much as good security is deemed essential.

REFERENCES

Andrews, D. A., & Bonta, J. (1994). *The psychology of criminal conduct.* Cincinnati, OH: Anderson.

Andrews, D. A., & Bonta, J. (2010). *The psychology of criminal conduct* (5th ed.). Cincinnati, OH: Anderson.

Andrews, D. A., Bonta, J., & Wormith, S. (2011). The risk–need–responsivity (RNR) model: Does adding the good lives model contribute to effective crime prevention? *Criminal Justice and Behavior, 38*(7), 735–755.

Andrews, D. A., Zinger, I., Hoge, R. D., Bonta, J., Gendreau, P., & Cullen, F. T. (1990). Does correctional treatment work?: A clinically relevant and psychologically informed meta-analysis. *Criminology, 28,* 369–404.

Beck, A. T., Freeman, A., Davis, D., & Associates. (2004). *Cognitive therapy of personality disorders.* New York: Guilford Press.

Blackburn, R. (1993). *The psychology of criminal conduct: theory, research and practice.* Chichester, UK: Wiley.

Bordin, E. S. (1994). Theory and research on the therapeutic working alliance: New directions. In A. O. Horvath & L. S. Greenberg (Eds.), *The working alliance* (pp. 13–37). New York: Wiley.

Bowers, L. (2002). *Dangerous and severe personality disorder: Responses and role of the psychiatric team.* New York: Routledge.

Cleckley, H. (1941). *The mask of sanity.* St. Louis, MO: Mosby.

Cooke, D. J., & Michie, C. (2001). Refining the concept of psychopathy: Towards a hierarchical model. *Psychological Assessment, 13,* 171–188.

Di Placido, C., Simon, T., Witte, T., Gu, D., & Wong, S. C. P. (2006). Treatment of gang members can reduce recidivism and institutional misconduct. *Law and Human Behavior, 30*(1), 93–114.

Doren, D. M. (1987). *Understanding and treating the psychopath.* Toronto, ON, Canada: Wiley.

Douglas, K. S., Strand, S., Belfrage, H., Fransson, G., & Levander, S. (2005). Reliability and validity evaluation of the Psychopathy Checklist: Screening Version

(PCL-R: SV) in Swedish correctional and forensic psychiatric samples. *Assessment, 12*(2), 145–161.

D'Silva, K., Duggan, C., & McCarthy, L. (2004). Does treatment really make psychopaths worse?: A review of the evidence. *Journal of Personality Disorders, 18*, 163–177.

Ellickson, P., & Petersilia, J. (1983). *Implementing new ideas in criminal justice.* Santa Monica, CA: Rand.

Fazel, S., & Danesh, J. (2002). Serious mental disorder in 23,000 prisoners: A systematic review of 62 surveys. *Lancet, 359*, 545–550.

Gabbard, G. O. (2004). *Long-term psychodynamic psychotherapy: A basic text.* Washington, DC: American Psychiatric Association Press.

Gendreau, P. (1996). The principles of effective intervention with offenders. In A. Harland (Ed.), *Choosing correctional options that work* (pp. 117–130). Thousand Oaks, CA: Sage.

Gendreau, P., & Andrews, D. A. (1994). *The Correctional Program Assessment Inventory* (6th ed.). Saint John, NB, Canada: University of New Brunswick.

Gendreau, P., & Ross, R. R. (1979). Effective correctional treatment: Bibliotherapy for the cynics. *Crime and Delinquency, 25*, 463–489.

Goldstein, A. P. (2004). Skillstreaming: The behavioral component. In A.P. Goldstein, R. Nensen, & B. Daleflod (Eds.), *New perspectives on aggression replacement training* (pp. 21–29). Chichester, UK: Wiley.

Gordon, A., & Wong, S. C. P. (2010). Offense analogue behaviours as indicators of criminogenic need and treatment progress in custodial settings. In M. Daffern, L. Jones, & J. Shine (Eds.), *Offence paralleling behaviour: An individualized approach to offender assessment and treatment* (pp. 171–184). Chichester, UK: Wiley.

Hare, R. D. (2003). *The Hare Psychopathy Checklist—Revised* (2nd ed.). Toronto, ON, Canada: Multi-Health Systems.

Harpur, T. J., & Hare, R. D. (1994). The assessment of psychopathy as a function of age. *Journal of Abnormal Psychology, 103*, 604–609.

Harris, G. T., & Rice, M. E. (2006). Treatment of psychopathy: A review of empirical findings. In C. J. Patrick (Ed.), *Handbook of psychopathy* (pp. 555–572). New York: Guilford Press.

Harris, P., & Smith, S. (1996). Developing community corrections. In A. Harland (Ed.), *Choosing correctional options that work* (pp. 183–222). Thousand Oaks, CA: Sage.

Hawes, S. W., Boccaccini, M. T., & Murrie, D. C. (2013). Psychopathy and the combination of psychopathy and sexual deviance as predictors of sexual recidivism: Meta-analytic findings using the Psychopathy Checklist—Revised. *Psychological Assessment, 25*(1), 233–243.

Henggeler, S. W., Schoenwald, S. K., Borduin, C. M., Rowland, M. D., & Cunningham, P. B. (1998). *Multisystemic treatment of antisocial behavior in children and adolescents.* New York: Guilford Press.

Hobson, J., Shine, J., & Roberts, R. (2000). How do psychopaths behave in a prison therapeutic community? *Psychology, Law, and Crime, 6*, 139–154.

Hollin, C. R. (2008). Evaluating offending behaviour programmes: Does only randomization glister? *Criminology and Criminal Justice, 8*, 89–106.

Jesness, C., Allison, T., McCormick, P. M., Wedge, R. F., & Young, M. L. (1975). *Cooperative Behavior Demonstration Project: Final Report.* Sacramento, CA: Office of Criminal Justice Planning.

Hughes, G., Hogue, T., Hollin, C., & Champion, H. (1997). First-stage evaluation of a treatment programme for personality disordered offenders. *Journal of Forensic Psychiatry, 8*, 515–527.

Kennealy, P. J., Skeem, J. L., Walters, G. D., & Camp, J. (2010). Do core interpersonal and affective traits of PCL-R psychopathy interact with antisocial behavior and disinhibition to predict violence? *Psychological Assessment, 22*(3), 569–580.

Kowalski, R. M., Limber, S. P., Patricia, W., & Agatston, P. W. (2007). *Cyber bullying: Bullying in the digital age*. Malden, MA: Blackwell.

Laws, R. (1998). *Relapse prevention with sex offenders*. New York: Guilford Press.

Leichsenring, F. (2010). Evidence for psychodynamic psychotherapy in personality disorders: A review. In J. F. Clarkin, P. Fonagy, & G. O. Gabbard (Eds.), *Psychodynamic psychotherapy for personality disorder: A clinical handbook* (pp. 421–437). Washington, DC: American Psychiatric Association Press.

Leichsenring, F., & Leibing, E. (2003). The effectiveness of psychodynamic psychotherapy and cognitive-behavioral therapy in personality disorder: A meta-analysis. *American Journal of Psychiatry, 160*, 1223–1232.

Lewis, K., Olver, M., & Wong, S. C. P. (2012). The Violence Risk Scale: Predictive validity and linking changes in risk with violent recidivism in a sample of high-risk offenders with psychopathic traits. *Assessment, 20*(2), 150–164.

Lilienfeld, S. O., & Fowler, K. A. (2006). The self-report assessment of psychopathy. In C. J. Patrick (Ed.), *Handbook of psychopathy* (pp. 107–132). New York: Guilford Press.

Linehan, M. M. (1993). *Cognitive-behavioral treatment of borderline personality disorder*. New York: Guilford Press.

Lipsey, M. W. (2009). The primary factors that characterize effective interventions with juvenile offenders: A meta-analytic overview. *Victims and Offenders, 4*, 124–147.

Lipsey, M. W., & Cullen, F. T. (2007). The effectiveness of correctional rehabilitation: A review of systematic reviews. *Annual Review of Law and Social Science, 3*, 279–320.

Lipsey, M. W., & Wilson, D. B. (1998). Effective intervention for serious juvenile offenders: A synthesis of research. In R. Loeber & D. Farrington (Eds.), *Serious and violent juvenile offenders: Risk factors and successful interventions* (pp. 313–345). Thousand Oaks, CA: Sage.

Livesley, W. J. (2003). *Practical management of personality disorder*. New York: Guilford Press.

Livesley, W. J. (2007a). Common elements of effective treatment. In B. van Luyn, S. Akhtar, & J. Livesley (Eds.), *Severe personality disorder* (pp. 211–239). New York: Cambridge University Press.

Livesley, W. J. (2007b). The relevance of an integrated approach to the treatment of personality disordered offenders. *Psychology, Crime and Law, 13*(1), 27–46.

Marlatt, G. A., & Gordon, J. R. (1985). *Relapse prevention: Maintenance and strategies in the treatment of addictive behaviors*. New York: Guilford Press.

Martinson, R. (1974). What works?: Questions and answers about prison reform. *Public Interest, 35*, 22–54.

McCord, W., & McCord, J. (1964). *The psychopath: An essay on the criminal mind*. Princeton, NJ: Van Nostrand.

McGuire, J. (2008). A review of effective interventions for reducing aggression and violence. *Philosophical Transactions of the Royal Society of London: B. Biological Sciences, 363*, 2577–2597.

Miller, W. R., & Rollnick, S. (2012). *Motivational interviewing: Helping people change* (3rd ed.). New York: Guilford Press.

National Institute for Health and Care Excellence. (2009). *Antisocial personality disorder: Treatment, management and prevention.* London: National Collaborating Centre for Mental Health.

Nicholaichuk, T., Gordon, A., Gu, D., & Wong, S. C. P. (2000). Outcome of an institutional sexual offender treatment program: A comparison between treated and matched untreated offenders. *Sexual Abuse: A Journal of Research and Treatment, 12*(2), 137–153.

Ogloff, R. P., Wong, S., & Greenwood, A. (1990). Treating criminal psychopaths in a therapeutic community program. *Behavioral Sciences and the Law, 8,* 181–190.

Olver, M. E., Lewis, K., & Wong, S. C. P. (2013). Risk reduction treatment of high-risk psychopathic offenders: The relationship of psychopathy and treatment change to violent recidivism. *Personality Disorders: Theory, Research, and Treatment, 4,* 160–167.

Olver, M. E., Neumann, C. S., Wong, S. C. P., & Hare, R. D. (2013). The structural and predictive properties of the Psychopathy Checklist—Revised in Canadian aboriginal and non-aboriginal offenders. *Psychological Assessment, 25*(1), 167–179.

Olver, M., & Wong, S. C. P. (2009). Therapeutic responses of psychopathic sexual offenders: Treatment attrition, therapeutic change, and long term recidivism. *Journal of Consulting and Clinical Psychology, 77*(2), 328–336.

Olver, M., & Wong, S. C. P. (2011). Predictors of sex offender treatment dropout: Psychopathy, sex offender risk, and responsivity implications. *Psychology, Crime and Law, 17,* 457–471.

Olver, M. & Wong, S. C. P. (2013). A description and research review of the Clearwater Sex Offender Treatment Programme. *Psychology, Crime and Law, 19*(5–6), 477–492.

Olver, M., & Wong, S. C. P. (2014). Short and long-term recidivism prediction of the PCL-R and the effects of age: A 24-year follow-up. *Personality Disorder: Theory, Research and Treatment, 6*(1), 97–105.

Olver, M. E., Wong, S. C. P., & Nicholaichuk, T. (2009). Outcome evaluation of a high intensity sex offender treatment program. *Journal of Interpersonal Violence, 24,* 522–536.

Palmer, T. (1996). Programmatic and nonprogrammatic aspects of successful intervention. In A. T. Harland (Ed.), *Choosing correctional options that work* (pp. 131–182). Thousand Oaks, CA: Sage.

Patrick C. J. (Ed.). (2006). *Handbook of psychopathy.* New York: Guilford Press.

Petersilia, J. (1990). Conditions that permit intensive supervision programs to survive. *Crime and Delinquency, 36,* 126–145.

Polaschek, D. (2014). Adult criminals with psychopathy: Common beliefs about treatability and change have little empirical support. *Current Directions in Psychological Science, 23*(4), 296–301.

Pouls, C., & Jeandarme, I. (2014). Psychopathy in offenders with intellectual disabilities: A comparison of the PCL-R and PCL-SV. *International Journal of Forensic Mental Health, 13*(3), 207–216.

Prochaska, J. O., DiClemente, C. C., & Norcross, J. C. (1992). In search of how people change: Applications to addictive behaviors. *American Psychologist, 47,* 1102–1114.

Rice, M. E., Harris, G. T., & Cormier, C. A. (1989). *An evaluation of a maximum security therapeutic community for psychopathic and nonpsychopathic mentally disordered offenders.* Penetanguishene, ON, Canada: Mental Health Centre.

Rice, M. E., Harris, G. T., & Cormier, C. A. (1992). An evaluation of a maximum security therapeutic community for psychopaths and other mentally disordered offenders. *Law and Human Behavior, 16*, 399–412.

Rothwell, P. M. (2005) External validity of randomized controlled trials: To whom do the results of this trial apply? *Lancet, 365*, 82–92.

Salekin, R. (2002). Psychopathy and therapeutic pessimism: Clinical lore or clinical reality? *Clinical Psychology Review, 22*, 79–112.

Salekin, R., Worley, C., & Grimes, R. D. (2010). Treatment of psychopathy: A review and brief introduction to the mental model approach for psychopathy. *Behavioral Science and the Law, 28*(2), 235–266.

Stone, M. H. (2010). Treatability of personality disorder: Possibilities and limitations. In J. F. Clarkin, P. Fonagy, & G. O. Gabbard (Eds.), *Psychodynamic psychotherapy for personality disorders: A clinical handbook* (pp. 391–418). Washington, DC: American Psychiatric Association Press.

U.S. Department of Justice (1997). *Uniform Crime Reports.* Washington, DC: U.S. Government Printing Office.

Walters, G. D. (2003). Predicting institutional adjustment and recidivism with the Psychopathy Checklist factor scores: A meta-analysis. *Law and Human Behavior, 27*, 541–558.

Walters, G. D., Wilson, N. J., & Glover, A. J. (2011). Predicting recidivism with the Psychopathy Checklist: Are factor scores composites really necessary? *Psychological Assessments, 23*(2), 552–557.

Ward, T., & Brown, M. (2004). The good lives model and conceptual issues in offender rehabilitation. *Psychology, Crime and Law, 10*, 243–257.

Widiger, T., Simonsen, E., Sirovatka, A., & Regier, D. (2006). *Dimensional models of personality disorder.* Washington, DC: American Psychiatric Association..

Wong, S. C. P. (2000). Psychopathic offenders. In S. Hodgins & R. Muller-Isberner (Eds.), *Violence, crime and mentally disordered offenders: Concepts and methods for effective treatment and prevention* (pp. 87–112). Chichester, UK: Wiley.

Wong, S. C. P. (2013). Treatment of psychopathy in correctional settings. In O. Thienhaus & M. Piasecki (Eds.), *Textbook on correctional psychiatry* (pp. 6-1–6-28). Kingston, NJ: Civic Research Press.

Wong, S. C. P., & Gordon, A. (1999–2003). *The Violence Risk Scale.* Unpublished manuscript.

Wong, S. C. P., & Gordon, A. (2004). A risk-readiness model of post-treatment risk management. *Issues in Forensic Psychology. 5*, 152–163.

Wong, S. C. P., & Gordon, A. (2006). The validity and reliability of the Violence Risk Scale: A treatment-friendly violence risk assessment scale. *Psychology, Public Policy and Law, 12*(3), 279–309.

Wong, S. C. P., & Gordon, A. (2013). The Violence Reduction Program: A treatment program for high risk violence prone offenders. *Psychology, Crime and Law.* 19(5–6), 461–475.

Wong, S. C. P., Gordon, A., & Gu, D. (2007). The assessment and treatment of violence-prone forensic clients: An integrated approach. *British Journal of Psychiatry, 190*, S66–S74.

Wong, S. C. P., Gordon, A., Gu, D., Lewis, K. & Olver, M. E. (2012). The effectiveness of violence reduction treatment for psychopathic offenders: empirical evidence and a treatment model. *International Journal of Forensic Mental Health, 11*(4), 336–349.

Wong, S. C. P., & Hare, R. D. (2005). *Guidelines for a psychopathy treatment program*. Toronto, ON, Canada: Multihealth Systems.

Wong, S. C. P., & Olver, M. (2015). Risk reduction treatment of psychopathy and applications to mentally disordered offenders. *CNS Spectrums, 20*, 303–310.

Wong, S. C. P., Van der Veen, S., Leis, T., Denkhaus, H., Gu, D., Liber, E., et al. (2005). Reintegrating seriously violent and personality disordered offenders from a super-maximum security institution into the general offender population. *International Journal of Offender Therapy and Comparative Criminology, 49*(4), 362–375.

Woody, G. E., McLellan, A. T., Luborsky, L., & O'Brien, C. P. (1985). Sociopathy and psychotherapy outcome. *Archive of General Psychiatry, 42*, 1081–1086.

Yang, M., Wong, S. C. P., & Coid, J. (2010). The efficacy of violence prediction: A meta-analytic comparison of nine risk assessment instruments. *Psychological Bulletin, 136*(5), 740–767.

chapter 17

Enriching Self-Narratives

Advanced Phases of Treatment

Giancarlo Dimaggio, Raffaele Popolo, Antonino Carcione,
Giampaolo Salvatore, and William B. Stiles

Patients with personality disorders often live frustrating lives in which their goals are unmet and their ambitions thwarted by inner barriers. They lack a guiding vision for how to adapt themselves to a complex and ever-changing environment. For treatment to be successful, therapists need to help these people form richer self-narratives that make sense of their aspirations and shortcomings and provide them with a sense of purpose and direction in life. An effective self-narrative should be a detailed map of the relational world that guides social action and allows people to explore their environment and search for new opportunities to fulfill innermost wishes and adapt to social life (Angus & McLeod, 2004; Hermans & Dimaggio, 2004).

THE NEED FOR A LIFE SCRIPT

Humans encode information about relevant aspects of social life in a story format (Bruner, 1990; Neimeyer, 2000). Self-narratives are meaning bridges that link, organize, and give smooth access to our life experiences (Stiles, 2011). Events and meanings that are within the narrative are part of the self, available as resources. Those left out may be foreign or inaccessible. Thus effective self-narratives highlight important information from the stream of people's social interactions. They allow people to reflect on past experiences, focus on what they long for, and draw on what they have experienced to live a satisfying life in the present.

Self-narratives are useful heuristics for forecasting how others will act because the scripts they generate specify and explain how others are likely to behave under specific circumstances. Scripts enable quick guesses about others' possible actions that can nevertheless be revised during ongoing interactions as the intentions underlying the others' actions become clearer. Full, accurate scripts allow the person to understand others' intentions and respond appropriately to influence them in a predictable manner. This understanding permits the formation of shared plans and facilitates conflict resolution.

For example, a man needing a romantic partner in order to feel worthy and fulfilled has to follow a script in order to court a person he likes. Typically this might include representations of (1) an awareness that he is longing for a partner; (2) an end state, such as he and the partner kissing each other; (3) the actions typically needed to arouse the other's interest based on a knowledge of what is likely to attract a woman of that age, culture, and background; and (4) anticipation of actions to be avoided and how to overcome stalled situations or repair conflicts and negotiate when goals differ.

To understand clearly what the client's prototype script is, the therapist needs to ground his or her understanding on specific events rather than generalized statements. For example, the typical life script of a person with narcissism, as he tells it during the first sessions, sounds like: "I wish for admiration and special status, but if others get too close to me they will discover I am no more than a charade. When I seek to reach my goals, dull and hostile persons will hinder me, which drives me mad, so I prefer working alone." This is a typical example of what could be termed a life theme or prototypical life script (McAdams, 2001). It contains an all-embracing plot with a conscious account, a working model to guide action. Nevertheless, it is hard for the clinician to plan treatment from such a generalized statement (Dimaggio & Attinà, 2012; Dimaggio, Salvatore, Fiore, et al., 2012). Specific details are required to concretize the general theme—for example, information about what a person wishes in a specific interaction with relevant others, the feeling evoked by expectations about how others will react, the feeling evoked by the actual reactions, and the coping strategies enacted when a wish is unachieved and causes suffering or maladaptive behaviors.

THE NEED FOR MULTIPLE LIFE SCRIPTS

A full life requires a self-narrative that can generate a rich variety of scripts. Stories must be woven around a wide array of wishes and must yield strategies for achieving them, along with reasonable expectations about how others could be allies in building bridges toward a brighter future. The same man who seeks a romantic partner is also driven by the quest for achievement and status, a social domain with different rules and strategies. A different script is needed to guide action in this new domain, as the actions typically needed to form and sustain a romantic relationship are not the same as those needed to apply for a job, to behave convincingly during an interview, and to work cooperatively with colleagues.

Each map must be suited to a specific territory; narratives and the scripts they generate therefore need to be tailored to the social motive they serve (Gilbert, 2005) and to the circumstances and context in which they occur. Adaptation requires multiple narratives (Dimaggio, Hermans, & Lysaker, 2010). We need stories about how to obtain care from our caregivers when we feel weak and distressed. We need a totally different script dealing with social rank motivation when we are searching for a new job. And, in the group inclusion domain, we need scripts on how to catch up with friends and maintain bonds.

DYSFUNCTIONS IN LIFE SCRIPTS IN PERSONALITY DISORDERS

In comparison with fully functioning people, those with personality disorder typically have few such scripts, and they are less open to rewriting those they have (Dimaggio, Salvatore, Popolo, & Lysaker, 2012; Gonçalves, Matos, & Santos, 2009; Gonçalves et al., 2012; Salvatore, Dimaggio, & Semerari, 2004). Therefore, if their scripts always read like, "When you want to have success others will try to stop you and be malevolent toward you, therefore be ready to fight or flee," the patient will not be able to realize that alternative interpretations of others' behavior are possible, and as a consequence no strategies alternative to fight or flight will be enacted. Another element in personality disorder pathology is a paucity of representation of inner life in the self-narrative and therefore a lack of access to innermost wishes. Many patients do not realize that they can be guided by passion, and as a consequence they are passive and flat and do not start pursuing goals in autonomy; this state is described as a deficient sense of agency (Adler, Chin, Kolisetty, & Oltmans, 2012). Deprived as they are of access to their own potential passions, they experience emptiness, boredom, a sense of apathy, and the feeling that life is not worth living.

SELF-NARRATIVES AS A TARGET FOR PSYCHOTHERAPY

As life scripts are impoverished and rigid in personality disorder, psychotherapy must include strategies to enrich them and make them more flexible. A desired goal is to form new scripts that then become part of a patient's self-narrative. Eliciting specific autobiographical memories can enrich and broaden the narrative and lead to a more stable sense of identity. The more persons can retrieve specific memories, and the more they recall them in session, the more information they have available for self-recognition.

After observing themselves acting in a variety of situations, patients progressively discover wishes, needs, and typical reactions that are part of who they are, a process that enriches their self-concepts. Moreover, once their awareness of who they are increases and becomes more stable, they can plan actions to enrich their life scripts. As the narrative expands, they find that they can wish for something different and enlarge the set of actions they perform. They can allow themselves to attain goals they previously did not attempt, even though those goals had been within their reach.

Techniques are available to help patients passing from a narrow to a broader and more flexible life script. For example, a therapist should try to get a patient with narcissism to access goals other than those aimed at sustaining the grandiose self, to build narratives in which self-aggrandizing is not the main action engine. A healthy self-narrative can arise from a review of multiple specific autobiographical episodes recounted during sessions, with discrepancies from early expectations being noted and integrated into a revised plot. For example, a new narrative by a patient with narcissism, after successful treatment, might be: "I strive for success and am still somewhat of a perfectionist, but I realize that I also want to enjoy life, spending time with friends and appreciating small, everyday things. I acknowledge that working in a group is difficult but rewarding, and I see opportunities to achieve things together with others."

Other examples of desirable therapeutic approaches are promoting stories based on agency and autonomy in persons with dependent traits and exposing persons with avoidant personality disorder to feared social contacts so that they form a more benevolent representation of self and others and become able to share experiences with peers.

Enriching the self-narrative involves broadening the script repertoire, pursuing multiple goals, and overcoming the power of maladaptive dominant narratives—for example, a woman's scripts dictating her to surrender to an abusive husband because reacting would entail abandonment or punishment (Gonçalves et al., 2012). It also involves achieving the metaunderstanding that one can be the author of one's own life.

Enriching self-narratives is a completely different affair from dismantling schemas or treating symptoms; it requires time, as it consists of a true process of construction of the mental structures and behavioral skills required to enact new plans, building meaning bridges with previously disregarded life experiences, as well as experiences during therapy. We contend that this is one of the reasons that treating personality disorder takes time: It is necessary to go over the same problem repeatedly and tackle the same deficits until new aspects of the cognitive–affective personality system (Clarkin, Yeomans, De Panfilis, & Levy, Chapter 18, this volume) are built up and fully functional and able to take over control from preexisting dysfunctional patterns. Such new behaviors become fluid only after many attempts.

WHEN TO TRY TO ENRICH THE SELF-NARRATIVE

The enrichment of the self and the construction of a more adaptive sense of identity are necessarily the work of the later stages of long-term therapy for two reasons. First, patients need to have achieved a sufficient degree of metacognitive differentiation (Dimaggio & Lysaker, 2010), that is, the ability to question their own beliefs and understand that their experience is subjective and that their ideas and expectations do not dictate reality. Achieving differentiation means understanding that relational problems and distress are often created by dysfunctional anticipation of events and not by the external world and learning to distinguish these dysfunctional anticipations from actual traumas such as loss, violence, or abuse. Awareness of recurring internalized relational patterns is especially important. For example, a woman with dependent personality disorder may complain that when she seeks attention and support the other will react with criticism and by denying help. Such a description cannot promote actions aimed at changing internal attitudes. The patient needs to be aware that it is not that others refuse to help but that she expects that they will neglect or criticize her. She must come to recognize her attentional bias toward seeing signs of lack of attention and harsh judgment as likely to reinforce her expectation and hamper exploration of alternative hypotheses about others' actions. Having achieved this understanding, the patient is more likely to realize that her reactions to anticipated criticism, such as avoidance/withdrawal, are not necessary because the expected criticism or neglect is unlikely to be forthcoming.

Patients must come to realize that such negative expectations about how others will react to their needs and wishes hinder their chances of realizing these needs and wishes because they do not either plan or perform effective actions. It is important to help patients to broaden their ability to make social encounters meaningful so that they can respond more flexibly to social problems.

With the therapist's help, patients must first plan new actions, then perform them, and finally reflect on what happened that was new. Through this process, patients integrate new knowledge into a revised life script. Intellectually understanding the causes of problems does not automatically breed change. Patients and therapists arrive at an understanding that engaging in new action is a key to change (Gonçalves et al., 2012). Patients need to be aware that without such a behavioral commitment, change is unlikely, and their social dysfunctions are likely to persist. At this stage, in spite of an emerging cognitive appraisal of the ways in which their usual self-narratives are dysfunctional, the restrictive scripts still dictate action in the direction of avoidance, fight-or-flight strategies, and inhibition of the exploratory system. Without behavioral experiments, the insidious effects of such automatic patterns is likely to persist. As they assimilate the new patterns, however, patients come to consider themselves as agents who can influence the world and be influenced by it in more ways than they had previously realized. They realize that there are aspects of the self that can potentially take control of action and generate new experiences that enrich their understanding of the social world with maps, tools, strategies, and new meanings (Stiles, 1999, 2011).

Once patients have achieved the required metacognitive differentiation and recognized their own agency, therapists and patients need to reformulate the therapy contract to plan the joint activities they need to perform in order to foster change (see Links, Mercer, & Novick, Chapter 5, this volume).

NEGOTIATING A REVISED TREATMENT CONTRACT

When the key therapy goals become to pass from increased self-awareness to behavioral change and restructuring of the life script, the therapy contract will need to be revised. Clarity about how the patient should contribute to making change happen is essential. In an open and totally nonconfrontational manner, a therapist should help the patient focus on treatment expectations and figure out possible cause-and-effect links between new actions and desired outcomes. A patient must realize that without social exposure her or his aloneness will never disappear. A typical reformulation of the contract would sound as follows:

> "Well, we now realize how you see yourself as awkward and inept, and that's why you feel ashamed and avoid meeting persons you might like and with whom you could form bonds. You know this is the way you see yourself and not who you actually are. On the other hand, you still have a big fear of being in the limelight because you don't know what to do in that situation. You don't understand how others might react, and you are still afraid of their reactions, which means a part of you still holds a negative view of yourself vis-à-vis critical and rejecting others. For treatment to be helpful, we need to make some attempt at doing something new outside the therapy room and increase social contacts. For example, we could plan together that you phone your friend and ask him to go out with you on Friday night. Would you agree to that? It is important to say that that is not my goal. It is just a reasonable expectation about whether, and under what conditions, therapy can, from now on, help you connect with others and have a relationship with a girl, which is something you long for. If you feel willing to do it, we can make a plan. If you feel it is too much for you, we just need to be aware of the limited healing power the therapy will have in the future, with less chances of providing you with an avenue toward satisfaction and adaptation. Can we shake hands to show you agree, so that we can decide what the next move is?"

PROMOTING ENRICHED SELF-NARRATIVES: BEHAVIORAL EXPOSURE AND METACOGNITIVE REFLECTION

The iterative procedures aimed at enriching self-narratives consist of: (1) *planning* new behaviors and forming forecasts about the possible states that will be experienced, while foreseeing positive and negative consequences; (2) actual *behavioral exposure/exploration* of new social avenues and roles; (3) *ongoing reflection* about new experiences and *integration* of emerging mental states into the self-system.

Forming enriched narratives requires a multilevel process:

1. Offering a reformulation of what has been achieved in therapy and gathering feedback from the client until agreement is obtained. This reformulation must include an idea of what else is still needed in order to achieve further change.

2. Providing a rationale for why change requires new action and highlighting the importance of patients' engagement in new actions aimed at reaching the desired outcomes.

3. Establishing a new contract based on the understanding that change requires new action and that the patient needs to be willing to follow this plan. The therapist should state that new behaviors are not the desired outcome in themselves, though of course adaptive behaviors leading to goal satisfaction are welcome! Action is the context that allows the mind to make contact with new experiences and to integrate formerly disavowed parts of the self into the identity; new behaviors elicit residual negative patterns and provide a context for new learning and fresh experience for meaning making. The formation of new meanings and a broader sense of an agentic and fulfilling social life is the actual goal.

4. Mandatorily providing validation. Attempting to form a new narrative is highly demanding, as patients are asked to do things that sound dangerous, unknown, and unpredictable to them. The therapist should therefore validate any new adaptive action and be attentive to and understanding of any fear or hesitation requiring encouragement. According to Semerari (2010, p. 277), validation may be both cognitive and emotional: "(cognitive) *validation* means confirming the sense of the forecasts and evaluations that a person constructs: 'I understand that you can have this point of view about the world.' (Emotional) *Validation* . . . is a therapist stressing the comprehensible and acceptable nature of at least a part of . . . patients' dysfunctional experience: 'I understand how you can feel like that.' "

5. Therapy must convey a sense of hope that results will be rewarding and a realistic confidence that the patient will be able to perform the required actions. Again, feedback from the patient should be continuously elicited in order to gauge whether his or her sense of safety is overly threatened or self-efficacy drops.

Each of the former elements is necessary but not sufficient for constructing a broadened self-narrative. *Planning* behavioral experiments makes new situations predictable and fosters agency because patients decide what they are willing and able to attempt; they can gauge what they can tolerate and be motivated by the positive expected consequences. *Behavioral exposure/*

exploration makes change happen and makes it possible for patients to act as embodied agents engaged in an exploration of landscapes they never sensed before. After experiencing the well-modulated and safe session environment, patients are now able to and need to engage in *ongoing reflection*, which allows them to keep the new knowledge of what they have just experienced in their working memories and integrate aspects of the self that they were previously unaware of in the broader self-image (Gonçalves et al., 2012; Stiles, 2011). Patients should mentalize things they have seen, touched, heard, sensed, and smelled and understand how they are different from their previous negative expectations.

PLANNING BEHAVIORAL EXPERIMENTS

Planning behavioral experiments in order to promote innovation in the life script requires a focus on patients' unfulfilled wishes and an understanding that without their fulfillment life will not be rewarding and will continue to lack purpose. Expected negative responses from others should then be evaluated. Patients should be made aware of their usual safety strategies and how these prevent them from reaching life goals. A joint evaluation of the resources that patients possess but are not using is very important. A forecast of the likely states of mind that they will experience when performing new actions should now be made. This will make the unforeseen future more predictable and allow patients to face the feared scenario with a more realistic and optimistic stance. Patients will be less fearful about trying new ways of behaving if the clinician helps them to accept that these actions may give rise to positive feelings of activity, vitality, and freedom and that, if these actions lead to negative experiences, they will be no more painful than usual and that these feelings can be tolerated.

Finally, it is important to assess the skills needed to fulfill wishes. This aspect has a pragmatic slant: Although the ultimate aim of the phase of therapy described here is to broaden the self-narrative, action is the key ingredient. Typical examples of actions that can be discussed during session, negotiated, and then carried out include doing the housework, getting a driving license, acquiring new acquaintances, dating potential partners, writing a resume, applying for a job interview, and starting new training programs.

> In the case of Lucien, a patient with narcissistic personality disorder, perfectionism, and social avoidance (see Dimaggio & Attinà, 2012, for a thorough description of the therapy), planning experiments involved an awareness that his wishes for autonomy and exploration were met with parental criticism and rejection, resulting in a life script in which any attempt at autonomy led to loneliness and feeling despicable. Because this meant that his innermost wishes were suppressed and unrecognized, planning involved his becoming aware that his work as an assistant in his

brother-in-law's law firm was unrewarding and uninteresting and that he kept it primarily to avoid criticism. He also had to overcome his moralistic tendencies, which prevented him from leaving the job because he did not want to offend a relative. The therapist and patient then discovered that a potential vocational area consistent with his wish for autonomy was nested in the patient's passion for studying ancient history. Together, they planned that he should try to fulfill this wish. Lucien then had to confront his parents' perceived and actual negative reaction to his desire to study archaeology. Finally, the therapist and patient foresaw how going to the campus, talking with the staff in the university offices, and conversing with other students would be extremely demanding tasks for him, so that each had to be handled with great care. Thanks to this assessment, a new plan was formed that enabled Lucien to enroll in a new university program.

Planning contributes to the ultimate goal of obtaining a revised and enriched life script. In the case of Lucien, formulating the plan became something like: "I am a person capable of working and having friends. I find pleasure in sustaining bonds. I am still concerned with the recognition issue and somewhat fear criticism, but I am able to carry on with my actions even when others are not praising me." Such a narrative must be grounded on actual autobiographical episodes discussed during sessions to avoid becoming an intellectualization. Arriving at such a narrative involved Lucien's first realizing how his wishes for autonomy were matched with expectations of being criticized and rejected by his parents, both actual and internalized. He then decided to face the pain of the expected rejection, supported by the therapist's faith that he could tolerate such distress. This helped him to find the courage to leave the job with his brother-in-law. Finally, he spent time exploring the university grounds and the library, overcame his parents' skepticism about his ability to do so, and faced up to all the related difficulties, both internal and external.

We now provide details about the aims of what can actually be the most important aspect of enriching the self-narrative: *exploration/behavioral change*.

THREE AVENUES TO ENRICHED SELF-NARRATIVES: THE AIMS OF EXPLORATION/BEHAVIORAL EXPOSURE

As therapists, we want patients to activate the exploratory system, to become curious and open-minded, creating the conditions for enriching their self-narrative's set of experiences. Curiosity and exploration need an object to prepare the cognitive–affective system to integrate experiences different from the previous dominant and barren life scripts (Stiles, 1999, 2011). To illustrate: A young man with avoidant personality disorder needs to actually court a woman both to challenge his anticipation that he will be inept and deserve rejection and to experience making love, giving and receiving tenderness, and negotiating conflicts. Without the actual experience of dating a woman and sleeping with her, the self-system stays impoverished and barren even after the patient, at a cognitive level, fully understands the reasons for his problems. The actual experience enables the man to reason about what happened, mentalize the feelings he had, make sense of the dialogue with the woman and the associated sensory experience, and thus enrich his self-narrative with new meanings. For example, emptiness and shame may alternate with a sense of purpose in continuing the relationship. Thanks to this new set of experiences, parts of the self that were formerly overshadowed will flourish, for example, a sense of oneself as being funny and able to make other people smile. At the same time, self-aspects formerly considered problems can acquire new meanings and be integrated into the self-system as useful resources (Stiles, 2011): A certain degree of shyness may be appreciated by a partner who considers a man delicate and gentle instead of awkward and inept.

Exploration/behavioral exposure has three different aims, which can be intertwined with each other and yet need to be distinguished in order to adjust the way actions aimed at promoting change are planned and enacted:

1. Becoming aware of overlooked healthy self-aspects and integrating them into the self-system.
2. Eliciting and confronting maladaptive scripts through exposure to formerly avoided situations; overcoming behavioral avoidance of socially feared situations.
3. Acting as the healthy self in the social arena and broadening the life script.

The overarching aim is to enrich the self-narrative; these three subgoals are the stairs leading to the top floor.

Becoming Aware of Overlooked Healthy Self-Aspects and Integrating Them into the Self-System

Enriching self-narratives involves accessing healthy self-aspects that patients with personality disorder systematically overlook, broadening the space they have in consciousness and giving them a chance to guide behavior and eventually be integrated into the identity. Healthy experiences include agency, autonomy, sensuality, playfulness, self-esteem, and mutuality. These experiences, once accessed, need to be kept in the working memory—mostly in session—long enough to be progressively stored in autobiographical memory and become a part of identity. As the patient has now entered the exploratory mode, the stage is set for searching for previously unattended, warded-off, suppressed, or dissociated material. Clinicians can help the patient access healthy self-aspects in two ways. The first is, as noted, during session. They should pay the greatest attention to any nonverbal markers signaling that there are positive aspects that the patient is not attending to in the experiences nested in the narrative episode just told. A patient with dependent features can describe herself as inadequate and inferior but then display a lively facial expression and a twinge of enthusiasm in her voice while describing herself performing a task at work. In such a case, the clinician should usually stop the discourse and signal the discrepancy between the self-concept "I'm inept" and the nonverbal behavior pointing to aspects of self-efficacy and self-esteem.

Clinicians should be aware here of the level of severity of personality disorder. Some patients barely display healthy self-aspects in their everyday lives, which feature only emptiness, anger, resentment, loneliness, and social withdrawal. With such patients the *in vivo* experience of positive self-aspects creates the embryo of a renewed identity. In other patients, healthy aspects may be present but overshadowed by dysfunctional narratives that make them unable to see that they are functioning better than they believe. In one case, a clinician tried to get a young man with severe avoidant personality disorder with passive–aggressive, schizoid, and covert narcissism traits to observe himself with words something like: "You feel uninterested in pursuing anything in your life. You say you are detached and life has no meaning for you. But when you describe the way you guide the team during your Internet simulation games, you are full of energy. You describe how you want to lead the team, are able to motivate others and devise a strategy, and feel like sharing in something with others." After repeated observations like these, the therapist of this patient was able to motivate him to ask his fellow team members out for a pizza, which was the first real peer contact he had had in years.

In other cases things are easier, and therapy is more about getting patients to become aware of experiences they have had outside sessions during everyday life but that they have not attended to. Rather than leaving these to disappear, therapists can use them to fuel a positive self-image and motivate goal-directed action.

Whether they are achieved during sessions at a blossoming stage or usually experienced in everyday life, positive experiences will not stick unless they are practiced, a point we return to later (Gonçalves et al., 2012). The therapist should create a context in which new actions and reflections can be used to enrich the patient's self-narrative, with new scripts based on feelings of agency and autonomy, thus fostering a sense of self-efficacy and self-esteem. Accessing the healthy self-aspects—and later giving them room in patients' lives—goes side by side with the reemerging of dysfunctional narratives, which need to be seen from a different angle and not taken as true. The processes of (1) promoting healthy self-narratives and (2) taking a critical distance from dysfunctional life scripts occur in parallel. During the same session, therapists can swing from one process to the other.

FURTHER ELICITING MALADAPTIVE SCRIPTS AND OVERCOMING BEHAVIORAL AVOIDANCE

During behavioral exposure, old patterns surface again, trying to take control. Along with making room for new aspects of experience, these patterns need to be elicited and revised repeatedly. During this process patients become aware of the affective and implicit aspect of their meaning-making constructions, which are usually harder to change than are the cognitive–semantic aspects.

At this point, it is important to encourage both the ego-dystonic and the ego-syntonic aspects to surface and become objects of reflection. Patients with narcissism need to tackle their tendencies to be spiteful, to resort to an ivory tower, and to enter into fights filled with frozen anger with partners and colleagues. Patients with paranoid features need to become aware of how much their attributions of malevolence to others come mostly from an inner perception of feeling vulnerable, inadequate, and subjugated; they must slowly recognize that their vulnerability is not an objective truth but a mental image they hold of themselves (Salvatore et al., 2012).

One typical condition in which old patterns surface during behavioral experience/exploration is facing fear of social rejection. Patients with fear of social rejection and criticism, for example with a mixture of avoidant and obsessive–compulsive features, realize how they sense impending criticism deep within their bodies. They come to realize how this is an internalized attributional style, even in the absence of external cues.

> One patient, 26-year-old Geneva, had a very severe personality disorder with borderline, avoidant, and passive–aggressive features, perfectionism, co-occurring eating disorders, and depersonalization. She repeatedly stated that she felt unable to study in her university library because people would criticize her. After a difficult negotiation, she tried to expose herself to this environment, and she still reported being criticized, even if she acknowledged that no one displayed any sign of rejection. It took more than 1 year of repeated exposure and reflection, both in individual and group sessions, for Geneva to understand that this pattern was automatic and not in line with signals coming from outside. Only recently has Geneva been able to date a man and sleep with him, bearing in mind both what she thought beforehand—"I'm fat, ugly, and stupid, and he'll laugh at me"—and the actual sensations she felt: "It was hard to face the situation, but eventually I felt fine. He was kind to me. Now it's up to me to do something different rather than disappearing as usual through fear of being rejected." When, for example, Geneva decided to go to study in the university library and in the next group session reported that she had not done this, the therapists validated the positivity of her focusing on the task and discovering that she held a self-image so negative that she could not even face social contact. This helped foster self-reflection and let her realize further how that was mostly an internalized image.

A first good outcome of such an exploratory attitude, even when actual exposure fails, has the patient becoming involved in focusing on the beliefs and feelings leading to not facing a particular situation. Once awareness of how maladaptive scripts still dictate actions at an automatic-procedural level, the next therapy step is to engage patients in actions aimed at overcoming avoidance.

Overcoming avoidance requires that the patient and therapist agree on what situations the patient does not want to face and form a plan for exposure to these. The approach is similar to CBT for anxiety disorders: The less distressing and/or more desirable situation must be explored first. Standards for successful performance are kept very low; what the therapist should expect is simply the patient's commitment to thinking about what to attempt and then reflecting about what happened.

When behavioral exposure is successful, patient and therapist should reflect on what happened in recent narrative episodes and explore the sensations and ideas the patient had during any interpersonal situations. Usually there is a mixture of old feelings, reappearance of maladaptive narrative, and new elements of subjective experience. This is the moment at which to note any discrepancy between patients' actions, ideas, and emotions during the episode and their usual script-driven states of mind.

Passing from an increased awareness of how avoidance was triggered by her negative self-image to overcoming avoidance was the next step in Geneva's therapy.

> After months of struggling with her negative self-image, Geneva accepted an invitation to go out with a couple of friends and a man she had not met before. In the session she tended toward refusing the invitation, as her fear of being ridiculous once again appeared, but then after a brief discussion with the therapists and other group members, she agreed to try and accept the rendezvous because she was tired of surrendering to the negative view she held of herself. At the start of the encounter, she was prey to ideas consistent with her negative self-image: The man was only interested in having sex with her and would despise her soon afterward, discovering how stupid she was. She anticipated in her mind how inept and nerd-like her behavior would seem, and she felt tempted to go straight home to stop the bad movie that was playing in her mind becoming true. However, she recalled the conversations in therapy and was able to stop herself from going offstage. After a while she noticed how she was attracted to the man and guessed he reciprocated. Some days later she was invited again by the same couple of friends and the guy. She was extremely anxious about the situation, and the idea of refusing to go out surfaced again. The topic was discussed during a session, and she accepted the rendezvous, acknowledging that this new encounter could have an open-ended outcome. Before watching a movie at a cinema, she felt hungry and had a slice of pizza. She criticized herself for her disordered eating and was extremely ashamed about eating something she actually did not need. She noticed her girlfriend laughing with her own fiancé and was convinced that they were laughing at her, that her friends were commenting about her eating disorder. She was both ashamed and angry, but this time she realized that this could be just an opinion, her usual rumination. After the movie she slept with the man and was happy to have done so. She acknowledged that he was kind and gentle and wanted to see her again. She also realized that the problem to tackle now was not being rejected

> but the way her avoidant behaviors usually led her to disappear. After several weeks she was still dating the man.

We underscore that the aim of eliciting maladaptive scripts is not to challenge them as being unrealistic. The aim is to show the patient how negative memories are triggered, filled with intense and often distressing emotions, and built around scripts that hamper adaptation. Patients are not asked to refute their constructions of reality but rather to commit to actions based on different postulates, to explore their subjective experience when they do something new. In any case, at this moment, there is usually some reappraisal of old self-representations, as the patient critically questions his or her formerly firmly held, maladaptive beliefs (see Leahy, Chapter 12, this volume, for a more systematic way of changing cognitive schemas for self and others).

Even cautious exploration of formerly forbidden avenues bears some risk. No matter how careful the therapist is in explaining that success is not performing a specific behavior but just adopting a stance of curiosity and openness and then discussing any related state of mind during sessions, patients can focus on performance failures. Negative forecasts, filled with hopelessness and passivity, also come to the fore. Moreover, patients often forget that performing new actions was not an imposition by their therapists but a shared decision and thus attack their therapists or say they want to terminate treatment.

At such moments the focus must swiftly switch to the therapy relationship: The therapist needs to adopt a mentalistic stance, inquire about any negative reaction the patient might have felt, and provide a safe place for exploration of negative feelings such as shame, impotence, frustration, or desperation. There must be validation: The clinician should constantly recall that the actual aim was to explore the patient's inner world over and above succeeding in performing new actions, and therefore the negative states appearing are a sign of how the patient is committed to the therapy. It is useful here for the therapist to keep a balance between optimism and remembering that change does not come easily. Reframing one's way of seeing oneself in the world is a difficult task, which requires time and practice. In parallel, the therapist must engage in tactful exploration of the therapy relationship and metacommunication about it in order to repair ruptures. The focus must be kept on the therapy relationship until cooperation and the alliance are restored (see Dimaggio, Salvatore, Fiore, et al., 2012; Tufekcioglu & Muran, Chapter 6, this volume).

A problem we only marginally address here for the sake of space is that patients may have problems in rewriting their life histories because they lack social skills or because these skills activate such negative interpersonal cycles in real life that their relations remain stuck and no true progress is made. This is often the case in persons with hostility, negativism, and extreme agency impairment traits. Clinicians must be warned that therapy is much longer in such instances. They will have to work hard to engage with such patients when they are participating in behavioral experiments. They should provide coaching about appropriate ways to behave in demanding interpersonal contacts and review narrative episodes with a stress on both providing validation and helping patients change those dysfunctional attitudes that elicit negative responses from others. Here, too, very careful attention needs to be paid to the therapy relationship (Dimaggio et al., 2010). The relationship can provide an important learning experience. In advanced therapy stages, clinicians can offer an insight into the negative reactions the patient elicits in him- or herself by explaining that this is what can happen in everyday life. The therapist can also validate any moments of mutuality and reciprocal understanding in the relationship, which the patient should later be invited to export into real-life exchanges. For such clients, the therapy relationship itself is typically the ground on which new narratives are formed (Summers, 2012).

Acting According to the Healthy Self in the Social Arena and Broadening the Life Script

As DSM-5 notes, key features of personality disorder are lack of agency, goal-directedness, and autonomy, low capacity for intimacy, and negative or unstable self-esteem. The capacity to experience pleasure in everyday life activity is low as well. Once patients start becoming aware that they can act according to their own will and can take charge of their own personal fulfillment instead of portraying themselves as victims or as unable to influence events, the clinician should negotiate with them about how to act in view of these new sensations. The sense of agency and purpose is the pillar on which to build this aspect of therapy. The patient should be asked to focus on what she or he feels like wanting to pursue and actively engage her- or himself in actions aimed at reaching these goals. Therapists help also patients focus on their strength, resilience, and positive qualities and act according to those (Padesky, 2012). Then, during sessions, an ongoing reflection on the details of the narrative episodes, grounded in pursuing the patient's utmost wishes, should be started. Therapists should pay the greatest attention to any script-discrepant feelings or thoughts in order to show patients that there is material inside them that could lead them both to change their self-conception and to pursue more adaptive avenues in which their positive qualities can be used and that the skills they have in one domain may be generalized to others (Padesky, 2012).

The overall stance of this therapy aspect is that the stress should be less on challenging maladaptive beliefs about oneself and others and more on promoting different perspectives and related committed actions. In other words, this therapy aspect is not about asking persons with narcissism to challenge their grandiose self-images or patients with paranoia to convince themselves the world is a benevolent place (which is not actually true!). Instead, we ask them to try to focus on different aspects of what they experience when interacting with others and to pay attention to previously unattended material. They may, for example, discover that, in a very specific episode, the other person was not malicious but was seeking attention or that acting without the goal of supporting grandiosity may lead to relaxing and taking pleasure in spending time having fun with friends. Awareness and the pursuit of a healthy self-aspect as an enrichment and integration of the self-system are much more the goals of therapy at this stage than is challenging maladaptive scripts. Note that taking a critical distance from the hardcore negative beliefs forming the cognitive nucleus of the self-narrative is still an important part of personality disorder therapy (see Leahy, Chapter 12, this volume).

In the case of narcissistic disorders, for example, patients need to focus on wishes that are not aimed at sustaining grandiosity and to pursue them for the sake of experiencing pleasure and opening their senses to what comes from the outer world (Dimaggio & Attinà, 2012). A patient treated by one of us was unable to perform any physical exercise without measuring all his bodily parameters with a view to reaching perfect harmony. The therapist disclosed to him how he walked through the same woods where the patient usually ran, lining a beautiful beach in Tuscany, and how he felt those woods had something magical. The patient agreed with these observations and was surprised at how he himself was usually unable to pay attention to his environment, whereas he had been able to when he was a university student. This opened up the path to a life less built on striving for social rank and more open to pleasure and relaxation (Dimaggio et al., 2010).

> A very severely ill patient, Bianca, a woman in her early 20s with passive–aggressive tendencies and dependent, avoidant, and borderline personality disorders with severe Axis I co-occurrence, including depression, social anxiety, and obsessive–compulsive disorder (OCD), started therapy in a state in which she was barely able to get out of bed. After years of struggle, she joined group therapy. When in a negative mood she was violently self-effacing, her sense of agency completely disappeared, and she became clinging, asking the therapists to decide what to do on her behalf. If the individual and group therapists suggested any activity, such as making her bed, changing her wardrobe around, or even just taking a shower, she became harshly self-critical and felt a sense of coercion. Her passive–aggressive traits came to the fore, and she refused to perform any tasks, as she felt driven by outer alien forces (Bateman & Fonagy, 2004). Once she refused to perform actions, she fell into self-deprecation and insulted both herself for not being able to do anything and the therapist for not helping her. She skipped many sessions because she felt unable to talk, but soon after each session she started phoning and sending text messages to the therapists. After careful management of countertransference, which ranged from guilt to worry about her suicidal threats (she never made any real attempts), and intense anger at both her passivity and her insults, the therapists decided to reformulate the contract. It was made crystal clear that participation in sessions was mandatory and that phone calls or messages would not be answered if she skipped the session. Then the therapists asked her to take her time and decide what her therapy goals were and, most of all, what she thought she could achieve. Together they gauged the implications in terms of agency, self-esteem, and autonomy of

each of the scenarios she considered. The therapists systematically denied any preference for the scenarios she portrayed in order to avoid her becoming passive and shutting her mind off (something she was able to do in a few seconds when shifting from active pursuit of goals to asking the therapists' opinions). She firmly protested for months, made numerous calls and sent an infinity of text messages, and insulted the therapists a few times, but after this struggle she started to focus on being in charge of her life and had to decide what to do. She considered that dropping out of the university would be detrimental to her self-esteem, but on the other hand she had no real internal drive to continue studying. She was just complying with abstract expectations about being a university student as the sole path worth following. She decided first to study nail makeup. She took a 5-month course and completed it with success. During the course she experienced a sense of agency. She felt self-efficacy when doing her first practical exercise and noticed during group role play how she was surprised at finding her hands active and skilled. This experience bolstered her self-esteem. The next year she started attending a 2-year beautician course. The first year was distressing, as her perfectionistic standards coupled with loss of self-efficacy were taken to the extreme. She skipped many lessons and had many ups and downs during the 2 years, but her adherence to the contract was stabilized by the therapists. She was always reminded that she only had to choose between staying or leaving and that it was not the therapists' will but her own that had made her take the course. This helped her overcome a sense of coercion and practice her free will. Eventually she completed the first year with success and is now finding the second year less distressing. Her OCD, depression, and social anxiety have dramatically improved.

As Bianca's case highlights, building up new self-narratives is possible when patients learn new ways to reach goals in their social lives and expand their range of actions and associated skills. Patients need to be helped and, in the most severe cases, sometimes coached in focusing on what to do in order to meet their goals.

ONGOING REFLECTION AND INTEGRATION OF NEW MATERIAL IN THE SELF-NARRATIVE

The integration of new experiences into the self-narrative is a later therapy step that is probably necessary for therapy outcomes to be sustained over time. The therapist should engage the patient in a prolonged reflection about the experiences emerging at the exploration stage or in sessions. The aim is mostly to move memories of the healthy self from working memory to long-term autobiographical memories. The therapist should try to steer patients' attention to memories of agency, autonomy, positive self-esteem, and self-efficacy and to the capacity for mutual respect and recognition and to show how these experiences are now part of their patients' lives.

A patient is thus able to see how repeated experiences of agency have led to positive outcomes, unlike earlier forecasts of failure or of being blamed, attacked, and rejected. The therapist should here promote an integrated understanding of the functional and dysfunctional elements in the patient's meaning-making style and of how the self-narrative is complex and multifaceted. Some patients can realize that even if some tendencies, such as self-derogation, are still present, they no longer need to dictate actions. Instead, a new sense of purpose in, for example, joining or belonging to a group or being a devoted parent is built up. A sense of dependency may now be less entwined with feelings of worthlessness and tendencies to become submissive. Instead, dependency may link more with a sense of warmth in sustaining bonds, though now alternating with a sense of self-efficacy at work and the ability to pursue one's own career.

This is the moment at which many aspects of a former problematic self-narrative are revised and integrated into a bird's-eye view of the self in a new life script, in which there are more avenues to be followed, granting more choice and freedom and the ability to overcome traumatic experiences (Gonçalves et al., 2012; Neimeyer, 2012; Stiles, 2011). The therapist at this stage should provide a sort of metacognitive scaffolding, helping the patient to swiftly recognize which different aspects of the self are called into action and to build the capacity to leave problematic aspects aside in order to let, whenever possible, the more adaptive scripts take the lead (Ribeiro, Ribeiro, Gonçalves, Horvath, & Stiles, 2013). Patients at this phase typically face the ups and downs of daily life and react to stressors with an alternating of good and poor functioning. When they fail to pass a test, maladaptive scripts surface again, filled with contents of mistrust toward others ("they want me to fail"), narcissism ("they hamper my goals and don't understand my value"), social rejection ("I'm inept, so others will humiliate me"), and so on. Such scripts should be revised and memories of positive episodes recalled very quickly in sessions to help the patient achieve a more balanced identity. Stable tendencies (e.g., personality traits; see Livesley, Chapter 11, this volume) should be acknowledged to be personal styles, and the path should be toward acceptance of the self and its balance between limits and qualities.

CONCLUDING COMMENTS

Forming an integrated self-narrative is made possible with specific techniques such as writing diaries, assessing one's self-narratives, or using diagrams and reformulation letters, the topic of a specific chapter in this book (Salvatore, Popolo, & Dimaggio, Chapter 19). With these tools the set of life scripts, with their positive and negative facets, can be brought to the patient's attention for discussion and to increase awareness. When the actual outcome is an enriched life script and therapy fosters a richer sense of identity, patients gain an integrated sense of self in which they are aware of their innermost tendencies, skills, fears, and limitations and think of themselves of agents able to live a life with a purpose.

ACKNOWLEDGMENT

We thank Paul Lysaker and Miguel Gonçalves for their helpful comments on earlier versions of this chapter.

REFERENCES

Adler, J. M., Chin, E. D., Kolisetty, A. P., & Oltmans, T. F. (2012). The distinguishing characteristics of narrative identity in adults with features of borderline personality disorder: An empirical investigation. *Journal of Personality Disorders, 26,* 498–512.

Angus, L., & McLeod, J. (Eds.). (2004). *The handbook of narrative and psychotherapy: Practice, theory and research.* London: Sage.

Bateman, A., & Fonagy, P. (2004). *Psychotherapy for borderline personality disorder: Mentalization-based treatment.* Oxford, UK: Oxford University Press.

Bruner, J. S. (1990). *Acts of meaning.* Cambridge, MA: Harvard University Press.

Dimaggio, G., & Attinà, G. (2012). Metacognitive interpersonal therapy for narcissistic personality disorders with perfectionistic features: The case of Leonardo. *Journal of Clinical Psychology: In-Session, 68,* 922–934.

Dimaggio, G., Hermans, H. J. M., & Lysaker, P. H. (2010). Health and adaptation in a multiple self: The role of absence of dialogue and poor metacognition in clinical populations. *Theory and Psychology, 20,* 379–399.

Dimaggio, G., & Lysaker, P. H. (Eds.). (2010). *Metacognition and severe adult mental disorders: From basic research to treatment.* London: Routledge.

Dimaggio, G., Salvatore, G., Fiore, D., Carcione, A., Nicolò, G., & Semerari, A. (2012). General principles for treating the overconstricted personality disorder. Toward operationalizing technique. *Journal of Personality Disorders, 26,* 63–83.

Dimaggio, G., Salvatore, G., Popolo, R., & Lysaker, P. H. (2012). Autobiographical memory dysfunctions and poor understanding of mental states in personality disorders and schizophrenia: Clinical implications. *Frontiers in Cognition, 3,* 529.

Gilbert, P. (2005). Compassion and cruelty: A biopsychosocial approach. In P. Gilbert (Ed.), *Compassion: Conceptualisations, research and use in psychotherapy* (pp. 9–74). London: Routledge.

Gonçalves, M. M., Matos, M., & Santos, A. (2009). Narrative therapy and the nature of "innovative moments" in the construction of change. *Journal of Constructivist Psychology, 22,* 1–23.

Gonçalves, M. M., Mendes, I., Cruz, G., Ribeiro, A. P., Sousa, I., Angus, L., et al. (2012). Innovative moments and change in client-centered therapy. *Psychotherapy Research, 22,* 389–401.

Hermans, H. J. M., & Dimaggio, G. (2004). *The dialogical self in psychotherapy.* London: Brunner-Routledge.

McAdams, D. P. (2001). The psychology of life stories. *Review of General Psychology, 5,* 100–122.

Neimeyer, R. A. (2000). Narrative disruptions in the construction of self. In R. A. Neimeyer & J. D. Raskin (Eds.), *Constructions of disorder: Meaning making frameworks for psychotherapy* (pp. 207–241). Washington, DC: American Psychological Association.

Neimeyer, R. A. (2012). Reconstructing the self in the wake of loss: A dialogical contribution. In H. J. M Hermans & T. Gieser (Eds.), *Handbook of dialogical self theory* (pp. 374–389). Cambridge, UK: Cambridge University Press.

Padesky, C. A. (2012). Strengths-based cognitive-behavioral therapy: A four-step model to build resilience. *Clinical Psychology and Psychotherapy, 19*, 283–290.

Ribeiro, E., Ribeiro, A. P., Gonçalves, M. M., Horvath, A. O., & Stiles, W. B. (2013). How collaboration in therapy becomes therapeutic: The therapeutic collaboration coding system. *Psychology and Psychotherapy: Theory, Research and Practice, 86*(3), 294–314.

Salvatore, G., Dimaggio, G., & Semerari, A. (2004). A model of narrative development: Implications for understanding psychopathology and guiding therapy implication for clinical practice. *Psychology and Psychotherapy: Theory, Research and Practice, 77*, 231–254.

Salvatore, G., Lysaker, P. H., Procacci, M., Carcione, A., Popolo, R., & Dimaggio, G. (2012). Vulnerable self, poor understanding of others' minds, threat anticipation and cognitive biases as triggers for delusional experience in schizophrenia: A theoretical model. *Clinical Psychology and Psychotherapy, 19*, 247–259.

Semerari, A. (2010). The impact of metacognitive dysfunctions in personality disorders on the therapeutic relationship and intervention technique. In G. Dimaggio & P. H. Lysaker (Eds.), *Metacognition and severe adult mental disorders: From research to treatment* (pp. 269–284). London: Routledge.

Stiles, W. B. (1999). Signs and voices in psychotherapy. *Psychotherapy Research, 9*, 1–21.

Stiles, W. B. (2011). Coming to terms. *Psychotherapy Research, 21*, 367–384.

Summers, F. (2012). Creating new ways of being and relating. *Psychoanalytic Dialogues, 22*, 143–161.

chapter 18

Strategies for Constructing a More Adaptive Self-System

John F. Clarkin, Frank Yeomans, Chiara De Panfilis, and Kenneth N. Levy

There is growing consensus that the essential features of personality disorder involve difficulties with self-identity and interpersonal dysfunction (Bender & Skodol, 2007; Gunderson & Lyons-Ruth, 2008; Horowitz, 2004; Livesley, 2001; Pincus, 2005). This is a view that has long been espoused in object relations theory (Kernberg, 1984). These difficulties in identity and interpersonal functioning are intertwined, just as attention and memory contribute to conception of self and others and lead to the final common pathway of interpersonal behavior. In this chapter we describe aspects of a psychodynamic object relations approach (Caligor, Kernberg, & Clarkin, 2007; Clarkin, Yeomans, & Kernberg, 2006) to psychotherapy for patients' faulty conception of self and others, issues that are central to all personality disorders, and methods for exploring and modifying these internal representations. We are not advocating here the use of an object relations approach in the strict sense for all patients with personality disorder, as there are multiple empirically supported treatments, especially for patients with severe personality disorder, such as those with borderline personality disorder (BPD) (Bateman & Fonagy, 2008; Clarkin, Levy, et al., 2007; Linehan, Armstrong, Suarez, Allmon, & Heard, 1991). Rather, we are suggesting that in constructing an integrated treatment for patients with personality disorder—a treatment that addresses both disturbed behavior and disturbed internal world—concepts and procedures emphasized in our approach for the treatment of patients with personality disorder at various levels of severity could be useful for all therapists.

NORMAL AND PERSONALITY-DISTURBED REPRESENTATIONS

In describing personality disorder as involving dysfunctional mental representations of self and others, it is implied that individuals without personality disorder have accurate and integrated representations of self and others that enable them to interact productively, pleasurably, and flexibly with others. In contrast, patients with personality disorders manifest both observable behavior that is interpersonally disruptive and a pattern of internal symbolic representations of self and others that are dominated by extreme self-conceptions and intense affects—both overwhelmingly negative and unrealistically ideal—that interact with neurobiological aspects of the personality to affect their behavior (Lenzenweger, McClough, Clarkin, & Kernberg, 2012).

Cognitive–Affective Processing in Normal Personality Functioning

A prominent theory of normal personality that takes both enduring internal dispositions and particular environmental situations into account is the cognitive–affective processing system (CAPS) described by Mischel and Shoda (1995, 2008). CAPS theory conceives of personality in terms of distinct cognitive–affective units (CAUs) that describe an individual's encoding and construal of situations, beliefs about the world, affective tendencies, goals and values, and self-regulatory competencies (Mischel & Shoda, 1995). These cognitive–affective units are seen as distinct representations that exist in a structured network and mediate between the objective situation and the individual's behavioral response to it. The system itself is intrinsically interactional, so that its behavioral expressions are reflected in contextualized "if–then" patterns—the behavioral signatures of personality. Although the roots of this personality system are in the idiographic study of person–situation interactions (Mischel, 1973; Shoda, Mischel, & Wright, 1994), nomothetic research is also possible within CAPS based on particular structures and combinations of CAUs. In this manner, CAPS theory is able to capture intraindividual, interindividual, and group differences in personality (Eaton, South, & Krueger, 2009), making it a compelling model for personality dysfunction.

The CAPS model implicates an understanding of personality pathology in terms of various levels of severity in the impairment of interpersonal processing. When an individual processes situational features, his or her behavior is mediated by a set of CAUs, consisting of unique, specific mental representations of self and others, expectations, affects, and self-regulatory strategies such as attentional control. In this context, individuals' ability to regulate themselves under psychosocial stress constitutes a crucial ingredient for better functioning. More specifically, the effective regulation of negative arousal under conditions of interpersonal stress enables the inhibition of undesired, impulsive behaviors that may be elicited by the "automatic," "hot" activation of individual sets of CAUs (*self–other representations*). In turn, this may enable the impulse control, planning, and "cooling" operations that are basic for effective problem-solving strategies (Ayduk et al., 2000). An example of a dysfunctional CAU is rejection sensitivity, that is, the disposition to anxiously expect rejection. When these rejection-sensitive individuals encounter cues from the environment that they associate with rejection, expectations of rejection are activated, along with processing biases and intense emotional reactions that put a strain on the capacity for self-regulation. Under these conditions it is especially patients with BPD who lose sight of broader perspectives and long-term goals and react with rage (Berenson, Downey, Rafaeli, Coifman, & Paquin, 2011).

Object Relations Theory

The overall CAPS theory of personality functioning has a notable similarity to the object relations theory that we use (Clarkin et al., 2006; Kernberg & Caligor, 2005), as both place emphasis on mental representations accompanied by affective states that are activated by particular environmental situations. However, object relations theory utilizes observations from clinical therapeutic experiences to describe the dynamic action of the cognitive–affective units that are stimulated as the person interacts with the environment. Based on years of clinical experience with patients across a wide range of personality functioning, object relations theory focuses on the understanding of the internalized representations of self and others to levels of normal and abnormal personality functioning.

Object relations theory combines a dimension of severity of pathology with a categorical or prototypical classification based on a conception of personality organization (Clarkin et al., 2006; Kernberg & Caligor, 2005). This approach emphasizes both the severity of personality pathology by assessing the dimensions of identity, defensive operations, reality testing, aggression, and moral values and levels of personality organization captured in degrees of severity, going from high-level personality organization (i.e., neurotic organization) to mid- or borderline organization to severe or low-level borderline organization. The model attends in particular to the potential role of a stable but pathological sense of self, the extent to which pathology is influenced by aggression, the extent to which affective dispositions to depression or anxiety influence personality functioning, and the potential influence of a temperamental disposition to introversion or extroversion.

The object relations model posits four central structural aspects in the functioning of the normal personality (Kernberg, 2004). The normal individual's identity is composed of an integrated representation of self and representation of others. This internal, coherent sense of self and external behavior reflecting self-coherence enables the individual to function with balanced and realistic self-esteem, enjoyment, and zest for life. An integrated view of self ensures the capacity to use one's capacities to strive for one's goals and long-range commitments. An integrated view of others ensures the capacity to appropriately evaluate others, experience empathy, and invest emotionally in others in friendships and intimate relations without losing one's autonomy.

The second structural aspect of the normal personality is the broad range of emotional dispositions, capacity for affect modulation and impulse control, and capacity for investment in work and values. A third structural aspect of the normal personality is an internalization of a value system that is stable, abstract, and individualized. This moral structure is reflected in a sense of personal responsibility, capacity for realistic self-criticism, integrity and flexibility in dealing with ethical decision making, and commitment to values, ideals, and standards. A final structural aspect of the normal personality is appropriate and satisfying management of libidinal and aggressive impulses. This aspect is manifested in a capacity for a full expression of sensual and sexual needs, integrated with tenderness and emotional commitment, with a normal degree of idealization of the other. Aggression is expressed in the form of self-assertion and withstanding criticism or aggression from others without excessive reaction.

In the process of formulating a treatment plan for the individual patient, the severity of personality pathology is typically as important as the personality "type." This view is consistent with that of those who emphasize that severity of personality pathology is most relevant for treatment planning (e.g., Verheul et al., 2008). Object relations theory has developed in a clinical treatment setting with information and data from experience with patients.

SOCIAL-NEUROCOGNITIVE ADVANCES

Recent advances in social-cognitive neuroscience demonstrate that patients with personality disorder exhibit various degrees of impairment in social-cognitive abilities. Social cognition broadly refers to the ability to interpret and predict another's behavior in terms of beliefs, intentions, and desires and to use flexibly the representation of the relationship between oneself and others to guide social behavior. Underlying processes involved in social cognition capacities include basic neurocognitive functions (working memory, attention), emotion and face perception, self- and other representation, attachment systems, responses to social pain and rejection, empathy, theory of mind, and reflective functioning (see, e.g., Dimaggio, Semerari, Carcione, Procacci, & Nicolò, 2006). Clinically, an impairment in social cognition among people with personality disorder is reflected in their inaccurate social reality testing (i.e., the capacity to read and correctly interpret social cues and to tactfully respond to social situations; Caligor & Clarkin, 2010) and, ultimately, in their pervasive deficits in interpersonal functioning. Specifically, individuals who exhibit borderline personality organization (i.e., various degrees of personality pathology) tend to possess a hostile, paranoid world view that leads them to be preoccupied with negative information in the environment and to be suspicious of the intent of others (e.g., Kernberg, 1967). This characteristic may represent a failure in the ability to recognize that others may have different intent and perspectives than oneself and to correctly identify the nature of those perspectives (Selman, 1980). Social information-processing research has shown that children who fail to develop this ability at appropriate ages and who exhibit hostile attributional biases are at risk for serious concurrent and future adjustment patterns, such as peer rejection, aggressive behaviors, or to a lesser extent, avoidance/withdrawal (Crick & Dodge, 1994), as well as borderline features (Crick, Murray-Close, & Woods, 2005).

Rejection Sensitivity

The construct of rejection sensitivity (RS), which has emerged from CAP theory, is central to understanding difficulties in self–other representation and their relationship to disturbed interpersonal functioning among people with personality disorder. RS is conceptualized as a cognitive–affective processing disposition to anxiously expect, readily perceive, and react in an exaggerated manner to cues of rejection in the behavior of others. People high on RS focus extensively on anxious expectations of rejection and thus perceive intentional hurt in significant others' ambiguous or even innocuous behavior and respond to rejection with greater negativity. Thus they have difficulty encoding contextual information that may provide alternative explanations for others' behavior and facilitate taking others' perspectives. Rather, they interpret by default a social situation as confirming their rejection fears (Ayduk et al., 2000, 2008; Downey, Mougios, Ayduk, London, & Shoda, 2004; Romero-Canyas, Downey, Berenson, Ayduk, & Kang, 2010). This automatic, "hot," and reflexive ascription of negative dispositions to others accounts for increasing interpersonal conflicts, leading to a self-fulfilling prophecy of rejection (Ayduk et al., 2000; Ayduk, Mischel, & Downey, 2002; Downey & Feldman, 1996; Romero-Canyas, Downey, Berenson, et al., 2010). Therefore, individuals with high RS are vulnerable to developing poor self-esteem, flawed peer relationships, inability to cope with stress, lower educational attainment, and limited social adjustment (Ayduk et al., 2000; Mischel et al., 2011).

Consistently, RS is considered a core feature fostering the interpersonal difficulties of several groups of personality disorders, such as avoidant (characterized by extreme social avoidance), dependent (characterized by extreme social preoccupation) (Feldman & Downey, 1994), and BPD (characterized by a negative or hostile attitude toward others) (Ayduk et al., 2008; Staebler, Helbing, Rosenbach, & Renneberg, 2011; Staebler, Renneberg, et al., 2011). The relevance of RS for adjustment and personality psychopathology is not surprising. In order to successfully navigate the interpersonal world, individuals must be able to deal with trust and rejection-related or ambiguous challenges arising from social interactions in everyday life, and this is likely to require sophisticated social-cognitive skills.

The Paradox of Trust

Trusting and cooperating are always risky, given the unpredictability of the intentions of the partner in a social exchange. To build a trust relationship, partners must learn that they can depend on each other. Establishing expectations of others as trustworthy requires, first of all, the activation of the paracingulate cortex, a region involved in representing the mental states of other people, and subsequently of the septal area, a limbic region that has been demonstrated to modulate various aspects of social behavior, including social memory, learning, and attachment. This may suggest that during the building stage of trust partners must infer each other's intentions to determine whether to trust their partners and whether their partners will reciprocate their trust in the future. In turn, by developing "better" mental models, partners accumulate sufficient mutual trust to become socially attached to each other and to cooperate in advantageous ways (Krueger et al., 2007).

On the other hand, human beings are strongly motivated to avoid social rejection and maintain social bonds. Consistently, perceived social rejection is a powerful trigger for intrapsychic conflict. Specifically, both social pain and violations of acceptance expectations activate brain regions commonly associated with emotional and cognitive conflicts (namely, the ventral and the dorsal anterior cingulate cortex [ACC]). This "alarm" system functions to signal prefrontal areas (dorsolateral prefrontal cortex [LPFC]) so that the need to increase cognitive control in order to respond to and help interpret goal-incongruent events such as rejection (Bishop, Duncan, Brett, & Lawrence, 2004; Eisenberger, Lieberman, & Williams, 2003; Somerville, Heatherton, & Kelley, 2006). This additional recruitment of LPFC allows interpreting rejection-related stimuli in ways that minimize personal distress, making it possible to promote one's goal achievement and adjustment in spite of events that violated social motives and expectancies for affiliation and bonding (Kross, Egner, Ochsner, Hirsch, & Downey, 2007). Indeed, among individuals without clinical disorders, the ability to successfully resolve conflicts arising from perceived interpersonal rejection depends on the deployment of effortful attentional strategies subserved by LPFC activity (Hooker, Gyurak, Verosky, Miyakawa, & Ayduk, 2010). For instance, a strategy adopted after social exclusion may involve increased mentalizing for positive social cues and less mentalizing for the contents of negative social scenes (Powers, Wagner, Norris, & Heatherton, 2013). Furthermore, both successful self-regulation following an interpersonal conflict and the capacity to attribute independent mental states to others and to take into account others' beliefs when interpreting their behavior depend on the activity of those attentional control networks (Hooker et al., 2010; Lin, Keysar, & Epley, 2010). Thus such effortful social-cognitive processes are likely to be crucial to help inhibit one's own experience (e.g., perceived rejection) during the consideration of another's state of mind (e.g., perceived malevolence or untrustworthiness), and they favor the unbiased ascription of independent motivations to another person's behavior (e.g., neutral intention, context-dependent evaluation), ultimately promoting affect regulation, prosocial behavior, and adjustment (Lieberman, 2007). Interestingly, people with high RS show decreased activity in the PFC regions related to cognitive control after viewing rejection-themed images (Kross et al., 2007).

These insights into the neurocognitive underpinnings of trust and responses to social rejection are particularly relevant for personality disorder pathology, as available evidence suggests that these patients may differ dramatically from participants without disorders with respect to the strategies deployed to deal with rejection–trust dilemmas. Specifically, the capacity to "reflectively" deal with social rejection and trust issues seems to be grossly decreased in patients with personality disorders. For instance, low executive control abilities increase the risk of developing borderline features in individuals high in RS (Ayduk et al., 2008) and predict difficulties in decoding others' facial expressions of anger in people with high BPD traits (Gardner, Qualter, Stylianou, & Robinson, 2010). Furthermore, patients with BPD exhibit an "automatic" hypersensitivity to negative social cues (Koenigsberg, Siever, et al., 2009) coupled with deficits in perspective taking and increased personal distress (Dziobek et al., 2011). In other words, they show a marked tendency to adopt a self-referential processing and first-person perspective (i.e., a "reflexive" processing of human actions and assessment of intentions) when faced with social stimuli. Finally, patients with BPD also show atypical social norms in perception of social exchanges, consistent with pervasive social expectations of untrustworthiness, that eventually lead to the inability to benefit from cooperative exchange (Kings-Casas et al., 2008). Taken together, these findings suggest that patients with BPD do not deploy the attentional skills necessary to process interpersonal rejection–trust dilemmas in a "reflective" way, thereby increasing the likelihood of reacting in a self-centered and defensive manner and of developing interpersonal disturbances and uncooperative behaviors.

The Role of Negative Affect

Negative affect plays a major role in shaping the relationship between a reflexive social-cognition style and personality disorder psychopathology. According to a biased competition view of attention and cognitive resources (Desimone & Duncan, 1995; Heatherton & Wagner, 2011), competition among stimuli for neural representation is strongly influenced by bottom-up stimulus salience. Threat-related (i.e., negative affectively charged) stimuli are of high salience and are strong competitors for attention. Under such circumstances, increasing cognitive control skills are required to deal with the compelling issue of emotional and behavioral regulation. This might result in decreased availability of cognitive control resources to process rejection-related stimuli and to accurately infer others' perspective. In this regard, social exclusion in BPD is associated with increasing negative affect (Sadikaj, Russel, Moskowitz, & Paris, 2010), including negative emotions toward others (Renneberg et al., 2012; Staebler, Renneberg, et al., 2011), emotion dysregulation, and problem behaviors (Selby, Ward, & Joiner, 2010). Because under conditions of negative affect patients with BPD show an impairment in conflict resolution and cognitive control (Domes et al., 2006; Silbersweig et al., 2007), this mechanism might potentially explain why patients with BPD undergo difficulties in social problem solving after negative affect induced by social rejection (Dixon-Gordon, Chapman, Lovasz, & Walters, 2011).

Finally, the intensity of negative affect experienced by patients with personality disorders does not seem to be counterbalanced by top-down processes required to bias the competition among stimuli that would otherwise allow objects and tasks that are less salient (e.g., reflective social attributions or goal-directed behavior) to win attentional competition over emotionally salient stimuli/distractors (i.e., negative affect). For instance, trait anxiety is associated with decreased LPFC control over threat-related stimuli (Bishop et al., 2004), and patients with BPD show a relative inability in top-down control and reappraisal of negative affect (Koenigsberg, Fan, et al., 2009; Lang et al., 2011).

These considerations suggest that personality psychopathology may be viewed in part as a dysregulated, reflexive response to managing the rejection–trust dilemma in the interpersonal arena. Patients with personality disorders are constantly faced with an approach–avoidance dilemma posed by (1) desperately wanting to connect to others while (2) being intensely threatened by the prospect of rejection by them. However, they may show different types of maladaptive "solutions" to deal with this dilemma. For instance, rejection cues may foster anger, rage, and hostile reactions among patients with personality disorders when it is impossible to disengage from rejection-relevant cues (Berenson et al., 2011), but they may also be associated with attentional avoidance of social threats in an effort to regulate the experience of threat by reducing emotional arousal and distress in situations in which it is impossible or undesirable to flee (Berenson et al., 2009) or with the inhibition of actions that might elicit further exclusion and efforts to please the threat source when there is a viable possibility of acceptance (Romero-Canyas, Downey, Reddy, et al., 2010). Thus rejection could be a trigger of both prosocial and disrupted behavior, depending on the interpersonal context and the unique dispositional cognitive–affective processing of the individual.

Therefore, the RS dynamics represent a promising venue through which to explore the phenomenology of personality pathology. From the perspective of the CAPS system, RS is a dynamic pattern of interconnected expectations of self and others and related affects that is triggered by specific psychological features of the interpersonal situation and that, in turn, elicits intense reactions to rejection (Ayduk et al., 2000). Furthermore, recent findings from social-cognitive neuroscience converge to suggest that RS dynamics among patients with personality disorders are not buffered by the adoption of "controlled," "cooling" social-cognitive strategies, thus accounting for the increasing expectations of rejections and untrustworthiness, negative affect in response to social cues, and consequent maladaptive responses. Finally, the diverse behavioral and defensive strategies that patients adopt to deal with expected or perceived rejection from significant others may play a major role in shaping PD phenomenology and severity.

THERAPEUTIC APPROACHES TO REPRESENTATIONS OF SELF AND OTHERS

Clinicians across diverse treatment orientations, including cognitive (Pretzer & Beck, 2004), metacognitive (Dimaggio & Lysaker, 2010), interpersonal (Benjamin, 2005; Cain & Pincus, Chapter 14, this volume), attachment (Levy, 2005; Meyer & Pilkonis, 2005), and object relations (Clarkin, Lenzenweger, et al., 2007; Clarkin, Levy, et al., 2007) perspectives emphasize therapeutic intervention focused on the patients' representations of self and others. These internal representations of self and others are variously referred to as *CAUs*, *schemas*, *interpersonal copies*, *internal working models*, and *internalized object relations dyads* (which is our preferred term) and in process terms such as *reflective functioning*. Interpersonal behavior is guided by cognitive–affective representations of self and others (see Mischel & Shoda, 2008). These self–other representations constantly appear in therapy exchanges in which patients describe their relationship patterns with others to the therapist and in patients' descriptions of their feelings and thoughts about the therapist.

In the object relations orientation, the severity of the personality disorganization is as important to treatment planning as the specific type of personality disorder as described in DSM-5. Severity of personality disorder is related to dimensional measures of degree of identity diffusion, quality of object relations, defenses, reality testing, amount and degree of aggression, and the level of internalized moral values (see Caligor & Clarkin, 2010). Table 18.1 describes levels of severity of self-representations, representations of others, and interpersonal functioning. Patients with personality disorders with mild levels of severity have a complex and realistic internalized representation of self and others that enables them, albeit with some conflicts, to realistically relate to others and to control their affect in interpersonal relations. In contrast, patients at the moderate level of personality disorder severity have a biased internal representation of self and others, which leaves them with difficulties in goal-oriented self-direction and challenges in accurately perceiving the motivations of others. Patients with severe personality disorder not only have identity diffusion—that is, polarized and distorted perceptions of self and others—but also more aggressive temperament, lack of clear goals, and minimal internal moral coherence. In our experience, treatment planning depends in a major way on the severity level of personality dysfunction in

TABLE 18.1. Representations of Self and Others and Object Relations: Degrees of Health and Severity of Dysfunction

Self-representation	Representation of other	Interpersonal relations
Self-experience and life goals are coherent and continuous across time and situation	Stable, integrated, realistic representations of others	Strong, durable, realistic, nuanced, and satisfying relations with others; able to form and sustain friendships and intimate relations
Self-experience and life goals are somewhat coherent	Clear, reflective picture of others that is integrated and relatively stable though somewhat superficial	Attachments are generally strong and durable; some degree of impairment in intimate/sexual relations
Self-experience and life goals are somewhat poorly integrated, superficial, discontinuous	Representations of others are unstable, vague, or superficial, may be self-referential	Attachments are superficial, brittle, and flawed; tendency to view relationships in terms of need fulfillment; limited capacity for empathy with others' needs
Self-experience is poorly integrated, unstable, superficial; life goals unclear, unstable, and/or unrealistic	A rudimentary description of others but contradictory, unstable	Attachments are few and flawed; sees relationships largely in terms of need fulfillment; little capacity for empathy with others' needs independent of those of the self
Unintegrated and chaotic self-experience; no sense of a coherent self or life goals	Superficial, chaotic representations of others that are largely defined by own anxieties, defenses, and needs	Severe paucity of attachments; sees relationships entirely in terms of need fulfillment; no capacity for empathy; no capacity to sustain interest in others

conjunction with the particular personality disorder(s) the patient manifests. The research on severe personality disorder suggests that treatment is effective in significantly reducing symptoms but that differentiated effects of specific treatments are elusive. Furthermore, the mechanisms by which the treatments achieve their effects, although hypothesized by the various treatment orientations, have not been convincingly demonstrated.

The integrated treatment approach espoused in this book builds on the knowledge that common factors across treatments must be involved in significant change. An integrated treatment approach openly faces the clinical reality that in those situations in which one standard treatment is applied (e.g., dialectical behavior therapy [DBT]), there are important nuances in the specific relationship between patient and therapist. It could be that common factors are most operative and effective with mild personality disorder severity and that skilled use of specific approaches are required in the moderate to severe cases of personality disorder.

We have outlined a range of treatment strategies (Caligor et al., 2007; Clarkin et al., 2006) that enable the clinician to examine with the patient his or her mental representations of self and others as they are activated in the ongoing relationship with the therapist. We suggest that from the very beginning of clinical assessment a consistent and structured approach be used toward defining the responsibilities of both patient and therapist if the treatment is to be successful. The behaviors required for consistent and systematic treatment engagement are the beginnings of some self-responsible attitudes and related behavior. In the contract setting phase of treatment, we negotiate with the patient some form of volunteer or paid part-time or full-time work activity. In the process of negotiating this aspect of the treatment, the patient must call upon previous work activities and known capabilities to choose a suitable work activity during the treatment. The choice of a work activity is an essential process in the accruing sense of self-identity and putting some of that into action. In addition, treatment activity focused on a patient's current interpersonal relations with the therapist and with social contacts in the patient's current life environment can correct distortions in the patient's perception of these interchanges.

We have found that the therapeutic discussion between patient and therapist activates the patient's habitual and characteristic mental representations of self, other, and relationship patterns not only in the content of their discourse but even more so in the interaction with the therapist. In these approaches, it is assumed that the patient exhibits in the relationship with the therapist some of the same interpersonal difficulties that plague his or her daily life. Examination and understanding of these difficulties in the therapeutic relationship can help patients make needed adjustments to improve other relationships in their lives.

An ill-informed stereotypical view of dynamic treatments, including transference-focused psychotherapy (TFP), is that they focus exclusively on internal experience without attention to behavior and behavior change. In this chapter, we hope to show that change in identity and self-functioning is intertwined with change in self-representation combined with change in behavior. For example, patients with BPD at the most defective end of identity diffusion also manifest related behavioral patterns of lack of investment in work and leisure activities and difficulties in intimacy, interdependence, and gratification in both intimate and social relations (see Table 18.1). As described in the clinical case in this chapter, TFP begins with a treatment contracting process that addresses the individual patient's current work capacity and activity. In our estimation, many of these patients are not working, are living off parents or the welfare system, but are capable of some form of part-time or full-time work activity. This is not just an issue of parasitism and lack of work productivity, but in real terms this is an issue of identity and self-definition. The self-identity or self-representation is activated most in terms of work activities and intimate relations. In the treatment process, there is an interactional process between changing self-representations and improvement in work, social, and intimate interpersonal functioning.

From an integrationist view, it is important to note that most of the empirically supported treatments for BPD focus to varying degrees on the relationship between patient and therapist. DBT focuses on the patient–therapist relationship when the relationship is seen as interfering with the treatment (see McMain & Wiebe, 2013). In such circumstances, the therapist is encouraged to reveal his or her personal reactions to the patient and thus overcome the interference with the treatment process. In contrast, mentalizing-based therapy (MBT; see Bateman & Fonagy, Chapter 7, this volume), interpersonal therapy (see Cain & Pincus, Chapter 14, and Tufekcioglu & Muran, Chapter 6, this volume), and TFP place more central importance on understanding the relationship between patient and therapist as directly therapeutic.

One cannot conceptualize techniques of treatment that can be applied to patients with personality disorders irrespective of the context in which these therapist interventions are utilized. In our clinical experience with patients with personality disorder of moderate to severe levels, there are three major contexts in which the utilization of psychodynamic strategies and techniques are useful in advancing the patient's conception of self and others. These three situations can be described as follows:

1. Moments of intense affect demonstrated by the patient toward the therapist and/or the treatment. These moments test the therapist's ability to stay in role and begin to help the patient understand and accept her or his own intense affects as related to momentary perceptions of self and other.
2. Moments in the treatment when there is an opportunity for the therapist to help the patient understand how intense affects that overwhelm his or her cognitive efforts can be rooted in the experience of self and others.
3. The therapist's ability to draw the patient's attention to ways in which his or her characteristic ways of experiencing self and other get played out in behaviors and life choices that undermine the patient's options for finding satisfaction in work and relationships.

The following case example depicts instances of all three of these events as they unfold in the treatment.

CASE EXAMPLE

A 23-year-old woman began therapy after 7 years of prior treatment for depression, anxiety, and self-destructive and suicidal behaviors. Her diagnoses had included bipolar illness, recurrent major depression, and BPD. At the time of referral, BPD was the primary diagnosis. Prior treatments included supportive psychotherapies, medication (antidepressants, mood stabilizers, anxiolytics, and low-dose neuroleptics), and a number of hospitalizations.

The patient was married and unemployed at the beginning of treatment. She did not work or attend classes because of her fear that others would be critical and rejecting of her. Her prior therapist had considered her the victim of neglectful parents and offered her extra contact outside of sessions in an attempt to soothe the patient's feelings of loneliness and emptiness. This strategy did not help, as the patient's symptoms continued, and she was hospitalized after another suicide attempt.

The patient's initial response/transference to her new therapist was to experience him as a cold, uncaring robot. The trigger for this was the therapist's beginning the treatment with more emphasis on the treatment frame than had existed in the prior therapy. One element of this frame was that phone contact between sessions was limited to calling about practical arrangements or true emergencies (in contrast to the patient's chronic distress, chaos, and wish for immediate but fleeting support). The therapist worked on helping the patient see that her particular perception of and response to the treatment frame might provide valuable information about her automatic way of experiencing herself as the object of the uncaring neglect of others and to use this observation of her automatic tendency to more accurately appraise her encounters with others. However, as happens in these cases, the patient's affective experience temporarily took precedence over her ability to understand, appreciate, and apply the ideas being discussed. Her internal world flooded the treatment situation, as is expected and can be worked with. In sessions the patient began to report thoughts about dangerous acting out. The therapist experienced anxiety and discomfort as he listened to these reports, but the patient maintained a calm tone.

The therapist hypothesized that this part of their interaction might be an expression in action of another set of internal representations of self and other: in addition to the neglected–neglecter dyad, the patient's internal world seemed to be populated by a persecutor–victim dyad. The therapist attempted to engage the patient's attention in considering the possible impact on the therapist of her apparently carefree urges to hurt herself. He suggested that, in addition to the intrapersonal relief that the patient reported from harming herself, there might be an interpersonal element, such as trying to engage more active involvement from him or trying to show that she was stronger than he. However, the patient's reports of urges to hurt herself increased to the point that she went to the emergency room one evening. Because the emergency room staff was familiar with her capacity for self-destructive behavior, they placed her on "one-to-one observation" with a security guard. In that setting, she took a razor blade she had hidden and cut both wrists without the guard's immediate notice. She was then hospitalized.

Her therapist arranged a session with her in the hospital. His focus was on understanding the patient's experience rather than more directly changing her behavior. In her narrative of the events leading to the hospitalization, the patient described her being able to cut herself in the presence of the guard with a visible pleasure. The therapist stopped the patient in narrative and asked if she were aware of her affect. She was not. When he pointed out that she appeared to experience some pleasure at her ability to cut herself in front of the guard and thereby humiliate him, the patient responded with indignation, accusing the therapist of labeling her as a sadist and angrily denouncing his cruelty in suggesting such a thing. The therapist observed the patient's discomfort with that term and wondered whether she found it difficult to consider that she might find some pleasure in aggressive impulses, as many people do. The patient was discharged from the hospital, and the next sessions continued this exploration of her relationship to her aggressive side. She came to understand that those emotions constituted a part of her that she had always been very uncomfortable acknowledging. She had typically dealt with them in one of two ways. She most often confused the source of the aggressive affect in a relationship and experienced it as present in others rather than in herself, as she had done in accusing her therapist of cruelty in talking about her aggressive affect. Her perception camouflaged her anxiety about working, studying, or otherwise interacting with others, whom she tended automatically to see as aggressive. The second way she dealt with aggressive affect was to put it into an action without a conscious awareness that it involved aggression; for instance, although she was very sensitive to and objected to any display of aggression on the part of others (e.g., boys "roughhousing" in the park), she did not consider that there was any aggression—either to herself or to those who cared about her—in her cutting or otherwise harming herself.

This discussion of the patient's aggressive affects appeared to help her acknowledge and integrate this part of herself that she had traditionally experienced as part of a relationship rather than being within herself. In other words, one aspect of her experience of self had traditionally been that of the victim of others' judgments, criticisms, and aggression. This view of self and other existed *within* her and guided her perception of herself in relation to others and her behavior in relation to others. She was wary and avoidant of others, anticipating negative responses. Nevertheless, she also identified with the persecutor side of the victim–persecutor relationship dyad, enacting the persecutor (1) in relation to herself by means of judgments, criticisms, and, at times, self-destructive actions and (2) in her relations with others, as seen in the example in the emergency room and in her tendency to cause pain in others through her attacks on herself.

The therapist's help succeeded in getting the patient to know and symbolically represent and reflect on her aggressive affects and had a positive impact in reducing her self-destructive acting out in that the patient stopped self-cutting and overdosing, the two principal problems for a number of years. However, even without those dramatic problems, she continued to experience difficulties in her life, especially in the form of anxiety in relation to others. As part of the treatment contract (which included an agreement to engage in school or work), the patient began to attend college courses to complete her undergraduate degree. The most common theme in sessions became her conviction that the other students disliked and disapproved of her. Symptoms of anxiety and depressive affect were associated with this. Exploration of the extent of her feelings revealed that she secretly harbored very critical views of her classmates. The problem in her life once again appeared to be based on a view of self and others in terms of the paradigm of the aggressed–criticized and the aggressor–critic. This paradigm was somewhat attenuated now in contrast to its earlier manifestation in physical acting out. Once again, bringing the patient to an increased level of awareness of her views of self and other helped diminish her symptoms.

After a year and a half of therapy, the patient decided she was stable enough to have a child, and she became a mother less than a year later. She suspended her therapy for a number of months to stay at home with her baby boy. Although she managed reasonably well, she was not without some symptoms of anxiety, loneliness, and difficulties with self-esteem. She returned to therapy to work on these. As her child grew into his second year, the patient became preoccupied with the anxiety that one of the doormen in her apartment building harbored illicit sexual feelings toward the boy. She based this suspicion on certain looks she perceived and minor interactions. The challenge in therapy was to distinguish between "internal" anxieties based within the patient and the possibility that her anxieties represented an accurate reading of a real situation. At this point the therapist wondered about the views of self and other that emerged in relation to sexual and sensual feelings. The patient's parents had been somewhat loose with boundaries in the home as the patient was growing up (e.g., walking around the house naked). As the therapist helped the patient explore her thoughts about sexual feelings that might be experienced in the context of the physical sensations involved in mothering, her anxieties about the doorman resolved. At this point, the views of self and other that were activated had more to do with libidinal than aggressive feelings and involved becoming comfortable with certain feelings and fantasies that can be part of a natural bond rather than necessarily perverse.

Toward the end of her therapy, the patient moved from the city to a suburb. As she settled into the new environment, she experienced some recrudescence of the anxiety that others—her new neighbors, in this case—were critical and rejecting of her. This represented a repetition of the less disturbing but still present view of self and others that was based on negative critical affects. Knowing the theme well by now, the patient and therapist were able to explore the ambiguous situations that the patient perceived as rejecting to distinguish between situations in which the experience of rejection may have a base in reality and those that appeared to be based on what remained of her internal images and to help her enter more quickly into the more objective, less threatening reality of her new environment. It should be noted that the patient's anxiety about relations diminished in intensity as her acceptance and mastery of her own aggressive feelings proceeded. Part of this process was the development of more socially acceptable forms of expressing aggression, such as irony and humor. Another part of the process was that the decrease in projection allowed her to engage in social activities that she had often previously avoided. This increased engagement with others provided data that the world was generally more benign than the earlier internal images that guided her. She was able to take in this more objective data only when she became consciously aware of the power and location of those internal images.

CONCLUDING COMMENTS

Psychotherapeutic intervention for individuals with various levels of personality pathology should be based on sound theoretical conceptions of normal personality functioning that becomes distorted in abnormal personality functioning. There is a convergence of interest in the real-time functioning of individuals across CAPS theory, object relations theory, and social neurocognitive research. It is most specifically the question of how individuals in real time interact socially with other human beings that captures the essence of both normal and abnormal personality functioning. Both internal representations of self and others with related affects and behavioral manifestations of these internal states are essential to understanding human social behavior. In normal human functioning, the individual has a need to relate to others, and this need is carried out with some basic sense of security by anticipating acceptance by others and a trust in mutual cooperation. This basic sense of acceptance and trust is disturbed in individuals with personality pathology. Just as theory and research focus on the real-time functioning of the individual, psychotherapy can utilize an in-depth examination of the real-time functioning in the interaction between patient and therapist.

The case example described in this chapter concerns one individual, but this individual is typical of many patients with personality disorder and related comorbid conditions in our empirical efforts. In reference to levels of personality disorder severity, she was at the high level of severity, as she reported both high levels of subjective anger and self-destructive behavior. She was suspicious of others (in analytic conceptions, she projected her own aggression onto others and perceived it as coming at her from the outside), and was high in rejection sensitivity. We have examined in this chapter the neurocognitive underpinnings of rejection sensitivity and the various ways (e.g., avoidance, rage) that it can be handled.

The therapist structured the treatment with a verbal contract at the beginning, eliciting the patient's effort to control self-destructive behavior. The self-destructive behavior and its relationship to the interpersonal realm (i.e., the impact of her self-destructive behavior on the relationship with the therapist) were highlighted in this approach. Once the self-destructive behavior was acknowledged by the patient in the relationship with the therapist, it decreased as the affects associated with it were explored, and this provided space for investigating the patient's self–other perception in the major areas of relationship in her life. Both a gratification in being critical–aggressive and also rejection sensitivity were paramount in the patient's experience of classmates, the doorman, and new neighbors. One can conceive of this treatment progression as going from aggression expressed in the form of suicidal and self-destructive behavior to serious suspicions of others to cautious expansion of her interpersonal world while becoming more aware of the inaccurate expectation of rejection. This progression was accomplished in the context of a conflicted but consistent and gradually safer relationship with a therapist who could tolerate the aggression and tactfully point out the aggression to the patient, while staying in the therapeutic role without attacking or abandoning the patient.

In the case of severe personality disorder described here, this therapist's drawing attention to the patient's aggression toward others and toward him (the therapist) enabled the patient to both more fully acknowledge her own aggression (without just blaming others) and to modify the expression of the aggression. Aggressive behavior decreased, but perception of aggression from others, whether real or imagined, remained, with concomitant feelings of anxiety and fear of rejection by others perceived as critical and aggressive. This, in turn, was explored as it surfaced concerning the doorman, neighbors, and so forth. As representations of self and others changed, she took steps to further her education and become a parent, behavioral activities that both activate and enhance a growing, positive sense of self.

The case example illustrates: (1) the impact of internal experiences of self and other on the individual's life and symptoms and (2) the utility of working with these images in helping a patient improve symptomatically, behaviorally, and in his or her appreciation of life. The process of change involves:

- Experiencing the patient's sense of self both with the therapist and in other settings.
- Helping the patient become more aware of the interplay between her internal affect states and her experience of self and others.
- A dialectic between change in the patient's awareness of aspects of her own affective experience and her experiences in the world; the patient's learning to question and modify her views of self and others within the therapy leads to a change in perception of experiences in the world—and then to a change in the nature of those experiences—that further contributes to the change process.

REFERENCES

Ayduk, O., Mendoza-Denton, R., Mischel, W., Downey, G., Peake, P. K., & Rodriguez, M. (2000). Regulating the interpersonal self: Strategic self-regulation for coping with rejection sensitivity. *Journal of Personality and Social Psychology, 79*, 776–792.

Ayduk, O., Mischel, W., & Downey, G. (2002). Attentional mechanisms linking rejection to hostile reactivity: The role of "hot" versus "cool" focus. *Psychological Science, 13,* 443–448.

Ayduk, O., Zayas, V., Downey, G., Cole, A. B., Shoda, Y., & Mischel, W. (2008). Rejection sensitivity and executive control: Joint predictors of borderline personality features. *Journal of Research in Personality, 42,* 151–168.

Bateman, A., & Fonagy, P. (2000). Effectiveness of psychotherapeutic treatment of personality disorder. *British Journal of Psychiatry, 177,* 138–143.

Bateman, A., & Fonagy, P. (2008). 8-year follow-up of patients treated for borderline personality disorder: Mentalization-based treatment versus treatment as usual. *American Journal of Psychiatry, 165,* 631–638.

Bender, D. S., & Skodol, A. E. (2007). Borderline personality as self–other representational disturbance, *Journal of Personality Disorders, 21,* 500–517.

Benjamin, L. S. (2005). Interpersonal theory of personality disorders: The structural analysis of social behavior and interpersonal reconstructive therapy. In M. F. Lenzenweger & J. F. Clarkin (Eds.), *Major theories of personality disorder* (2nd ed., pp. 157–230). New York: Guilford Press.

Berenson, K. R., Downey, G., Rafaeli, E., Coifman, K. G., & Paquin, N. L. (2011). The rejection-rage contingency in borderline personality disorder. *Journal of Abnormal Psychology, 120,* 681–690.

Berenson, K. R., Gyurak, A., Ayduk, O., Downey, G., Garner, M. J., Mogg, K., et al. (2009). Rejection sensitivity and disruption of attention by social threats cues. *Journal of Research in Personality, 43,* 1064–1072.

Bishop, S., Duncan, J., Brett, M., & Lawrence, A. D. (2004). Prefrontal cortical function and anxiety: Controlling attention to threat-related stimuli. *Nature Neuroscience, 7,* 184–188.

Caligor, E., & Clarkin, J. F. (2010). An object relations model of personality and personality pathology. In J. F. Clarkin, P. Fonagy, & G. O. Gabbard (Eds.), *Psychodynamic psychotherapy for personality disorders: A clinical handbook* (pp. 3–35). Washington, DC: American Psychiatric Publishing.

Caligor, E., Kernberg, O. F., & Clarkin, J. F. (2007). *Handbook of dynamic psychotherapy for higher level personality pathology.* Washington, DC: American Psychiatric Publishing.

Clarkin, J. F., Lenzenweger, M. F., Yeomans, F., Levy, K. N., & Kernberg, O. F. (2007). An object relations model of borderline pathology. *Journal of Personality Disorders, 21,* 474–499.

Clarkin, J. F., Levy, K. N., Lenzenweger, M. F., & Kernberg, O. F. (2007). Evaluating three treatments for borderline personality disorder: A multiwave study. *American Journal of Psychiatry, 164,* 922–928.

Clarkin, J. F., Yeomans, F. E., & Kernberg, O. F. (2006). *Psychotherapy for borderline personality: Focusing on object relations.* Washington, DC: American Psychiatric Publishing.

Crick, N. R., & Dodge, K. A. (1994). A review and reformulation of social information processing mechanisms in children's social adjustment. *Psychological Bulletin, 115,* 74–101.

Crick, N. R., Murray-Close, D., & Woods, K. (2005). Borderline personality features in childhood: A short-term longitudinal study. *Development and Psychopathology, 17,* 1051–1070.

Desimone, R., & Duncan, J. (1995). Neural mechanisms of selective attention. *Annual Review of Neurosciences, 18,* 193–222.

Dimaggio, G., & Lysaker, P. H. (Eds.). (2010). *Metacognition and severe adult mental disorders: From research to treatment.* New York: Routledge.

Dimaggio, G., Semerari, A., Carcione, A., Procacci, M., & Nicolò, G. (2006). Toward a model of self pathology underlying personality disorders: Narratives, metacognition, interpersonal cycles and decision-making processes. *Journal of Personality Disorders, 20,* 597–617.

Dixon-Gordon, K. L., Chapman, A. L., Lovasz, N., & Walters, K. (2011). Too upset to think: The interplay of borderline personality features, negative emotions, and social problem solving in the laboratory. *Personality Disorders: Theory, Research, and Treatment, 2,* 243–260.

Domes, G., Winter, B., Schnell, K., Vohs, K., Fast, K., & Herpertz, S. C. (2006). The influence of emotions on inhibitory functioning in borderline personality disorder. *Psychological Medicine, 36,* 1163–1172.

Downey, G., & Feldman, S. I. (1996). Implications of rejection sensitivity for intimate relationships. *Journal of Personality and Social Psychology, 6,* 1327–1343.

Downey, G., Mougios, V., Ayduk, O., London, B. E., & Shoda, Y. (2004). Rejection sensitivity and the defensive motivational system: Insights from the startle response to rejection cues. *Psychological Science, 15,* 668–673.

Dziobek, I., Preissler, S., Grozdanovic, Z., Heuser, I., Heekeren, H. R., & Roepke, S. (2011). Neuronal correlates of altered empathy and social cognition in borderline personality disorder. *NeuroImage, 57,* 539–548.

Eaton, N. R., South, S. C., & Krueger, R. F. (2009). The cognitive-affective processing system (CAPS) approach to personality and the concept of personality disorder: Integrating clinical and social-cognitive research. *Journal of Research in Personality, 43,* 208–217.

Eisenberger, N. I., Lieberman, M. D., & Williams, K. D. (2003). Does rejection hurt?: An fMRI study of social exclusion. *Science, 302,* 290–292.

Feldman, S., & Downey, G. (1994). Rejection sensitivity as a mediator of the impact of childhood exposure to family violence on adult attachment behavior. *Development and Psychopathology, 6,* 231–247.

Gardner, K. J., Qualter, P., Stylianou, M., & Robinson, A. J. (2010). Facial affect recognition in non-clinical adults with borderline personality features: The role of effortful control and rejection sensitivity, *Personality and Individual Differences, 49,* 799–804.

Gunderson, J. G., & Lyons-Ruth, K. (2008). BPD's interpersonal hypersensitivity phenotype. *Journal of Personality Disorders, 22,* 22–41.

Heatherton, T. F., & Wagner, D. D. (2011). Cognitive neuroscience of self-regulation failure. *Trends in Cognitive Sciences, 15,* 132–139.

Hooker, C. I., Gyurak, A., Verosky, S. C., Miyakawa, A., & Ayduk, O. (2010). Neural activity to a partner's facial expression predicts self-regulation after conflict. *Biological Psychiatry, 67,* 406–413.

Horowitz, L. M. (2004). *Interpersonal foundations of psychopathology.* Washington, DC: American Psychological Association.

Kernberg, O. F. (1967). Borderline personality organization. *Journal of the American Psychoanalytic Association, 15,* 641–685.

Kernberg, O. F. (1984). *Severe personality disorders: Psychotherapeutic strategies.* New Haven, CT: Yale University Press.

Kernberg, O. F. (2004). *Aggressivity, narcissism, and self-destructiveness in the psychotherapeutic relationship.* New Haven, CT: Yale University Press.

Kernberg, O. F., & Caligor, E. (2005). A psychoanalytic theory of personality disorders. In M. F. Lenzenweger & J. F. Clarkin (Eds.), *Major theories of personality disorder* (2nd ed., pp. 114–156). New York: Guilford Press.

Kings-Casas, B., Sharp, C., Lomax-Bream, L., Lohrenz, T., Fonagy, P., & Montague, P. R. (2008). The rupture and repair of cooperation in borderline personality disorder. *Science, 321,* 806–809.

Koenigsberg, H. W., Fan, J., Ochsner, K. N., Liu, X., Guise, K. G., Pizzarello, S., et al. (2009). Neural correlates of the use of psychological distancing to regulate responses to negative social cues: A study of patients with borderline personality disorder. *Biological Psychiatry, 66,* 854–863.

Koenigsberg, H. W., Siever, L. J., Lee, H., Pizzarello, S., New, A. S., Goodman, M., et al. (2009). Neural correlates of emotion processing in borderline personality disorder. *Psychiatry Research: Neuroimaging, 172,* 192–199.

Kross, E., Egner, T., Ochsner, K., Hirsch, J., & Downey, G. (2007). Neural dynamics of rejection sensitivity. *Journal of Cognitive Neuroscience, 19,* 945–956.

Krueger, F., McCabe, K., Moll, J., Kriegeskorte, N., Zahn, R., Strenziok, M., et al. (2007). Neural correlates of trust. *Proceedings of the National Academy of Sciences of the USA, 104,* 20084–20089.

Lang, S., Kotchoubey, B., Frick, C., Spitzer, C., Grabe, H. J., & Barnow, S. (2011). Cognitive reappraisal in trauma-exposed women with borderline personality disorder. *NeuroImage, 59*(2), 1727–1734.

Lenzenweger, M. F., McClough, J. F., Clarkin, J. F., & Kernberg, O. F. (2012). Exploring the interface of neurobehaviorally linked personality dimensions and personality organization in borderline personality disorder: The Multidimensional Personality Questionnaire and Inventory of Personality Organization. *Journal of Personality Disorders, 26,* 902–918.

Levy, K. N. (2005). The implications of attachment theory and research for understanding borderline personality disorder. *Development and Psychopathology, 17,* 959–986.

Lieberman, M. D. (2007). Social cognitive neuroscience: a review of core processes. *Annual Review of Psychology, 58,* 259–289.

Lin, S., Keysar, B., & Epley, N. (2010). Reflexively mindblind: Using theory of mind to interpret behavior requires effortful attention. *Journal of Experimental Social Psychology, 46,* 551–556.

Linehan, M. M., Armstrong, H. E., Suarez, A., Allmon, D., & Heard, H. L. (1991). Cognitive-behavioral treatment of chronically parasuicidal borderline patients. *Archives of General Psychiatry, 48,* 1060–1064.

Livesley, W. J. (2001). Conceptual and taxonomic issues. In W. J. Livesley (Ed.), *Handbook of personality disorders: Theory, research, and treatment* (pp. 3–38). New York: Guilford Press.

McMain, S., & Wiebe, C. (2013). Therapist compassion: A dialectical behavior therapy perspective. In A. W. Wolf, M. R. Goldfried, & J. C. Muran (Eds.), *Transforming negative reactions to clients: From frustration to compassion* (pp. 163–174). Washington, DC: American Psychological Association.

Meyer, B., & Pilkonis, P. A. (2005). An attachment model of personality disorders. In M. F. Lenzenweger & J. F. Clarkin (Eds.), *Major theories of personality disorder* (2nd ed., pp. 231–281). New York: Guilford Press.

Mischel, W. (1973). Toward a cognitive social learning reconceptualization of personality. *Psychological Review, 80,* 252–283.

Mischel, W., Ayduk, O., Berman, M. G., Casey, B. J., Gotlib, I. H., Jonides, J., et al. (2011). "Willpower" over the life span: Decomposing self-regulation. *Social Cognitive and Affective Neuroscience, 6,* 252–256.

Mischel, W., & Shoda, Y. (1995). A cognitive–affective system theory of personality: Reconceptualizing situations, dispositions, dynamics, and invariance in personality structure. *Psychological Review, 102,* 246–268.

Mischel, W., & Shoda, Y. (2008). Toward a unified theory of personality: Integrating dispositions and processing dynamics within the cognitive–affective processing system. In O. P. John, R. W. Robins, & L. A. Pervin (Eds.), *Handbook of personality: Theory and research* (3rd ed., pp. 208–241). New York: Guilford Press.

Pincus, A. L. (2005). A contemporary interpersonal theory of personality disorders. In M. F. Lenzenweger & J. F. Clarkin (Eds.), *Major theories of personality disorder* (2nd ed., pp. 282–331). New York: Guilford Press.

Powers, K. E., Wagner, D. D., Norris, C. J., & Heatherton, T. F. (2013). Socially excluded individuals fail to recruit medial prefrontal cortex for negative social scenes. *Social Cognitive and Affective Neuroscience, 8*(2), 151–157.

Pretzer, J. L., & Beck, A. T. (2004). A cognitive theory of personality disorders. In M. F. Lenzenweger & J. F. Clarkin (Eds.), *Major theories of personality disorder* (2nd ed., pp. 36–105). New York: Guilford Press.

Renneberg, B., Herm, K., Hahn, A., Staebler, K., Lammers, C.-H., & Roepke, S. (2012). Perception of social participation in borderline personality disorder. *Clinical Psychology and Psychotherapy, 19*(6), 473–480.

Romero-Canyas, R., Downey, G., Berenson, K., Ayduk, O., & Kang, N. J. (2010). Rejection sensitivity and the rejection–hostility link in romantic relationships. *Journal of Personality, 78,* 119–148.

Romero-Canyas, R., Downey, G., Reddy, K. S., Rodriguez, S., Cavanaugh, T. J., & Pelayo, R. (2010). Paying to belong: When does rejection trigger ingratiation? *Journal of Personality and Social Psychology, 99,* 802–823.

Sadikaj, G., Russel, J. J., Moskowitz, D. S., & Paris, J. (2010). Affect dysregulation in individuals with borderline personality disorder: Persistence and interpersonal triggers. *Journal of Personality Assessment, 92,* 490–500.

Selby, E. A., Ward, A. C., & Joiner, T. E. (2010). Dysregulated eating behaviors in borderline personality disorder: Are rejection sensitivity and emotion dysregulation linking mechanisms? *International Journal of Eating Disorders, 43,* 667–670.

Selman, R. L. (1980). *The growth of interpersonal understanding.* Orlando, FL: Academic Press.

Shoda, Y., Mischel, W., & Wright, J. C. (1994). Intraindividual stability in the organization and patterning of behavior: Incorporating psychological situations into the idiographic analysis of personality. *Journal of Personality and Social Psychology, 67,* 674–687.

Silbersweig, D., Clarkin, J., Goldstein, M., Kernberg, O., Tuescher, O., Levy, K., et al. (2007). Failure of fronto-limbic inhibitory function in the context of negative emotion in borderline personality disorder. *American Journal of Psychiatry, 164,* 1832–1841.

Somerville, L. H., Heatherton, T. F., & Kelley, W. M. (2006). Anterior cingulated cortex responds differentially to expectancy violation and social rejection. *Nature Neuroscience, 9,* 1007–1008.

Staebler, K., Helbing, E., Rosenbach, C., & Renneberg, B. (2011). Rejection sensitivity and borderline personality disorder. *Clinical Psychology and Psychotherapy, 18,* 275–283.

Staebler, K., Renneberg, B., Stopsack, M., Fiedler, P., Weiler, M., & Roepke, S. (2011). Facial emotional expression in reaction to social exclusion in borderline personality disorder. *Psychological Medicine, 41,* 1929–1938.

Verheul, R., Andrea, H., Berghout, C. C., Dolan, C., Busschbach, J. J. V., van der Kroft, P. J. A., et al. (2008). Severity Indices of Personality Problems (SIPP-118): Development, factor structure, reliability, and validity. *Psychological Assessment, 20,* 23–34.

chapter 19

Promoting Integration between Different Self-States through Ongoing Reformulation

Giampaolo Salvatore, Raffaele Popolo,
and Giancarlo Dimaggio

LACK OF DIFFERENT SELF-STATES IN PERSONALITY DISORDERS

Many patients with personality disorder lack a coherent image of themselves—an overall view that integrates different facets of the self into a picture that makes sense to them. As a result, they are often surprised by abrupt shifts between different self-states (Horowitz, 2012) that occur for reasons that they are unable to grasp. Such individuals swing from transitory calm states to suddenly feeling anxious or edgy without being aware of what triggered the shift. They can be prey to intensely disturbing somatic sensations, such as stomach pains or headache, which can ignite panic attacks or health anxiety, and they are incapable of perceiving what relational causes trigger their heightened negative arousal. Such patients typically feel puzzled about happens during the flow of everyday relationships and uncertain about their feelings toward others: "If I swing from moments in which I feel fine to other moments when I feel constricted or dominated by my girlfriend and would like to be alone, does this mean I don't love her anymore?" The lack of a coherent self-image often leaves patients alarmed by differences in their presentation and behavior from one situation to another and confused about what course of action to pursue.

Elisa, a patient suffering from obsessive–compulsive personality disorder with significant narcissistic traits, passive–aggressive features, and prominent perfectionism and pessimism shifted from moments in which she felt in love with her boyfriend to others in which she felt nervous and alone. At such times, she questioned her love for him and doubted whether she wanted to continue the relationship. Over time, her therapist helped her to realize that her moments of edginess and her wish to be alone started after feeling rejected by him or when he was silent for a long time because he was watching a football match on TV. This helped her realize that she actually loved him and hence felt bad when she felt rejected. This was a sign that she wanted to be closer to him, so that, when she withdrew or questioned her love for him, this was generally a reaction to feeling abandoned.

PROMOTING COHERENCE AMONG SELF-STATES IN THE PSYCHOTHERAPY OF PERSONALITY DISORDERS

Promoting a coherent self-image (Clarkin, Kernberg, & Yeomans, 1999) is one of the key targets in any personality disorder therapy. Patients need to gradually build up a comprehensive and integrated view of themselves that captures all aspects of their personalities, including strengths and weaknesses and differences in behavior and feelings across situations. A consistent self-image is an important stabilizing force that consolidates one's identity and allows patients to recognize the different aspects of themselves while also feeling themselves to be a *self* and able to occupy different psychological positions flexibly and securely (Stiles, 2011). For example, one can feel one is a good parent, even if one has had problems at work: The momentary wavering in self-esteem due to work setbacks should not affect one's self-esteem as a parent, and overall one is able to maintain a sense of a positive personal value because failures are considered to be of marginal importance when the overall picture is positive. In this chapter, we discuss ways to construct a more integrated sense of self and identity through an ongoing process of reformulation using diagrams to depict the relationship between different self-states and the links between these states and self-schemas. We argue that the process begins immediately after assessment with the development of a collaborative formulation that is progressively revised during treatment.

The construction of a case formulation following assessment is an important step that not only forms a blueprint for therapy but is also the basis for the subsequent development of an integrated sense of self. Showing patients the links among their mental states and the underlying interpersonal schemas provides them with tools for tracing the suffering experienced in real-life situations to forms of functioning that can be identified and foreseen. In this way, patients acquire knowledge of and control over their own mental functioning rather than being overwhelmed by it. For example, the therapist may help the patient pass from a self-description such as "At times I am depressed, lose motivation with no real cause, and this is frustrating, I can't do anything in life as I am unpredictable" to "When I ask for care and people who are important to me neglect me, I think I will be abandoned forever, and then I become depressed and feel unworthy and inept. This is something I always was vulnerable to, as I often felt not supported by my parents." With such a formulation, the patient is no longer frightened by states of depression coming abruptly, as he or she makes sense of the reasons underlying the mental state transition.

In this chapter we describe how to promote integration among different self-states, at the end of the assessment, during shared case formulation, and during psychotherapy, in order to help the patient figure out how he or she is changing during psychotherapy. With the help of the therapy and the strategies described here, the patients will be able to form a more comprehensive picture of who they are and have a sense of unity, notwithstanding the shifts among different aspects of the self they may experience (Dimaggio, Hermans, & Lysaker, 2010b).

FORMULATION AND REFORMULATION

Our approach is consistent with the core conflictual relationship theme template (CCRT; Luborsky & Crits-Christoph, 1990). The CCRT identifies interpersonal schemas on the basis of what is the goal—*wish*—that a patient pursues and fears will be disappointed on account of others' responses. Therefore, once the wish is activated, the patient expects a *response from the other*, and typically this is followed by a *response from the self* to the other's response. The self-image underlying the wish is deduced from the associated schema. For example, a patient might wish to be cared for, expect that the other will reject him or her, and react by withdrawing, getting depressed, and losing hope. This suggests that the self-image underlying the desire for attention was *self not deserving of love*. Thus, when the attachment motive gets reactivated, a patient expects a rejection that he or she believes to be deserved and behaves accordingly by avoiding asking for attention or by doing it in such a cautious manner that the other does not realize that he or she is asking. Alternatively, the patient might ask for help while already suffering in anticipation of a rejection or react with dysregulated emotions because a contingent rejection is a sign of the confirmation of a schema, leaving him or her without any hope of love (see Tufekcioglu & Muran, Chapter 6, this volume; Leahy, 2003 and Chapter 12, this volume). As well as the responses expected from the other, the identification of a pathogenic schema also includes internalized responses, that is, how a part of the self reacts to the desires expressed by another part of the self (Pokorny, 1984). For example, a patient might wish for independence but have internalized a critical voice that says "Acting independently would mean I'm selfish" (*internalized other's response to the wish*) and thus, of his own will, he criticizes his own plans without even taking account of what others would think about his goal.

The therapist should also try to understand how an interpersonal schema can be the source of a patient's mental state vis-à-vis the therapist. A patient might, for example, come to a session declaring that there is something wrong in the critical thoughts she has had about her elderly father; her face may display shame and her nonverbal behavior indicates defensive withdrawal. The therapist might hypothesize that the shame and withdrawal may indicate that she was expecting the therapist to be critical. Shame would thus correspond to the self's response to the response expected from the other.

Another factor influencing mental states is the impact that dysfunctional interpersonal schemas have on real relationships and vice versa. One of the dysfunctional schemas of Elisa, the patient described earlier, seemed to be *self wishing to be loved and helped*; the response expected from the other was *rejection and criticism*. In response the patient felt *inadequate* and reacted by asking ever more intensively for the other to provide an intimate and exclusive relationship. When the other felt pressured and withdrew, she felt even more rejected and angry. At this point, the state of malaise resulting from rejection led her to think she was not in love with her partner. At other times, when he was looking for intimacy and affection, she tended to feel he was restricting her freedom and wanted independence; she also interpreted her wish for autonomy as a sign that perhaps she did not love him any more. To dispel the reader's doubts about whether in fact Elisa really did not love her partner: After 7 years they are still together, and she is pregnant with their first child.

We stress that the schema also includes dysfunctional coping mechanisms. Usually coping mechanisms are the self's response to the other's response. For example, when Elisa felt rejected and unlovable, she would adopt perfectionist performance standards and become workaholic in an attempt to recoup a self-image that was positive and deserving of love. Understanding how her mental-state shifts depended on schemas helped Elisa to dispel lingering doubts about the importance of her relationship with her boyfriend and to grasp that her own mental state depended partly on how much she saw him as distant or close. The promotion of awareness of different self-states and the psychological factors linking them has been variously termed *promoting metacognitive integration* (Dimaggio, Semerari, Carcione, Nicolò, & Procacci, 2007; Semerari et al., 2005), *achieving the highest level of reflective functioning* (Bateman & Fonagy, 2004 and Chapter 7, this volume; Fonagy, Gergely, Jurist, & Target, 2002) and *establishing high levels of assimilation of problematic experiences* (Stiles, 2011).

The initial formulation should be expressed in language agreed on with the patient, be intelligible, and keep theories, technical expressions, and ungrounded inferences to the minimum possible. This kind of formulation with schemas is typical of cognitive analytic therapy (Ryle & Kerr, 2002) and plan analysis (Caspar & Ecker, 2008) or motive-oriented therapy (Kramer, Berthoud, Keller, & Caspar, 2014). It is important that the formulation is discussed with a patient in a collaborative way that allows the patient to amplify or modify it so that it is acceptable to him or her. The initial formulation can be presented either through a letter in the form of a conversation with the patient (Bateman & Fonagy, 2004; Ryle & Kerr, 2002) that summarizes key interpersonal patterns or by using diagrams to represent intrapsychic and relational variables. In our opinion, using diagrams to represent the relation between schemas and mental states makes it easier for both patients and therapists to recall case formulations. Even during assessment, a case formulation in diagram form stimulates patients' awareness of the functioning of their schemas and mental states, together with the mechanisms regulating interschema shifts.

The initial case formulation diagram should show the therapist's hypotheses about the relationships between mental states and interpersonal schemas. When discussing the formulation, the therapist and patient should together revise the diagram to show recurring mental states, the interpersonal schemas driving the patient's social actions, and the way shifts between mental states are driven by the patient's position within each schema. For example, a patient might describe herself as confused by her own swings between moments of anger and depression and her tendency toward isolation. With an analysis of a series of relational episodes, her clinician could help her to pinpoint how such states are activated and what triggers the transition from one state to the next. A therapist can help a patient to see how, before obtaining an opinion on his performance, the latter feels anxious and in need of approval, whereas once he has in fact obtained the opinion, he experiences depression, anger toward the person expressing it, and a desire to isolate himself. Consequently, when a patient's wish becomes activated but he is waiting for the other's response to his search for approval, he is in an anxious state; when, on the other hand, he is in the part of the schema in which he reacts to the other's response, the state is initially an angry one because the opinion is seen to be unfair, followed by depression at the idea of being unworthy. Fostering an understanding of what drives the shifts between mental states reduces patients' confusion, gives them a sense of mastery and control, and assists in joint treatment planning.

It is also helpful for the therapist to note areas of uncertainty and any metacognitive difficulties that hinder a full understanding of the patient's problems—for example, the exact nature of an ill-defined negative mental state that is activated by a negative response from the other—and that treatment will include attempts to improve awareness of subjective experience in those areas in which it is lacking, with the aim of further refining the case formulation. Once a patient and therapist have established what they are unable to understand about the patient's inner world, these gaps in self-knowledge should be the focus in the sessions that follow, with a joint attempt to improve metacognition (Dimaggio et al., 2007; Dimaggio, Popolo, Carcione, & Salvatore, Chapter 8, this volume) or mentalization (Bateman & Fonagy, 2004, Chapter 7, this volume). For example, if a patient feels depressed and in session declares that this depression is more acute at the end of a day's work but is unable to say why, it should be pointed out in the formulation that he needs to expand his knowledge of the relational and cognitive antecedents of his depressive state.

Subsequently, the initial formulation is modified in the light of new information uncovered in therapy. From time to time, the patient and therapist should jointly revise the formulation diagram to show how the patient was at the beginning of treatment and how he or she has changed. This makes it easier for both to see how the therapy is evolving and helps the patient to include emerging states, especially healthy and adaptive ones, in his or her self-image and to see that formerly feared self-aspects, such as acting independently from attachment figures and freely exploring one's environment, are not risky, as previously feared, but rather a vital resource.

This process fosters integration as, with diagrams or letters available in front of them, patients are provided with an image at a glance of the different self-states they experience, the triggers for the interstate shifts, and the typical interpersonal schemas underlying those shifts. The collaborative work between therapist and patient achieves a new understanding of the patient's inner experience, core self and interpersonal schema, and relationship patterns that extends the patient's self-knowledge.

This, in turn, forms the foundation for a more coherent self-system, as the patient now is able to realize that she is the same person when she feels inept before a social exposure; when her self-esteem rises after the performance has been completed and self-rated, with the therapist's help, as adequate; and when she discovers that she is a good mother thanks to the warm smiles she receives from her children.

We now illustrate with a case example how self-integration and a coherent self-image are built up in psychotherapy. We described how the formulation was constructed jointly at the end of the assessment process and how it was revised in an advanced stage of treatment. Diagrams of self-states were adopted in order to help the patient readily figure out what the main self-states and interpersonal schemas were and what the triggers for the shift among mental states were.

CASE EXAMPLE

Sally was 24 years old, had a literature degree, and lived with her parents. She met Axis I DSM-IV-TR criteria for an "eating disorder not otherwise specified" (EDNOS) and Axis II DSM-IV-TR criteria for obsessive–compulsive and dependent personality disorders. The assessment and weekly therapy took place in a private outpatient clinic using metacognitive interpersonal therapy (MIT) for personality disorders (Dimaggio et al., 2007, 2012; Dimaggio, Carcione, Salvatore, Semerari, & Nicolò, 2010) with one of us (Salvatore). Therapy lasted 3 years, with a further 1-year step-down (one session per month for 6 months and then one session every 2 months). At the beginning of therapy, Sally was limiting her calorie intake, had lost about 22 pounds in weight, and had amenorrhea. She would practice dancing for hours and ignore any signs of tiredness. Her identity was fragmented, and she said she felt "confused" because she could see "ongoing changes inside herself" and "rapid changes in mood" without managing to "get them organized." She was skeptical as to whether the therapy could help her to understand anything about herself. For this reason, the therapist agreed with her that the goal in the first four to five sessions should be to arrive at an agreed understanding and a labeling of the various mental states involving the suffering that she was experiencing. They were also to try to understand the characteristics of and reasons behind her shifts from one state to another. Furthermore, the therapist announced to Sally that at the end of this stage he would put a recapitulative diagram on the blackboard and ask her to make any corrections she might think necessary. The therapist explained that in this way they would arrive at a formulation of her problems that was "not theoretical" and "as close as possible to the reality of what was going on in Sally's mind." Sally felt encouraged by this work program, and her confidence in the therapy increased.

As noted by Dimaggio and colleagues (Chapter 8, this volume), the formulation of the schemas and the rules steering transitions between mental states should start with an analysis of detailed autobiographical memories to ensure that the diagrammatic formulation corresponds to the patient's raw experience rather than being a product of intellectualization. One of the first episodes Sally related concerned a dance lesson in which she felt she was fainting because she had not eaten and was very tired, but she could not pluck up the courage to tell the teacher because she would have been considered "an irresponsible and insufficiently committed pupil." Sally also recalled another episode with the same theme: She was at the dinner table—she was about 8 years old—and, while she was particularly relishing some food she was eating, her father "made her stop dead" by telling her that it formed part of her responsibilities to have an impeccable physical appearance and "never give one's fellow creatures the impression she did not know how to control her instincts," such as hunger. The therapist noted that on both occasions she had felt guilty and had seen herself as "a good-for-nothing" and "disappointing" in both her own and others' eyes. When asked by the therapist to recall similar episodes, Sally remembered that one evening, when she was a teenager, she had felt despair because she had spent "four hours looking at the same page of a book" and felt an enormous need to unburden herself with her father, to get his support for not going to school the day after, and to feel him hug her. However, when she found the courage to tell him that she had recently been experiencing problems at school, she suddenly felt "frozen by his stern look" and by the harsh words he used to "remind her of her responsibilities."

Sally seemed to have the following schema, typical of obsessive–compulsive personality disorder: The *wish* is to be understood and supported; the *other responds* by being incapable of understanding or giving support and instead criticizes, accuses, and draws attention to the person's moral duties. The *response* of the person is to feel guilty for transgressing ("I shouldn't have thought about not going to school"); as a result, Sally represses her request to be understood. In the end, she feels lonely and neglected but underrates these feelings, which are a sign of immorality. When it was formulated, this schema was termed the *responsibility schema* (Figure 19.1).

There were some characteristic and recurring mental states in this schema. Thanks to the formulation, Sally was now able to describe clearly (1) the state of self-efficacy characteristic when she felt her performance was perfect; (2) the anxious–doubtful–guilty state when she feared she had done her tasks wrong. Even checking calories and her body weight was tackled by Sally as a task that made her feel efficacious if conducted perfectly and guilty if she transgressed.

However, Sally was unable to comprehend that what she herself defined as "a general malaise" of both a physical and psychological nature was in reality a manifestation of feeling overloaded owing to the seriousness of the tasks she gave herself and her lack of access to the pleasure dimension. That Sally considered this malaise to be a sign of her "weak constitution," which, in her opinion, ought not "to be an obstacle" to her performance and could be "compensated for by willpower," was a further barrier to her awareness of this state.

Other dysfunctional aspects emerged in Sally's romantic relationships. Sally said that her last boyfriend, with whom the relationship had ended 1 year prior to her first meeting with the therapist, had many different interests that "kept him very busy." She related that on one occasion he had taken her to visit some caves in a village far away, and, so Sally declared, this "was an experience that was overall very stimulating" for her. The therapist invited her to describe in detail what happened, and Sally recalled certain particulars, for example, one moment at which she felt particularly cold. Precisely while she was relating this, all of a sudden the therapist saw a scarcely perceptible grimace of irritation on Sally's face, which seemed to jar with her words. He pointed out this impression of his to Sally, who smiled and admitted that in reality during the trip several things had "made her feel uneasy." Even though she felt happy at the idea that her boyfriend had wanted to share this experience with her, she had felt cold and bored. When she got home, this bored state "had gotten amplified, as it were," to the extent that it became "a sort of irritation and then anger," which she felt for several days afterward.

Sally recalled that she had also felt this same strange type of anger many times in her relationship with an earlier boyfriend, especially on an occasion on which she had stopped practicing dancing because one evening he said that her dancing took up too much time they could be using "for doing things together." She recalled that at that moment stopping her dancing had seemed something "automatic" and had not caused her any regrets. She had not seen giving it up as at all painful for her, but a few days later she had felt that same anger and had been "unmanageable at home with her parents."

Sally was thus able, with the therapist's help, to identify that in her romantic relationships she tended to comply with the other's wishes for fear

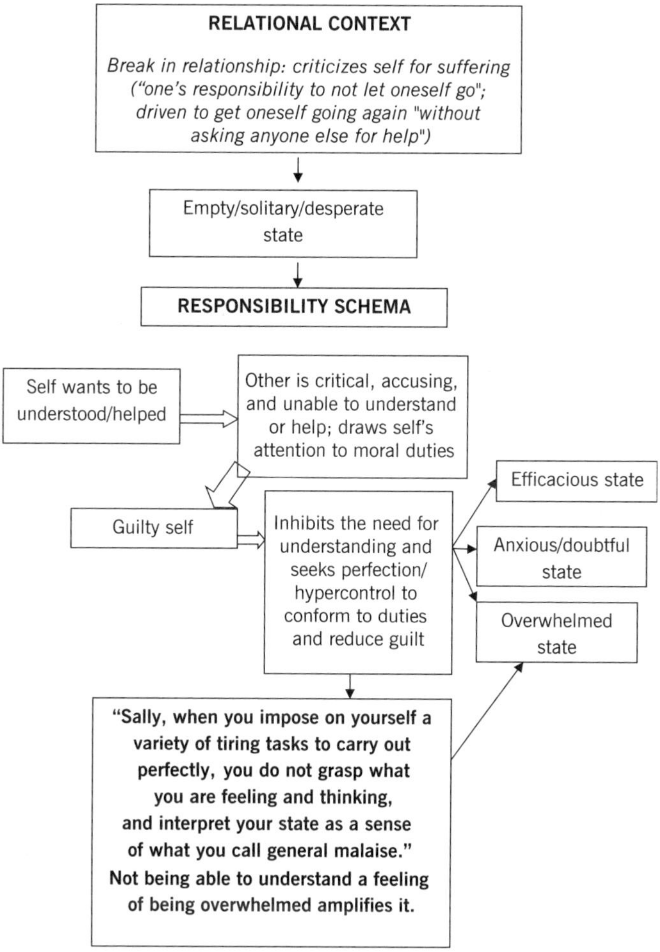

FIGURE 19.1. Responsibility schema.

of losing his attention and love but gave up pursuing her own desires; this, however, caused an anger in her, which Sally now, with the therapist, was able to encode as a sense of constriction.

Thanks to this realization, Sally was able to recall a prototypical episode from her childhood. Her mother was a very religious woman, who had taken Sally at a very early age to Sunday services and on various trips of a religious nature. On one occasion, when she was 9 years old, Sally told her mother that she wanted to go on a school trip instead of going to mass with her. Her mother's expression was of great disappointment and sorrow, and she did not speak to Sally for several hours, until, out of fear of having lost her love forever, Sally said that she would willingly forgo the trip. She felt "reborn" when her mother hugged her, and after that she never made other requests like it. However, during the days that followed, especially when she met friends who had gone on the trip and heard them sharing their experiences, she felt an "unexplainable" anger toward her mother.

This suggests the presence of a second dysfunctional schema: The self *wishes* its desires to be seen as valid and its independence respected; the *other* (e.g., her mother) *responds* by feeling disappointed and hurt and by denying love and attention; the *self's response* is fright at the idea of losing attention and love. The dysfunctional coping mechanism is to give up pursuing one's own independent plans in order to ensure the other's closeness. The *self-image* underlying the wish for independence is *unlovable*. At the moment of the formulation, the therapist called this the "dependency schema" (Figure 19.2). In the light of this schema, one could comprehend the joyful and vigorous mental state Sally experienced when she saw a significant other as being loving and attentive, her fear when she realized that she might disappoint the other and that there was the threat of the relationship breaking up, and her constriction when her own overmodulated wishes were contrary to those of the significant other and she systematically relinquished their satisfaction.

At this point, the therapist proposed a general formulation in the form of diagrams (see Figures 19.1 and 19.2). The two diagrams include an explanation of the role of Sally's metacognitive monitoring dysfunctions—that is, the difficulty in identifying one's own real desires and the causes at the root of certain emotions and negative states—in the maintenance of the schemas (Dimaggio, Semerari, Carcione, Procacci, & Nicolò, 2006; Dimaggio et al., 2007). In the responsibility state, Sally was often unable to identify what was making her feel overwhelmed. When in the dependency state, she was unaware that she felt constrained. Her metacognitive monitoring problems meant that Sally was unable to perceive that not pursuing her own wishes—not to go to the caves, to carry on with her dancing, and so forth—made her angry at being constrained.

Sally could fully recognize herself in this formulation and declared enthusiastically that she could now see that the *responsibility schema* was being activated in particular during stages in her life when she was not engaged in a romantic relationship, whereas the *dependency schema* was typically activated in the relationship with a partner.

At difficult moments in her current relationship, for example, when her boyfriend was away for work, Sally felt a very intense feeling of loss, a desire to cry or confide in a friend, but this immediately activated her feeling of guilt connected with the idea of being "one who does not know how to control her own instincts," in line with her father's internalized critical voice. On this basis she soothed her distress by reminding herself of "her duties" and intensified her training sessions to the point where, she now realized, she lost all pleasure in dancing and looked on it as a duty, one of those things in which she should be "perfect" as a way to overcome her instincts.

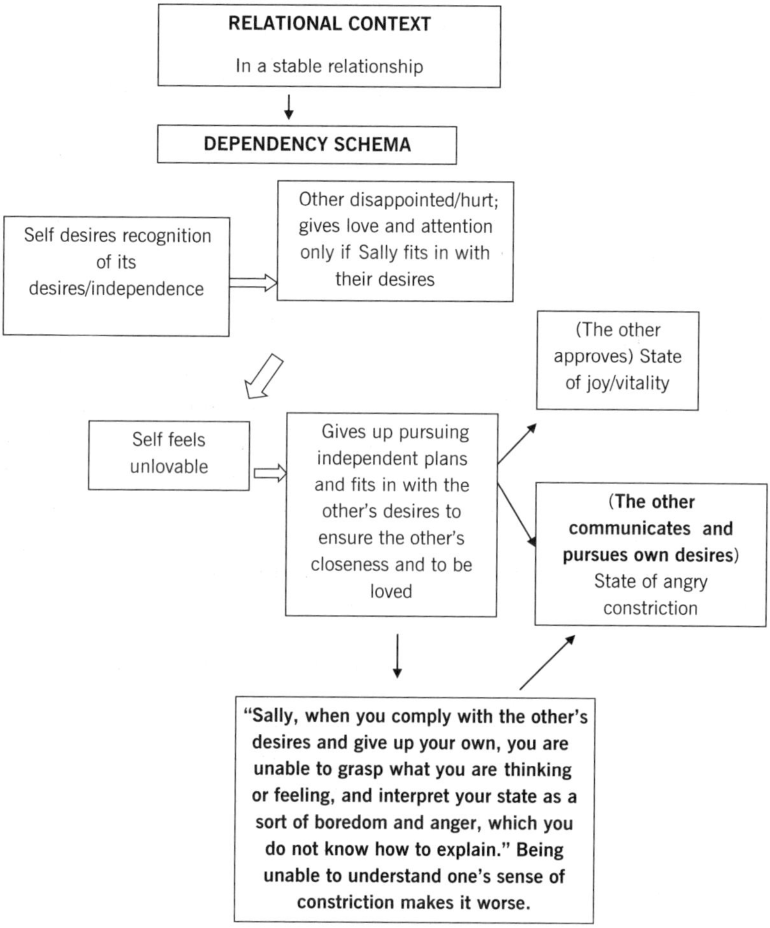

FIGURE 19.2. Dependency schema.

Sally added that when her partner who asked her to stop dancing broke up with her, she became enveloped in a sense of emptiness and despair. Sally now grasped that this had been one of the times at which she needed to be understood and supported, but—in line with the responsibility schema—she had "considered it her duty to not let herself go" and had taken up her dancing and her diet again in a perfectionistic manner. She, for example, remembered an occasion after breaking up with her boyfriend: She was "lying on her bed" and she suddenly recalled her father's strict expression. This was the decisive trigger for her to get moving again "without asking for help from anyone else."

On the basis of this formulation, it was possible for Sally and the therapist to work collaboratively to draw up the following treatment goals for her. The first was to improve her self-reflective ability to identify distressing mental states (e.g., being overwhelmed or constrained) and their close link to the activation of dysfunctional interpersonal schemas (Dimaggio et al., 2007 and Chapter 8, this volume). Second, she needed to learn to differentiate the contents of her schemas from reality. In other words, the goal was to realize that her fear of violating her responsibilities if she expressed a need for help (responsibility schema) and her fear of losing love and attention from a significant other if she expressed her own point of view and pursued independent plans (dependency schema) were the result of rigid schema-driven representations deeply rooted in her past relationships and were capable of guiding her actions while not actually reflecting what was happening at that moment.

To achieve this second goal, Sally needed help with challenging her schemas and experimenting with alternative behavior, such as expressing her own needs and point of view to the other or acting independently and then checking whether this triggered the criticism or abandonment she expected from the other. At the same time, the patient and therapist were together monitoring the sense of well-being, unexpected for Sally, that she felt when she behaved in new ways (Dimaggio et al., 2007 and Chapter 8, this volume; Leahy, 2003 and Chapter 12, this volume). This gradual attempt to challenge her negative schemas through behavioral experiments stimulated further, more short-term, goals, including improving access to her own desires and to pleasure in carrying out her own activities (eating, dancing); promoting the use of desires rather than moral duties and the pursuit of perfectionist standards of moral duty to guide her actions; and negotiating her desires in her relationships with others and finding alternatives to pleasing the other to manage the perceived threat of abandonment. The result of this work was that Sally gradually put together a more amiable self-image.

Therapeutic Change

Sally and her therapist pursued the first goal by working during sessions at exploring relationships with significant figures, especially her partner. For example, Sally identified that the "strange sensation" she had felt when one evening her partner told her to "Be sure this evening to get yourself ready at nine because we're going to the cinema to see that film" was anger at the idea of being constrained. She recognized that at such moments one of the thoughts that came automatically to mind was "If I tell him I've no wish to go and see that film because it doesn't attract me and I want instead to go out with my girlfriends, he'll go to the cinema alone and think he's had enough of me." The therapist went back to the diagram and pointed out to Sally that at that moment her partner was, in her eyes, embodying the role of the other who gets disappointed in her and withdraws his love if Sally openly expresses a contrary desire. She agreed. As a result of this work it became ever easier for Sally to reflect on her own mental states.

The therapist suggested that Sally use the diagram to understand when to attempt behavioral experiments to help her to satisfy her own needs within functioning relationships (see Dimaggio et al., 2007 and Chapter 8, this volume). The first aim of such experiments was to stimulate differentiation between fantasy and reality. Together they identified schema-dependent cognitions, such as "I'm afraid that if I say I won't go to the cinema, he'll leave me," and planned pattern-breaking behavior: "I'll try not going and see what happens." A second aim was to help Sally to focus on her own needs and wants and to use them to guide her in choices by negotiating them more assertively in relationships.

This therapeutic operation was hard for Sally because the fear of being abandoned was often too intense to carry out the experiment and the self-image of being abandoned was too distressing. The therapist handled this difficulty by validating Sally's fear and reminding her of the importance of "climbing this mountain together" in order to create the conditions for a lasting schema change. Constantly referring to the diagram helped Sally to remember that she was being influenced by her own schema-dependent convictions and that there were other episodes in which she had been accepted even without trying to please the other.

Thanks to these developments, in the second year of therapy, Sally was able to politely decline her boyfriend's suggestion that they visit another cave. She remembered the therapist's facial expression and reassuring words and the diagram they had drawn up together and was able to explain that it did not interest her. She said she experienced an agreeable sense of surprise and relief when her boyfriend, after thinking about it, gave up the idea of the trip because he preferred to spend the weekend with her.

The therapist proposed other behavioral experiments to weaken her perfectionist standards and allow herself to experience pleasure when eating and dancing. For example, she stopped weighing food and allowed herself 1 or 2 days' rest from training whenever she felt vaguely tired. These tasks also included the use of a copy of the diagram, which Sally took home with her. Each time she felt the impulse to weigh food or train without regard for her tiredness, she had to go back to the diagram, examine the responsibility schema, and acknowledge that her drive for perfectionism and hypercontrol was an acquired habit, born from her attempt not to feel guilty about violating the rules dictated by her father.

Formulation at an Advanced Stage of Treatment

After 2½ years of therapy, Sally and her therapist agreed that the goals drawn up had been successfully achieved. The therapist explained to Sally that, thanks to the increase in her ability to identify her own mental states and to the behavioral experiments for the construction of new schema-discrepant self-images, a new, adaptive, and functional part of her self-image had been created, which they called *lovable self*." This involved a substantial modification of the dependency schema. In this new schema, the other responds with love and attention to the self's desire to see its desires acknowledged, without this involving the loss of the other's closeness, and, as a result, the (lovable) self feels free to acknowledge and negotiate its desires and express its point of view. Sally had consequently improved substantially at identifying her own desires and explicitly communicating them to her partner. When she experienced a feeling of constriction, she was better at studying it and understanding that it depended on a failure to express her own desires and communicate them effectively.

Her checking of what she ate diminished to the extent that Sally was no longer diagnosed with EDNOS. Sally, however, agreed with the therapist that the responsibility schema was still partially active. She still had a tendency to control her performance when doing physical training. For example, she found it hard to miss a training session even when tired. During one session she referred to the diagram, which she had by now internalized, and said that perhaps there was still "a bit of the guilty self." However, as well as being able to recognize when this self-representation was activated, she was now capable of balancing her tendency to perfectionism with the pursuit of other desires and sources of pleasure. For example, one evening, after forcing herself to miss training because she was tired and bored, she organized going out for a pizza with some friends, and, as the evening unfolded, not only did she relax and enjoy herself but she "completely forgot about missing her training."

In one session at the start of her 3rd year of therapy, the therapist displayed these results with a new case formulation, shown in Figures 19.3 and 19.4.

The therapist proposed that the next course of treatment should aim at consolidating this functional schema so as to stabilize Sally's ability to acknowledge her own desires, authorize them for herself, and express them by negotiating them in interpersonal relationships. At the same time, they would concentrate further on an early identification of the signals that indicated entry into negative mental states and activation of dysfunctional schemas, especially the responsibility one, which was still partially active, to stop them developing and nip their pathogenic processes in the bud. Sally could

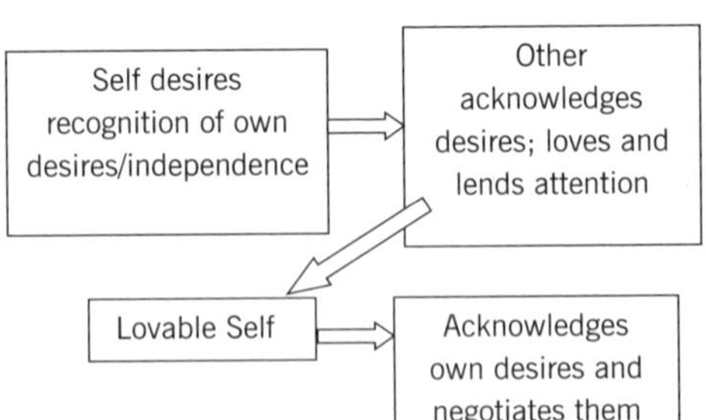

FIGURE 19.3. Trend in Sally's case after 2½ years of therapy: modification of dependency schema.

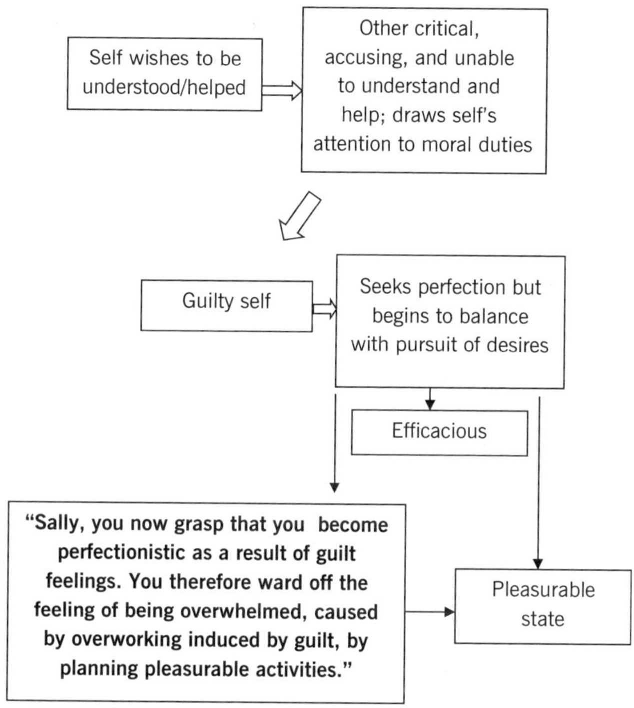

FIGURE 19.4. Trend in Sally's case after 2½ years of therapy: modification of responsibility schema.

fully identify herself in this formulation and was happy with it. Her self-efficacy and self-esteem increased further because she realized that the therapy was bearing results.

CONCLUDING COMMENTS

In this chapter we have shown how the use of explicit formulations, in the form of diagrams drawn up together with patients who are unaware of the workings of their own mental functioning, can promote integration of different self-states and self-representations. Such formulations promote an understanding of change and facilitate identification of the next steps in the change process. The use of diagrams helps patients to understand how states of subjective suffering are generated by maladaptive schemas and how difficulties in metacognition or mentalization prevent them from recognizing their schemas and how they trigger their behavior. Diagrams also help to explain how other people's negative responses contribute to maintaining vicious interpersonal cycles (Safran & Muran, 2000; Tufekcioglu & Muran, Chapter 6, this volume). Helping a patient to understand these issues strengthens the therapeutic relationship because patients can see how their insights are the result of a process in which they have played an active part. This understanding provides the common ground for negotiating treatment goals and for tracking therapeutic change.

The kind of written formulation that we have depicted provides patients with a useful tool for understanding and managing mental states and associated emotional experiences and interpersonal relationships. We consider this form of case formulation and reformulation a generalizable technical tool that not only promotes the integration of the self in therapy but also helps to maintain adaptive functioning and promote integration after therapy. A patient will not only see that she "has changed" but will be in a position to create, along with the therapist, a representation of the processes specific to her change, together with a labeling system that continues to be effective after treatment ends.

We do not think that the method described stands alone. Rather, it needs to be integrated with methods such as a constant and technically oriented attention toward the regulation of the therapeutic relationship, the prevention and immediate repair of ruptures in this relationship (Safran & Muran, 2000), the maintenance of a nonauthoritarian approach, and a predisposition to emotional validation (Dimaggio et al., 2007; Linehan, 2003). Nor do we think that the use of diagrams is the only way to approach formulation and reformulation. Earlier we discussed the use of reformulation letters (see Bateman & Fonagy, 2004; Ryle & Kerr, 2002). This is consistent with the approach we have used, and some patients and therapists prefer this approach. We believe that written or diagrammatic conceptualizations foster positive change in several ways: A patient is more likely to grasp the case formulation and to recall it during experiences, and it will be easier for both to plan goals if there is a clear, visible, and agreed starting point.

REFERENCES

Bateman, A. W., & Fonagy, P. (2004). *Psychotherapy for borderline personality disorder: Mentalization-based treatment.* Oxford, UK: Oxford University Press.

Caspar, F., & Ecker, S. (2008). Treatment of an avoidant patient with comorbid psychopathology: A plan analysis perspective. *Journal of Clinical Psychology, 64,* 139–153.

Clarkin, J. F., Kernberg, O. F., & Yeomans, F. (1999). *Transference-focused psychotherapy for borderline personality disorder patients.* New York: Guilford Press.

Dimaggio, G., Carcione, A., Salvatore, G., Semerari, A., & Nicolò, G. (2010). A rational model for maximizing the effect of regulating therapy relationship in personality disorders. *Psychology and Psychotherapy: Theory, Research and Practice, 83,* 363–384.

Dimaggio, G., Hermans, H. J. M., & Lysaker, P. H. (2010). Health and adaptation in a multiple self: The role of absence of dialogue and poor metacognition in clinical populations. *Theory and Psychology, 20,* 379–299.

Dimaggio, G., Salvatore, G., Fiore, D., Carcione, A., Nicolò, G., & Semerari, A. (2012). General principles for treating the overconstricted personality disorder: Toward operationalizing technique. *Journal of Personality Disorders, 26*, 63–83.

Dimaggio, G., Semerari, A., Carcione, A., Nicolò, G., & Procacci, M. (2007). *Psychotherapy of personality disorders Metacognition, states of mind and interpersonal cycles.* London: Routledge.

Dimaggio, G., Semerari, A., Carcione, A., Procacci, M., & Nicolò, G. (2006). Toward a model of self pathology underlying personality disorders: Narratives, metacognition, interpersonal cycles, and decision-making processes. *Journal of Personality Disorders, 20*, 597–617.

Fonagy, P., Gergely, G., Jurist, E., & Target, M. (2002). *Affect regulation, mentalization and the development of the self.* New York: Other Press.

Horowitz, M. J. (2012). Self-identity theory and research methods. *Journal of Research Practice, 8*(2). Available at *http://jrp.icaap.org/index.php/jrp/article/view/296/261.*

Kramer, U., Berthoud, L., Keller, S., & Caspar, F. (2014). Motive-oriented psychotherapeutic relationship facing a patient presenting with narcissistic personality disorder: A case study. *Journal of Contemporary Psychotherapy, 44*, 71–82.

Leahy, R. L. (2003). *Cognitive therapy techniques: A practitioner's guide.* New York: Guilford Press.

Linehan, M. M. (2003). *Cognitive-behavioral treatment of borderline personality disorder.* New York: Guilford Press.

Luborsky, L., & Crits-Christoph, P. (1990). *Understanding transference: The core conflictual relationship theme method.* New York: Basic Books.

Pokorny, M. R. (1984). Brief psychotherapy and the validation of psychodynamic theory. *British Journal of Psychotherapy, 1*, 68–76.

Ryle, A., & Kerr, I. B. (2002). *Introducing cognitive analytic therapy: Principles and practice.* Chichester, UK: Wiley.

Safran, J. D., & Muran, J. C. (2000). *Negotiating the therapeutic alliance: A relational treatment guide.* New York: Guilford Press.

Semerari, A., Carcione, A., Dimaggio, G., Nicoló, G., Pedone, R., & Procacci, M. (2005). Metarepresentative functions in borderline personality disorder. *Journal of Personality Disorders, 19*(6), 690–710.

Stiles W. B. (2011). Coming to terms. *Psychotherapy Research, 21*(4), 367–384.

part six

INTEGRATION

chapter 20

A Case Study of Integrated Treatment

John F. Clarkin, W. John Livesley, and Giancarlo Dimaggio

It is one thing to discuss abstractly and theoretically the process of matching the individual patient's particular domains of dysfunction to modules of treatment in a smooth and integrated way over a long period of time. It is another thing to apply this framework in a practical way. The process of therapy as it unfolds over time calls for the clinician to constantly observe the patient in the treatment interaction, inquire about his or her behavior and adjustment outside the treatment room, and continually adapt the treatment toward achieving the ultimate goal of a better adjustment for the patient. This vision of successful outcome (realistic in goal, hopeful of progress, and comprising techniques that can assist one to the goal) is more vivid in the therapist's mind than in the patient's at the beginning of treatment. In order to demonstrate this complex process, we present an actual case—the treatment of Sandra—that involved individual treatment over a period of 5 years. We discussed the assessment and formulation of Sandra's problems in Chapter 4 in this volume (Case Example 3).

ASSESSMENT

Sandra was 36 years old when she presented with the chief complaint of self-harming behavior and intense distress related to the recent abuse of her daughter by a neighbor whom Sandra had befriended. Briefly, Sandra was suffering dysphoria, had difficulty organizing her thoughts, and complained of a voice saying she was bad. The clinical picture immediately suggested a negative and fragmented conceptualization of self related to intense and unstable emotions that often poisoned her perceptions of others, leading to impaired and unstable interpersonal relations.

Sandra had been married for approximately 15 years. The relationship was highly conflicted, with frequent emotional outbursts. She complained that her husband was emotionally abusive and did not appreciate what she did for him and her three children, two boys with her husband and a teenage daughter from an earlier relationship. Sandra described growing up in a large dysfunctional and unstable family, with extensive emotional and physical abuse from her mother and her older siblings and extensive sexual abuse perpetrated by her mother's partner; her parents had separated when she was young.

Over the years, Sandra had been in therapy numerous times, and she rarely stayed in treatment more than a few months. She was mistrustful of therapists and often felt they were critical of her self-harming behavior.

In the clinical interview, Sandra showed characteristic features of personality disorder: She had a poorly developed sense of self and severely impaired interpersonal functioning. She found it hard to describe herself in psychological terms, and her sense of self changed markedly across situations. Sandra showed most traits in the emotionally dysregulated constellation, including emotional lability, anxiousness, submissive dependency, insecure attachment, and cognitive dysregulation. She also met criteria for categorical diagnoses of borderline and dependent personality disorder. Sandra was judged to have a severe personality disorder based on the presence of severe self-pathology and chronic interpersonal problems. It was judged that her problems could be managed in an individual treatment in an outpatient setting. However, the severity of her personality disorder led her clinician to prescribe sessions two times a week for the first year of treatment.

The therapist dedicated four sessions to a careful and detailed evaluation of Sandra and her individual characteristics in interaction with her particular environment. In the process, Sandra experienced the sustained attention of another individual who showed professional concern for her. (Later in treatment she spoke about how important and unusual it was for her to experience this kind of attention.) The therapist's paying careful attention to details of Sandra's troubled adjustment without criticism was reinforced by a summary of the evaluation that the therapist offered to Sandra and an invitation for her collaborative response to his summary. The evaluation interviews resulted in a therapeutic focus on four major domains of dysfunction in Sandra's life (see Table 20.1). In other words, Sandra's treatment began with a collaborative therapeutic alliance between her and her therapist. This collaboration began a helping relationship, even though interpersonal difficulties could well surface later that would cause ruptures in the alliance.

TABLE 20.1. Sandra: Domains of Dysfunction

Domain of dysfunction	Specifics	Treatment modules
Symptoms	Anxiety, depression, self-harming acts	Medication, functional analysis of stressful events
Emotion dysregulation		Use of affect regulation strategies
Interpersonal difficulties	Conflicts with mate, short-term relations not sustained, mistrustful	Pattern recognition in interpersonal scenarios; reflection about her role in conflicts
Identity problems	Fragmented sense of self, lack of goals, poor self-esteem	Encouragement of activities (e.g., work) that enhance self-esteem and self-concept

PHASES OF TREATMENT

Engagement and Containment Phase

The first 3 months of treatment were stormy, marked by incidents of deliberate self-harm usually triggered by disruptive incidents Sandra had with her husband and family. She was very distrustful during these sessions, finding it difficult to confide in the therapist, and she often expressed doubts about the value of the treatment. The therapist acknowledged these difficulties and tactfully explored Sandra's doubts while also noting that her difficulties with trust were understandable given her experiences. Most sessions were dominated by a description of the latest incidents with her husband and family. The therapist approached these issues with support and validation of feelings with the intent of fostering trust in the therapeutic alliance. Sandra was at risk for premature treatment termination, as this had been her pattern in the past.

Gradually, with the use of medication (selective serotonin reuptake inhibitor [SSRI], low-dose neuroleptic) and support, emotional lability and self-harming behavior decreased. The combination of medication and support seemed to improve Sandra's capacity to use cognitive strategies to self-manage her emotions and control impulses to harm herself. She was primarily focused on relief from intense distress, and this relief seemed to occur when she felt understood by the therapist.

Control and Regulation Phase

With the regularity of the sessions and the consistency of meeting twice weekly, Sandra became more comfortable with the therapist. With this progression, the therapist began to introduce cognitive and behavioral methods to improve emotion regulation and eliminate self-harm. With the use of functional analysis, Sandra began to recognize a pattern in her urges to cut herself and noted that they occurred whenever she felt intensely distressed because of vague feelings of being unappreciated. Sandra had been told by other clinicians and emergency room staff that her cutting was attention seeking; the therapist reframed the conception to an attempt on her part to manage distress. This surprised her. She commented that no one had ever told her that before. This reframing increased that alliance and made her more motivated to use emotion regulation strategies of distraction and self-soothing to combat urges to harm herself. Exercise and listening to soothing music were found to be helpful. These modest changes piqued the hopeful notion in Sandra that she could actually change.

With some growing control of destructive behavior, the therapist brought Sandra's attention to her thought processes that led to dysphoria. Upon reflection, she realized that she ruminated often about negative events. Even minor events were seen as catastrophic, and this reaction led to an escalation of distress. She began to realize that she could cognitively challenge her exaggerated reactions to events.

Sessions began to shift to a reflective focus on Sandra's problems in the present, usually interpersonal difficulties, and she was encouraged to review and gain some perspective. The therapeutic alliance was improving, probably as a result of multiple factors, including the therapist's consistent support, validation of Sandra's concerns and doubts, and reattribution of the causes of her self-harming behavior. This improvement enabled the therapist to introduce a simple relaxation exercise as a way to reduce anxiety. Sandra listened but was not motivated to use the relaxation exercises, explaining that she was angry at others who caused problems. It seemed very unfair to her that she was working hard to get better and that her abusers were not about to change. This dominant object relation conceptualization of herself as victim at the hands of victimizers had a history in her family of origin, in which the notion was conveyed that little could be done to change patterns of oppression.

The therapist perceived that Sandra's dependent-submissive interpersonal pattern with accompanying resentment was complicating the treatment itself. A focus on Sandra's submissiveness was brought into the treatment discussion (see Clarkin, Yeomans, De Panfilis, & Levy, Chapter 18, this volume). The therapist introduced a two-stage process to address and modulate her submissiveness. First, he highlighted the pattern of putting others' needs before her own, without assertion on her part, followed by resentment toward others. Second, the therapist encouraged Sandra to become more self-observant about how she acted in a subservient way in various interpersonal situations. Instead of reflexively reacting, she was encouraged to slow down her reactions and more closely monitor her own thoughts and feelings. She was encouraged to observe these patterns between sessions and to try out simple assertive moves.

These therapeutic efforts were gradually rewarded with Sandra's growing recognition that she sometimes contributed to the interpersonal disputes and that, in fact, at times she enjoyed the excitement of such a conflict. With these reflections, she began to realize that she could actively contribute to positive change in her relationships.

Throughout this period of the treatment Sandra mentioned somewhat obliquely that she was still bothered with memories of abuse that arose whenever she felt used and exploited. The therapist did not attempt to discuss early abuse in detail, but rather supported her and helped her deal with current emotional arousal when the memories surfaced. With more emotional control and fewer interpersonal crises in her current life, the treatment progressed to the next phase.

Exploration and Change Phase

Sandra's dependent-submissive pattern with others seemed to the therapist to be related to her severe childhood sexual abuse, which resulted in her passivity, proneness to see herself as the victim, and low motivation for change, although she was strongly motivated to help others, a need that was later to prove helpful in developing a sense of agency and constructing a meaningful life for herself. However, any attempt on the therapist's part to focus on abuse and its consequences were met with Sandra's momentary decompensation and dissociation. She was reluctant to change her style of being "a giving person" and trying "to please everyone" while feeling fragile, worthless, and bad herself. She had strong religious beliefs about being "a giving person" and valued being someone who always met others' requests even if inconvenient. Sandra continued to go out of her way to meet the demands of her extended family, even though she often felt pressured and exhausted by their almost incessant demands. Although the submissive-dependent pattern contributed to many of her difficulties, it was an important part of her sense of self and identity, deeply embedded in how Sandra saw herself that also contributed to what little self-esteem she felt.

Rather than focusing on attempts to restructure this pattern, the therapist introduced the idea of how Sandra could adopt a more structured and manageable way to help others. She found a volunteer position in a residential home and felt a lift in self-esteem in helping and caring for the residents there. This opportunity provided an outlet for Sandra's needs to care for others while at the same time containing these needs so that they were more manageable and made less demands on her time and resources. The therapist helped Sandra to establish some priorities among the demands made of her, placing high priority on the volunteer work. She found it easier to decline some of her family's demands because she wanted to feel rested when she was caring for people in the home so that she could give her best. These changes led to a substantial modulation in submissive-dependent tendencies.

During this time, Sandra reported flashbacks when she saw a man with features that reminded her of the man who had traumatized her when she was a teenager. The therapist introduced relaxation exercises that helped her counteract dissociative tendencies. These were augmented with an attention-regulating exercise (i.e., imagining a pleasant scene) to desensitize her to individuals that brought the past into mind.

Integration and Synthesis Phase

After 3 years of treatment in which Sandra's mood was less labile and with the absence of any self-harm behavior for over 1 year, she began to think about getting a job. This seemed an important development that suggested the emergence of a sense of autonomy and agency that differed substantially from her previous submissive dependency. The prospect of working excited Sandra, but she was also fearful of something she had not done for years. In fact, she had never had a full-time job that lasted more than a few months. Therapy focused on her concerns and doubts about her abilities, along with her fears of being independent and successful. Sandra's ambivalence was resolved by the offer of a part-time position in the residence where she was a volunteer. This met many of her needs, especially the need to be independent and less reliant on others and her need to care for others. This part-time position became a full-time position as the leadership recognized her enthusiasm and excellence in the work. In the face of work success, Sandra still complained of feeling like a "bad person" because she had been sexually abused and did nothing to stop it. However, she remained reluctant to discuss her self-perception at length, as she suspected the therapist would think badly of her. She also felt intense shame over what had happened. This was compounded by the fact that her mother and siblings blamed her for what happened because she was "too provocative." Nevertheless, Sandra felt she was now able to manage without the help of therapy; her work had led her to start a small business that was proving successful and taking more of her time.

What Sandra had done was to "get a life" for herself that was independent of her family, although she remained close to most family members. With the help of therapy, she had managed to create a personal niche that provided a constructive outlet for her values, needs, talents, and personality characteristics. As a result she felt more positive about herself and for the first time began to feel that she was in control of her own life and that she could shape her own destiny.

Of course, many things remained unresolved, but Sandra felt that she had achieved enough and that it was time to move on. The duration of the treatment was not predetermined at the time of assessment. Rather, the therapist and patient continued the treatment as long as both were motivated to engage in interaction that produced further change. So after about 5 years, the frequency of sessions was decreased and treatment gradually terminated.

During this process, Sandra observed that what had helped her most was the therapist's consistency, even though the consistency infuriated her at times to the extent that she tried to throw the therapist off track.

DISCUSSION

Because every case is unique, there are limits to what one can generalize from this particular patient–therapist pair over a treatment episode of 5 years. However, aspects of this case seem relevant to many cases, such as issues of treatment modules utilized in this case, the value of both diagnosis and severity levels, decisions regarding treatment intensity and duration, particular domains of dysfunction, and the sequences of interventions over time.

Treatment Modules Utilized

This example of integrated treatment of a patient in the severe range of personality pathology involved medication, skill development to manage symptoms, cognitive techniques to modulate ways of thinking about self and relationships with others, and dynamic techniques of focusing on beliefs about self and others in the relationship with the therapist. As important as the specific treatment modules utilized was the therapist's supportive, empathic stance, combined with a plan to help Sandra in domains of dysfunction as the issues unfolded in the process. The unstated but implied assumption was that Sandra could improve her condition in a careful, step-wise fashion.

The way the treatment unfolded over time is typical of treatment with individuals with severe personality disorders: a stormy beginning, with mistrust of the therapist and the therapy, and reporting of current crises with instances of self-harm. The therapist used support and validation of Sandra's feelings to begin to develop Sandra's trust and growing reliance on the therapeutic relationship. After about 3 months, she settled into treatment sufficiently to allow the focus to move to reduction of self-harm and emotion regulation. Events leading up to distress and self-harm were examined in detail, and alternatives to self-harm in managing her distress were discussed and considered. This naturally led to a more detailed discussion of Sandra's heightened emotional response to her cognitive understanding of the events. Sandra conceptualized herself as a victim of her husband's and extended family's many demands, to which she resentfully submitted. The therapist encouraged Sandra's expanding ability for self-observation and gradual self-assertion to modify her own submissiveness.

Throughout the treatment, Sandra's memories of childhood abuse emerged, with feelings of current and past exploitation. The therapist acknowledged these events and related feelings and provided support. Only toward the end of treatment were self-definitions of worthlessness and past abuse approached with caution, as she tended to dissociate and decompensate when these issues arose. This is an important clinical point on which we do not have relevant research, and the management of these phenomena demand clinical sensitivity and judgment. The treatment manuals vary on how cautiously (Bateman & Fonagy, 2006) and assertively (Clarkin, Yeomans, & Kernberg, 2006) one approaches a patient's fragmented and conflicted sense of self. Treatment manuals will never be able to address such individualized issues. Ultimately, it is the therapist in a relationship with the patient over time who has the best "feel" for how to manage these issues.

Diagnosis Combined with Severity and Domains of Dysfunction

This case illustrates the strategy of initial assessment and conception of the case not only around a diagnosis of personality disorder but also around four key areas of dysfunction: emotional dysregulation, dissocial or psychopathic behaviors, social withdrawal, and compulsivity. The severity range of personality pathology was established. The structure of the treatment was not made explicit but can be inferred as arising from the therapist's attention and consistency in the way Sandra settled into treatment following the stormy first 3 months. Sandra's experience was explored in detail, and change was introduced delicately in terms of suggestions for reconceptualizing the crises, using forms of self-regulation other than harmful self-cutting, and emotion reduction and enhanced self-observation with the introduction of new behaviors via assertiveness training. The therapist does not discuss his feelings toward Sandra. His steady concern and empathy with her struggles seems obvious between the lines, but there may have been moments when he had to contain his frustration regarding Sandra's limitations.

Treatment Intensity and Duration

In view of the severity of the personality disorder, the treatment began with an intensity of two sessions a week for 1 year. Two sessions a week provided close monitoring of Sandra's self-destructive behavior and created an atmosphere in which she could begin to include the therapist and the therapy into the support fabric of her life, which, without the treatment, consisted of a conflicted home life and no real friends. As Sandra's safety and emotional and behavioral containment and regulation increased, the therapy could go to once-a-week sessions until the fading down of the intensity at the end of 5 years.

Could the goals of treatment have been achieved in less time? The manualized treatments for borderline personality disorder are typically delivered over a 1-year period, but that is an arbitrary time frame, and different patients achieve various degrees of success at 1 year. The duration of Sandra's treatment was mutually determined by her and the therapist, with an eye toward her increasing improvement and a growing sense of what could be achieved.

Domains of Dysfunction

As this case illustrates, the domains of dysfunction that are the focus of treatment usually progress from dysfunctional behaviors to emotions and their regulation or dysregulation to cognitive–affective representations of self and others and how these representations drive interpersonal behavior and the individual's goals and strivings. No treatment is complete without attention to all levels of this multileveled situation. The advantage of an integrated modular approach is that it enables the therapist to be creative in applying different approaches to each of these complex domains of functioning.

Whereas most would agree that empirically investigated treatments that show effectiveness should be utilized, it has become clear that the existing data derived from randomized clinical trails have provided little useful information as the therapist faces the individual patient. Complex and specialized treatment packages (Bateman & Fonagy, 2006; Clarkin et al., 2006; Linehan, 1993) effectively reduce symptoms but do not show significant change across all the important domains of dysfunction. Furthermore, we know little about how these treatments actually work, and we do not know how specific modules of intervention are effective in specific domains of dysfunction. It is in this vacuum that clinical thinking must be used to help the individual patient.

The Smooth Direction of Intervention over Time

A major advantage of integration is the utilization of a range of strategies and techniques that can address the unfolding patient problem areas across time and the potential for shaping a unique combination of techniques for the individual patient. But what are the potential dangers or pitfalls in the process of integration?

Manualized treatments for severe personality disorders have a sequence and coherence based in one theoretical approach that is an advantage for the therapist but may not fit all patients. The clinician who is attempting to integrate strategies across treatment orientations and adapt them to a particular patient is making individual decisions throughout the treatment. This is not an easy task, especially with patients in the severe range of personality pathology who can stimulate intense feelings in the therapist, but it probably becomes easier for therapists as they gain experience with patients with personality disorder.

The central important point in this chapter is how this therapist used an integrative model and attitude applied to this particular patient to smoothly weave an ongoing intervention over 5 years that was always current with Sandra's relationship with the therapist, her dominant affective states, and the ongoing life issues in her environment outside the treatment room.

Probably the biggest integration threat is that an inexperienced therapist with the goal of integrating techniques from many schools of psychotherapy begins to be shaped in the process over time by the momentary and here-and-now behaviors of the patient. The more severe the personality pathology, the more likely it is that the patient has a fragmented and diffuse sense of self, with fluctuating affect-ridden momentary views of the therapy and the therapist. Patients with personality disorder without a coherent sense of self and related goals and investments in relationships and work can fluctuate, sometimes dramatically, from day to day in terms of their moods, likes and dislikes, and evaluation of others, including the therapist.

CONCLUDING COMMENTS

The advantage of a case report is that it provides a rich narrative of patient–therapist interaction over time. The disadvantage is subjective recall of the material and the limitations in generalizing from the particular case. Acknowledging the risks in generalization, we suggest that one can tentatively make some comments that are consistent with prior empirical work.

First of all, it seems paramount that, with patients with personality disorder, who by definition have difficulties in relationships, the therapist must be constantly attentive to the ongoing nature of the relationship between the two. Treatment modules will not work without the context of a productive relationship. The careful attention to the relationship in this treatment allowed Sandra to stay in treatment longer than in previous attempts. Second, Sandra's belief that change was possible and active motivation to work for change were central to treatment success. In Sandra's case, she was motivated by desire for relief from her symptoms, but only with some relief and a sense that treatment might work did she begin to actually believe that change was possible. It seems clear that the therapist must have a vision of possible change, and only gradually can the patient begin to adopt that vision and related motivation. Third, the ability of Sandra to go beyond her usual reactive mode of relating to her environment must be transformed slowly into a curiosity about and interest in reflecting on her own experience and how that guides her behavior (see Bateman & Fonagy, Chapter 7, this volume; Dimaggio, Popolo, Carcione, & Salvatore, Chapter 8, this volume). Sandra needed to create a life that she found worth living, and this involved a mental construction of herself and her own talents and desires and a crystallization of goals for herself that brought her some satisfaction (see Clarkin et al., Chapter 18 and Dimaggio et al., Chapter 8, this volume).

Two different loci of integration are central to Sandra's treatment. Given the complexities of clinical work with patients with personality disorder, a therapist's open-minded knowledge of the range of potential therapeutic techniques is a real advantage. A knowledge of and application of these techniques is not enough, however. The difference between a technician and a professional is that the latter integrates the techniques with the dominant relationship patterns of the patient, with timing geared to maximum impact, while fostering the patient's hope for change and encouraging new conceptions of self and others with healthier interpersonal behavior.

A second center of integration taking place during the therapy occurs in the patient. Referring once again to the cognitive–affective processing model of personality functioning (Mischel & Shoda, 2008), the patient with personality disorder suffers from both disturbances and distortions in the cognitive–affective units, which contribute to disturbed and disturbing interpersonal behavior. A thorough, integrated treatment will address both the disturbed behavior and the distortions in the cognitive–affective units. In this way, behavioral change is maintained over time. Treatment is an attempt to assist the patient in his or her smooth integration of balanced views of self and others with affective modulation and cooperative and satisfying interpersonal relations.

REFERENCES

Bateman, A., & Fonagy, P. (2006). *Mentalization-based treatment for borderline personality disorder.* Oxford, UK: Oxford University Press.

Clarkin, J. F., Yeomans, F. E., & Kernberg, O. F. (2006). *Psychotherapy for borderline personality: Focusing on object relations.* Washington, DC: American Psychiatric Publishing.

Linehan, M. M. (1993). *Cognitive-behavioral treatment of borderline personality disorder.* New York: Guilford Press.

Mischel, W., & Shoda, Y. (2008). Toward a unified theory of personality: Integrating dispositions and processing dynamics within the cognitive–affective processing system. In O. P. John, R. W. Robins, & L. A. Pervin (Eds.), *Handbook of personality: Theory and research* (3rd ed., pp. 208–241). New York: Guilford Press.

chapter 21

A Final Review of Integrated Modular Treatment for Personality Disorders

John F. Clarkin, W. John Livesley,
and Giancarlo Dimaggio

Empirical evaluations of manualized treatments for personality pathology are limited and largely confined to borderline personality disorder. That means there is modest information to guide clinicians about the best methods to employ, especially when working with individual patients who do not fit neatly into one personality disorder category. Nevertheless, we have argued that similarity in outcome across therapies and minimal differences between the outcome of specific personality disorder treatments and good clinical management provide solid empirical grounds for a unified approach. Faced with the paucity of outcome data, especially on the most effective interventions for treating different components of personality pathology, we have opted to gather together the treatment modules that expert clinicians have used to address different domains of dysfunction. The combination of domains of pathology and treatment modules espoused here is a form of technical eclecticism organized around a structure based on general change principles. We have called this *integrated modular treatment* (IMT) because it takes the clinician beyond the existing treatments by utilizing strategies and techniques from all major treatment schools and orientations. We do not claim originality for the guiding idea of integrated treatment because we have benefited from those who have advocated and utilized such an approach for many years (Norcross & Newman, 1992; Stricker, 2010).

Our approach has also been influenced by the ongoing debate about the best way to represent personality disorders and the advantages and disadvantages of categorical and dimensional approaches to diagnostic classification as a basis for treatment planning (Clarkin & Huprich, 2012). Although categories of personality disorder have a long clinical tradition that facilitates communication among clinicians, dimensional classification is better at accommodating the extensive heterogeneity observed among patients with the same categorical diagnosis and overlap among the categories. These considerations, along with strong empirical support for dimensional models of personality disorder, led us to adopt this way to represent clinically significant individual differences in personality pathology (see Livesley & Clarkin, Chapter 3, this volume). Dimensional classification is also more useful in treatment planning than global diagnoses because many emotional and interpersonal traits are closely related to actual therapeutic interventions. Besides trait dimensions, we have also stressed the importance of severity in determining treatment pathways and intensity. However, we have also argued that evaluations of severity and trait dimensions are not sufficient; the selection of treatment methods is also guided by evaluation of personality pathology in terms of commonly observed domains of dysfunction. This led us to articulate four domains of dysfunction based on clinical descriptions of personality disorder that cut across all forms of disorder that can be more directly related to treatment approaches: symptoms, regulation and modulation, interpersonal, and self/identity. A focus on functional impairment rather than more abstract diagnostic constructs also helped to tie assessment more closely to the selection and sequencing of interventions because domains form an approximate hierarchy of plasticity and amenability to change.

THE STRUCTURE OF INTEGRATED MODULAR TREATMENT

The conceptual framework for IMT that combines the common-factors and technical eclecticism approaches to psychotherapy integration led us to distinguish between general treatment modules that are utilized in every treatment and specific treatment modules that are targeted to specific domains of dysfunction that vary across individuals. This structure was also used to organize this volume. The early chapters describe the framework for unified treatment and the clinical assessment of the patient. These are followed by chapters related to the common factors—building and maintaining the alliance, enhancing metacognitive capacity, and establishing the treatment contract (see Table 21.1). The remaining chapters cover selected aspects of specific interventions.

The general treatment modules that operationalize the common factors as they apply to personality disorder treatment form the basic scaffolding that

TABLE 21.1. General Treatment Modules

Assessing personality pathology

- Assessment process (Livesley & Clarkin, Chapter 3)
- Focus on domains of dysfunction (Clarkin & Livesley, Chapter 4)

Structuring treatment

- Establishing a treatment framework (Links, Mercer, & Novick, Chapter 5)

Monitoring the relationship

- Resolving alliance ruptures (Tufekcioglu & Muran, Chapter 6)
- Validating the patient
- Therapist alert to indications of patient's positive–negative views of therapist/therapy
- Reciprocal communication strategies

Generic instrumental interventions

- Motivation (Livesley & Clarkin, Chapter 2)
- Mentalizing interventions (Bateman & Fonagy, Chapter 7)
- Metacognition (Dimaggio et al., Chapter 8)

helps to ensure coherent and coordinated therapy. Specific intervention modules are used only when the conditions created by these interventions are met. Thus, like several specific therapies for personality disorder, such as transference-focused psychotherapy (TFP) and dialectical behavior therapy (DBT), interventions used by IMT form a hierarchy: Interventions required to ensure the safety of the patient and others take priority other all other interventions. Once safety is ensured, general treatment modules take priority over specific treatment modules.

The hierarchical structure of therapy also extends to general modules. These modules address three basic components of effective treatment (see Livesley & Clarkin, Chapter 2, this volume). The structure module is primarily concerned with establishing the prerequisites to treatment: an explicit treatment model, the administrative conditions needed to treat personality disorder, a coherent formulation of the patient's problems and treatment plan, and a collaboratively established treatment contract. Although some aspects of structure are revised and reformulated as therapy progresses, the foundations of structure need to be in place before therapy begins. The second set of general modules dealing with the alliance, consistency, and validation form a second level of the hierarchy that focuses on building an effective treatment relationship and process. When the alliance is satisfactory, the more instrumental general modules dealing with motivation and self-reflection are used to build a commitment to change and the metacognitive processes (see Bateman & Fonagy, Chapter 7, and Dimaggio, Popolo, Carcione, & Salvatore, Chapter 8, this volume) needed for the patient to make effective use of more specific strategies.

We have emphasized the importance of maximizing the effects of common change mechanisms both because they make the most substantial contribution to change and because they offer an effective way to manage the core problems of personality disorder. We have also stressed the importance of performing a careful diagnostic assessment with a dual purpose of becoming allied with the patient in examining his or her life and in structuring a treatment with hope and motivation for positive change. Following a careful assessment (see Livesley & Clarkin, Chapter 3), the integration-oriented therapist must frame the treatment with a verbal agreement or contract that details the responsibilities of both parties in this treatment journey (see Links, Mercer, & Novick, Chapter 5, this volume). By definition, individuals with personality disorder have difficulties in relating to others, including difficulties in relating to a therapist. The therapist must make conscious and strategic efforts to relate to the individual with difficulties in relationships. Ruptures in the treatment alliance should not be seen in this context as unusual or crises but rather as expected opportunities for therapeutic intervention (see Tufekcioglu & Muran, Chapter 6, this volume). Thus a therapeutic attitude of expecting such ruptures in a calm, emotionally balanced manner is combined with a tactful approach to exploring with the patient the way he or she experienced the rupture, even if it involves criticism of the therapist.

The second component of therapy matches domains of personality dysfunction with specific treatment modules (see Table 21.2). To address this issue, we invited experts in the treatment of various aspects of personality disorder to contribute to this effort at integration. We emphasized to the prospective authors that we did not want descriptions of a stand-alone treatment approach but rather a description of how their treatment modules could be integrated into a more comprehensive approach. Although all initially agreed to this aim, we found that some of the authors had difficulty departing from their own approach as a stand-alone treatment. This experience in crafting the book is informative. There is a tendency among the leaders in the field to emphasize their approach to the exclusion of others. For them, integration is not natural and easy. In contrast, clinicians who are faced with complicated, unique patients are motivated to integrate, that is, to use any and all techniques that might help with the individual patient.

The specific domains of dysfunction vary with the individual patient, and these domains also have important differences in level of severity. A major result of this volume is a compilation of the domains of dysfunction in patients with personality disorder that have been identified and described by clinical writers. Each of these writers has experience with describing therapeutic approaches to the domains of dysfunction that they have observed. We think this approach is broader and more inclusive than simply reading manuals of empirically investigated treatments, as these are few in number and limited in their scope. We are not suggesting that we have exhausted the domains of dysfunction, but this book provides a guide to those that have been identified so far and may form a framework for future work.

TABLE 21.2. Specific Treatment Modules and Personality Pathology

Domain	Specific behaviors	Treatment modules	Authors and chapters
Patient safety	• Suicidal and self-destructive acts • Behavioral instability • Emotional instability • Quasi-psychotic thinking	• Medication • Structure and support • Crisis intervention • Brief hospitalization	• Links & Bergmans (Chapter 9) • Silk & Friedel (Chapter 10) • Wong (Chapter 16)
Containment	• Intense emotions • Dissociative behavior • Impaired cognitive functioning	• Medication • Structure and s upport	• Wong (Chapter 16)
Control and modulation	• Emotion dysregulation • Poor impulse control • Constriction and inhibition	• Functional analysis of chain of events • Growing awareness of functional links • Awareness of interpersonal triggers • Attitudes toward own emotions • Attention control • Self-soothing • Response prevention • Relaxation methods • Effective help seeking	• Leahy (Chapter 12) Salvatore et al. (Chapter 19) • Lynch, Hempel, & Clark (Chapter 15)
Exploration and change	• Cognitive–emotional schemas • Dysfunctional interpersonal patterns	• Awareness of interpersonal schemas, self-signatures, dominant object relations, self-narratives	• Bateman & Fonagy (Chapter 7) • Dimaggio et al. (Chapter 8) • Cain & Pincus (Chapter 14) • Clarkin et al. (Chapter 18) • Clarkin et al. (Chapter 20)
Integration and synthesis	• Incoherent sense of self • Distorted perceptions of others • Poor self-directedness • Lack of personal niche	• Construct a personal niche • Examine mental representations of self and others • Expand self and other curiosity	• Clarkin et al. (Chapter 18)

BARRIERS TO AN INTEGRATED TREATMENT

Although we think the case for an integrated approach is strong, we recognize that there are powerful obstacles to using integrated treatment. Now it seems appropriate to consider these barriers in the context of the conceptual framework we are proposing. A major barrier to implementation is that the way psychotherapy is taught and practiced tends to evoke allegiance to a specific theory of personality disorder and an associated treatment model that often limits the flexibility needed for integration. The dominant example at present is cognitive-behavioral theory and related treatments. Clinicians rally around such an orientation and form separate societies with journals focused almost exclusively on that orientation. This type of allegiance leads to knowledge being "stovepiped" in ways that hinder integration and clinical creativity. Allegiance to a specific form of therapy and the partisanship involved also encourages a focus on differences between therapies. In our terms, it leads to a focus on those specific interventions that differentiate therapies and neglect of common change mechanisms—the mechanisms that we consider the foundation for integrated treatment and which account for much of outcome change.

Second, the empirically supported treatment movement fosters the use of manualized therapies that show significant change in randomized clinical trials. This approach suggests at first glance that DBT should be used for all patients with BPD because it is the most investigated treatment. However, we do not consider such a conclusion clinically sound given that patients with a borderline diagnosis manifest different domains of dysfunction, not all of which are adequately addressed by DBT, and because other treatments also have empirical support. Why not utilize the best aspects out of each of the treatments that have been investigated and amplify them with clinical wisdom from clinical writers with experience with patients with personality disorder? This central idea led to the construction of this volume.

Third, a persistent barrier to integrated treatment is the seemingly unresolvable problems in the diagnostic classification of personality disorder and the continued emphasis within official diagnostic systems such as DSM-5 on categorical diagnoses. This implicitly fosters the idea that each category is associated with a single psychopathological impairment and hence that there is a specific treatment for each disorder, as opposed to more flexible treatment frameworks that are concerned with both treating the features common to all forms of personality disorder and accommodating the extensive heterogeneity neglected by categorical classifications.

But perhaps the most formidable barrier to integration is the demand it places on the individual clinician. In some respects, it is easier to utilize a one-size-fits-all treatment approach that rigidly specifies the use of treatment techniques, as the clinician does not have to use much judgment in this process. This procedure is especially comforting in the treatment of patients who are potentially suicidal or self-destructive in ways that raise anxieties in the therapist. However, the problem is more than a matter of comfort; there is also the substantial practical problem of how to coordinate and sequence an eclectic and diverse combination of treatment methods. The biggest threat to an integrated treatment is that the therapists' uncertainty of focus is often further confused by complexity of personality pathology, the clamor of multiple problems all vying for attention, and the patients' anxiety, need for attention, and attempt to find therapists' sympathy in daily crises. Without some clear indication of priorities in the treatment, the therapist will be at the whim and control of the day-to-day fluctuations in the patient's crises and current concerns. The crucial issue is how the therapist capitalizes on the advantages of having an extensive and eclectic repertoire of interventions without therapy becoming disorganized and confusing due to rapid changes in intervention strategy as the immediate concerns of patients change both within a session and across adjacent sessions. We discussed this issue in Chapter 2 in this volume and returned to it again in the case presentation in Chapter 20.

INTEGRATION AS A TREATMENT GOAL

Throughout this volume, integration has been viewed as the product of a mental process on the part of the therapist, who constructs a formulation of the clinical problems of the patient and uses a unified, transtheoretical approach to select interventions that are considered to be useful in treating these problems. There is, however, another aspect to integration to consider: integration as a treatment goal. Personality disorder involves impairments in the structure and organization of personality. The different components of personality do not function harmoniously together, creating difficulties in setting and achieving long-term goals and in constructing a coherent sense of self and a more adaptive life script. For these reasons, effective treatment not only involves promoting improved capacity to manage emotions and impulses and enhanced interpersonal abilities but also requires the development of more coherent personality functioning. As with operational integration, the locus of personality integration is also the mind of the therapist. It begins with the construction of a narrative case formulation that becomes the blueprint for developing a more adaptive autobiographical self. The challenge for the therapist is to find a way of translating his or her blueprint into treatment strategies that enable patients to construct a more coherent understanding of themselves. Unfortunately, there is a limited literature on how to promote personality integration and construct a more adaptive self-system. Only TFP addresses the problem in any systematic way. Consequently, we have included several chapters discussing different ways to help patients to synthesize a more adaptive sense of self.

An understanding of the broad integrative mechanisms of personality and the structure of the self-system makes it possible to use general treatment modules to foster integration. Important goals for longer-term treatment are to establish clearly delineated interpersonal boundaries, promote more integrated representations of self and others, increase autonomy and agency, and facilitate the development of an adaptive self. The raw material for constructing a sense of self and identity is self-knowledge and self-understanding. All treatments seek to increase self-knowledge in one way or another, and we have stressed the importance of building self-reflection and metacognitive capacity (see Bateman & Fonagy, Chapter 7, and Dimaggio et al., Chapter 8, this volume). Self-observation and self-reflection are important in the construction of the self because these processes transform self-experience into self-knowledge, examining and reorganizing these experiences. In the process, ideas about the self are differentiated, inconsistencies are reconciled, and a more integrated self-representation is constructed.

The integrative effects of improved self-observation are enhanced by encouraging patients to become curious about their own minds and the nature of their experience. As self-knowledge increases, the self is elaborated because aspects of self-knowledge that were suppressed often become more accessible, and integration is achieved through a treatment process that gradually imposes structure and organization onto self-experience by repetitively linking feelings, thoughts, and actions. At the same time, a consistent and stable treatment process promotes integration by providing a stable experience of the self in relationship with the therapist. A validating and empathic therapeutic stance helps to consolidate these developments by affirming and consolidating any changes that occur and by modulating tendencies to think in self-invalidating ways that hinder self-development.

Besides the indirect integrative consequences of generic treatment strategies, more specific interventions may also be needed to foster integration. Working with the patient to construct an initial formulation that is subsequently revised as new information is uncovered sets the process of constructing a self under way by helping to make problems and troublesome experiences meaningful. Integration can also be facilitated by working directly on understanding the relationship among different self-states and developing an understanding of the kinds of events that trigger the transition from one self-state to another (see Dimaggio, Popolo, Carcione, Salvatore, & Stiles, Chapter 17, and Salvatore, Popolo, & Dimaggio, Chapter 19, this volume).

An important part of facilitating personality integration is to help the patient to develop a way of living that is congenial to his or her personality characteristics—a process illustrated by the case we presented in Chapter 20. Psychotherapy is very attentive to environmental adversities that increase risk of personality pathology, but it often neglects the more positive benefits of an environment that promotes more adaptive functioning. However, when treating personality disorder, we need to recognize and make use of the important role that the environment plays in maintaining much of the structure and organization of behavior manifested in everyday action. Healthy individuals tend to construct an environmental niche for themselves that supports adaptive action and provides outlets for their interests, talents, abilities, and personal characteristics. Many patients with personality disorder fail to construct congenial personal niches of this type, creating instead life circumstances that help to maintain more dysfunctional patterns. With these patients, it is important at some point in treatment to raise the idea of constructing an adaptive niche and building a life worth living. Although many patients fail to articulate the issue for themselves, they intuitively recognize the problem; they often identify strongly with the need to "get a life," so when the matter is raised, they feel a sense of relief that therapy may address some significant issues leading to increased motivation and a sense of hope.

CONCLUDING COMMENTS

In proposing IMT, our goal was not to propose yet another therapy for personality disorder but rather to suggest an evidence-based alternative to reliance on a single-treatment model. Nor are we suggesting the need for randomly controlled trials that pit IMT against either treatment as usual or one or more of the specialized therapies for personality disorder. There does not seem to be much more to learn from such studies or from further evaluations of the overall efficacy of current therapies. To progress, the field needs a new generation of studies, usually referred to as dismantling studies, that seek to identify the effective elements of current treatments. Currently, we know that structured therapies for personality disorder work, but we have little idea about why they work. To improve outcomes, we need to identify the optimal way to operationalize common change mechanisms when treating personality disorder, interventions and strategies that are effective for each domain and subdomain of personality dysfunction, and the optimal way to match treatment methods with patient variables such as severity and trait constellations. The answers to these crucial questions will undoubtedly change the way personality disorder is treated. In advocating for integrated treatment, we seek to contribute to discussion on how best to move to the next stage in the development of effective treatment for personality disorder by proposing a conceptual framework that is sufficiently structured to ensure the consistent therapeutic process that is needed for successful treatment and that is also sufficiently flexible to accommodate new findings.

REFERENCES

Clarkin, J. F., & Huprich, S. K. (2012). Do DSM-5 personality disorder proposals meet criteria for clinical utility? *Journal of Personality Disorders, 25*, 192–205.

Norcross, J. C., & Newman, J. C. (1992). Psychotherapy integration: Setting the context. In J. C. Norcross & M. R. Goldfried (Eds.), *Handbook of psychotherapy integration* (pp. 3–45). New York: Basic Books.

Stricker, G. (2010). A second look at psychotherapy integration. *Journal of Psychotherapy Integration, 20*, 397.

Index

Page numbers followed by *f* indicate figure, *t* indicate table.

D

E

N

Q

R

S

T